IMMUNOLOGY AND IMMUNE SYSTEM DISORDERS

LUPUS

SYMPTOMS, TREATMENT AND POTENTIAL COMPLICATIONS

Immunology and Immune System Disorders

Additional books in this series can be found on Nova's website under the Series tab.

Additional e-books in this series can be found on Nova's website under the e-book tab.

Endocrinology Research and Clinical Developments

Additional books in this series can be found on Nova's website under the Series tab.

Additional e-books in this series can be found on Nova's website under the e-book tab.

IMMUNOLOGY AND IMMUNE SYSTEM DISORDERS

LUPUS

SYMPTOMS, TREATMENT AND POTENTIAL COMPLICATIONS

THIAGO DEVESA MARQUEZ
AND
DAVI URGEIRO NETO
EDITORS

Nova Science Publishers, Inc.
New York

For permission to use material from this book please contact us:
Telephone 631-231-7269; Fax 631-231-8175
Web Site: http://www.novapublishers.com

Library of Congress Cataloging-in-Publication Data

ISBN: 978-1-62081-078-1

Library of Congress Control Number: 2012931745

Published by Nova Science Publishers, Inc. † New York

Contents

Preface

Lupus is one of many disorders of the immune system known as autoimmune diseases, wherein the immune system attacks parts of the patient's body, leading to inflammation and injury in body tissues. This book presents current research in the study of the symptoms, treatment and potential complications of lupus. Topics include autoantibody-producing B cells and B cell therapy in systemic lupus erythematosus; neuropsychiatric and hematologic manifestations of systemic lupus erythematosus; pulmonary hypertension in systemic lupus erythematosus; dual roles for antibodies in lupus nephritis; and treatment of systemic lupus erythematosus with intravenous immunoglobulins.

Chapter I - *Context:* Lupus erythematosus is a chronic, inflammatory autoimmune disease that may affect multiple organ systems. *Aim of the review:* To provide a comprehensive, current summary of lupus epidemiology, diagnostic criteria, diagnostic techniques, pathophysiology and therapeutic modalities. *Methods:* We performed an extensive review of previous and current pertinent publications from the medical literature. *Conclusions*: The authors address multiple topics including a nosologic definition of lupus, incidence and prevalence, etiologic environmental factors and genetics, relevant autoantibodies, and laboratory diagnostic testing. Additional discussion includes pathophysiology relative to specific organ systems. Current treatment modalities, recommendations for patients and patient advocate groups are also reviewed.

Chapter II - A recent study has significantly improved the prognosis of systemic lupus erythematosus (SLE), a prototypic systemic autoimmune disease with multiple organ disorders. However, corticosteroids and immunosuppressive agents are still used in medical care. There are a significant proportion of patients with refractory disease and complications by the conventional drugs. In fact, few novel drugs have been approved for SLE during the past decades. Many studies suggest that the center in pathophysiology of SLE is autoreactive B cells producing autoantibodies. Therefore, B cell may be one of the most promising targets in therapies of SLE. Moreover, B cells would function as antigen-presenting cells, providers of pro-inflammatory cytokines, and activators of T cells other than function of effector cells that produce immunoglobulins in immune system. It is also evident that large population of abnormal B cells exists in active SLE. RP105 (CD180), one of the toll-like receptor associated molecules, is expressed on mature B cells. Previously, the authors found significantly increased population of RP105-negative B cells in SLE. Interestingly, phenotype of RP105(-) B cell subsets in SLE patients is greatly different from normal subjects and, importantly, RP105(-) B cells produce autoantibodies including anti-dsDNA antibodies. RP105(-) B cells are assigned as the B cell subsets in final stages of differentiation and may be one of the central B cells dysregulated in SLE. This review provides basic information of B cell biology and RP105(-) B cells in SLE and illustrates new insights of novel and alternative concept of B cell targeting therapies in SLE.

Chapter III - Systemic lupus erythematosus (SLE) is an autoimmune disorder that affects 0.1% of the world population. The disorder is characterized by systemic inflammation, auto-antibody production, and immune dysregulation, and it may lead to significant neurological and psychiatric morbidities. Both adults and children are diagnosed according to a set of clinical and laboratory criteria with a high sensitivity and specificity. A diagnosis of SLE in any age-group depends on excluding systemic infections or malignancies and the presence of at least 4 of 11 American College of Rheumatology (ACR) diagnostic criteria. Nephritis (leading to hypertension and renal dysfunction) and nervous system involvement are two of the more ominous manifestations in all age-groups. There are 19 case-based peripheral and central nervous syndromes that are postulated to be associated with SLE. Syndromes requiring prompt neurological evaluation include seizures, cerebrovascular accidents, demyelination, movement disorders, and peripheral neuropathies. Manifestations that may prompt psychiatric consultation include acute confusional state (delirium), affective disorders (anxiety and depression), cognitive impairment, and psychosis. Neuropsychiatric presentations may be caused by hypercoagulability in cerebral vessels (vasculopathy), proinflammatory cytokines, autoantibody effects on neuronal structures or receptors, and blood–brain barrier disruption. Alteration in the regulation of neurotransmitters such as dopamine and serotonin appear to play a role in behavioral changes seen in lupus-prone mice. The authors will review the prevalence, etiology and clinical presentation of neuropsychiatric manifestations in SLE. In addition, we will discuss treatment protocol for this serious manifestation in SLE.

Chapter IV - Systemic lupus erythematosus (SLE) is a prototypic inflammatory autoimmune disorder characterized by multisystem involvement and fluctuating disease activity. Symptoms range from rather mild manifestations such as rash or arthritis to life-threatening end-organ manifestations such as nephritis. Despite new and improved therapy having positively impacted the prognosis of SLE, a subgroup of patients do not response to therapy. Moreover, the risk of fatal outcomes and the damaging side effects of immunosuppressive therapies in SLE call for an improvement in the current therapeutic management of SLE. New therapeutic approaches are focused on B-cell targets, T-cell downregulation and co-stimulatory blockade, cytokine inhibition, or the modulation of complement. Several biological agents have been used in recent and ongoing studies, but this encouraging news follows several disappointments in trials of other biologic therapies. We will review potential therapeutics in SLE and reflect on where we stand, what we have learned, and what may lie ahead.

Chapter V - A chronic disorder with unknown etiology, systemic lupus erythematosus (SLE) is the most diverse autoimmune disorder with a relapsing and remitting course that may affect any organ in the body. SLE has a broad spectrum of clinical presentations with higher mortality than general population. These diverse clinical manifestations are mainly due to SLE complex immunopathology in which B cells produce autoantibodies against mainly intracellular auto antigen targets, and form complement fixing immune complex deposits resulting in irreversible organ damage. More than one hundred autoantibodies have been found in SLE, but only few of them are associated with the SLE manifestations. There are almost always autoantibodies against one or more cell components in the blood of SLE patients. Hematologic complications of SLE are among the most common manifestations of this disorder, and almost all patients have hematologic abnormality at some stage of the disease. In 1971, American college of rheumatology established the SLE criteria in which hemolytic anemia, leukopenia, and thrombocytopenia were the individual criterion.

Chapter VI - Interleukin-21 (IL-21) is a member of the γchain-dependent cytokine family and as such, its receptor (R) is made of the common γ chain associated to the IL-21R-specific α chain. This four α-helical bundle type I cytokine was first discovered in 2000 and since then, a large number of studies have evidenced its pleiotropic functions on the immune system. IL-21 seems to be a critical regulator of T cells since it induces the development of inflammatory Th17 cells while blocking the differentiation and counteracting the activity of regulatory T cells. It also modulates CD8+ T cell, natural killer cells, as well as dendritic cell functions. Moreover, IL-21 is involved in shaping the effector function and the fate of B cells and especially their final differentiation step in plasma cells, which implies that it may be central in immune diseases that have a major B cell component. Systemic lupus erythematosus (SLE) is one of these "B-cell mediated" disease, and numerous B cell abnormalities have been described, although T cells and many other immune mediators are also known to be altered. Lupus disease is indeed characterized by the production of autoantibodies (a lot of them being specific for nuclear components) and by the subsequent formation of inflammatory immune complexes. Some of them play a crucial role in associated cutaneous lesions and in glomerulonephritis, which can in turn be fatal. Therefore, B lymphocytes are undoubtedly key players in lupus disease. As such, they constitute a privileged objective for the development of new specific biologics and every molecule that affects their function, such as IL-21, may be a valuable therapeutic target in SLE. In this review, we will provide an overview of the role of IL-21 in B cell physiology and lupus pathology, and we will discuss the possible targeting of this cytokine to treat SLE.

Chapter VII - Systemic lupus erythematosus (SLE) is a chronic, multisystemic autoimmune disease predominantly affecting women of childbearing age. The impact of coronary heart disease (CHD) on morbidity and mortality in patients with established SLE has assumed increasing importance in their long-term management. Classic CHD risk factors and lupus-specific factors, such as antiphospholipid antibodies and nephrotic proteinuria, seem to be important in determining long-term cardiovascular risk, but the role of metabolic derangement, specifically the metabolic syndrome (MetS), is gaining increasing prominence in the literature. One very important aspects of classical cytokines derived from inflammatory cells is their importance in the pathogenesis of the metabolic syndrome. A generally enhanced adipose tissue-derived cytokine expression may be one plausible mechanism for the inflammation–MetS relationship. MetS can be associated with increased risk of develop autoimmune inflammatory diseases like SLE. The best treatment to MetS in SLE patients is maximizing lifestyle therapies. Statins treatment are used to reduction levels of low-density lipoprotein cholesterol (LDL-c) and one of the various immunomodulatory functions realized by statins, is to be able to reduce atherosclerotic vascular disease in SLE by lowering immune activation in the arterial wall and by attenuating SLE activity, but this result is not unanimous. In this chapter the authors will review the prevalence and importance of Mets in SLE and its implication in mortality in SLE.

Chapter VIII - Pulmonary arterial hypertension (PAH) is defined as a sustained elevation of pulmonary arterial pressure to more than 25 mm Hg at rest or to more than 30 mm Hg with exercise, with a mean pulmonary-capillary wedge pressure and left ventricular end-diastolic pressure of less than 15 mm Hg.

Chapter IX - Pathogenic antibodies in Systemic Lupus Erythematosus (SLE) are known to play a major role in initiating and exacerbating the disease through the formation of immune complexes that are deposited in kidney glomeruli. It is apparent that the IgG isotype and an antibody specificity to nuclear components, particularly double-stranded DNA, is associated with increased pathogenesis of autoantibodies. The role of autoreactive IgM is less clear. Through a series of experiments, we have demonstrated that IgM is not only not pathogenic in mice with a lupus-like syndrome (MRL/lpr) but that it is actually protective. Passive transfer experiments using anti-dsDNA IgM antibodies prevented development of lupus nephritis in these mice. The cells secreting protective antibodies displayed a different repertoire of immunoglobulin heavy chain variable region usage, suggesting the possibility of a distinct population of B cells that secrete these antibodies. The possibility of IgM therapy or differential activation of a putative B cell population secreting protective antibodies is discussed.

Chapter X - Systemic lupus erythematosus (SLE) is an autoimmune disease with a varied clinic picture, chronic course and exacerbation tendency as well as many complications resulting from the underlying disease and the immunosuppressive therapy administered. In case of an insufficient effect of immunosuppressive treatment or its contraindication other therapeutic processes are searched that would enable mastering the disease activity. In the paper authors describe two case reports of female patients with SLE with polyorgan involvement and infectious complications that were successfully treated by administering intravenous immunoglobulins.

Chapter XI - Diffuse alveolar hemorrhage (DAH), is a rare pulmonary complication of collagen-vascular diseases, including systemic lupus erythematosus (SLE). As the pathogenetic mechanism of DAH remains unclear, no established treatment is available. However, DAH is potentially fatal. Similar to adult respiratory distress syndrome (ARDS), DAH patients develop severe hypoxemia caused by wide alveolar collapse. Patients may require management with mechanical ventilation in the intensive care unit. The properties of the alveolar-capillary barrier are abnormal during acute lung injury, such as DAH. DAH patients develop severe hypoxemia. It is generally treated with immunosuppressive agents. However, the effects take several weeks. Therefore, mechanical ventilation is used to support these patients until the treatments are effective. DAH lungs include healthy tissue, recruitable tissue, and diseased tissue that are unresponsive to pressure changes. Most of the ventilation used during conventional management of these patients may be directed at recruitable and probably healthier units, resulting in their over-distention, which is thought to be one of the causes of ventilator-associated lung injury. Airway pressure release ventilation (APRV) is one mode of ventilation that may achieve recruitment and improve oxygenation while maintaining acceptable peak airway pressures. APRV applies a continuous airway pressure (P_{high}) identical to continuous positive airway pressure (CPAP) to maintain adequate lung volume and promote alveolar recruitment. APRV adds a time-cycled release phase to a lower set pressure (P_{low}). In addition, spontaneous breathing can be integrated and is independent of the ventilator cycle. By allowing patients to breathe spontaneously during APRV, dependent lung regions may be preferentially recruited without the need to raise the applied airway pressure. APRV has been used to treat acute lung injury, such as ARDS.

In: Lupus: Symptoms, Treatment and Potential Complications ISBN: 978-1-62081-078-1
Editors: T. D. Marquez and D. U. Neto

Chapter I

Lupus Erythematosus: A Comprehensive Review

Ana Maria Abreu Velez*[*] *and Michael S. Howard
Georgia Dermatopathology Associates, Atlanta, Georgia, US

Abstract

Context: Lupus erythematosus is a chronic, inflammatory autoimmune disease that may affect multiple organ systems.

Aim of the review: To provide a comprehensive, current summary of lupus epidemiology, diagnostic criteria, diagnostic techniques, pathophysiology and therapeutic modalities.

Methods: We performed an extensive review of previous and current pertinent publications from the medical literature.

Conclusions: We address multiple topics including a nosologic definition of lupus, incidence and prevalence, etiologic environmental factors and genetics, relevant autoantibodies, and laboratory diagnostic testing. Additional discussion includes pathophysiology relative to specific organ systems. Current treatment modalities, recommendations for patients and patient advocate groups are also reviewed.

Keywords: Lupus

Abbreviations

SLE	Systemic lupus erythematosus
NIAMS	National Institute of Arthritis and Musculoskeletal and Skin Diseases

[*] Correspondence to: Ana Maria Abreu Velez, M.D., Ph.D., Georgia Dermatopathology Associates, 1534 North Decatur Road, NE; Suite 206, Atlanta, Georgia 30307-1000, USA, Telephone: (404) 371-0077, Fax: (404) 371-1900. Email: abreuvelez@yahoo.com

NIH	U.S. Department of Health and Human Services National Institutes of Health
DLE	discoid lupus erythematosus
SCLE	subacute cutaneous lupus erythematosus
DIL	Drug-induced lupus
NSAID	nonsteroidal anti-inflammatory drug
ANA	antinuclear antibody
UV	ultraviolet light
BUN	blood urea nitrogen
eGFR	estimated glomerular filtration rate
APS	antiphospholipid antibody syndrome, or Hughes syndrome
ACR	American College of Rheumatology
PGA	Physician's Global Assessment
SLEDAI	SLE Disease Activity Index; modified to exclude anti-dsDNA and complement)
CTD	connective tissue disease
SSc	systemic sclerosis

Defining Lupus

Lupus is one of many disorders of the immune system known as autoimmune diseases. In autoimmune diseases, the immune system attacks parts of the patient's body, leading to inflammation and injury in body tissues. Lupus may affect many areas of the body, especially in systemic lupus erythematosus (SLE); potential areas of involvement include the joints, skin, kidneys, heart, lungs, blood vessels, and brain. Although people with the disease may present with variable symptoms, some of the most frequent ones include fatigue, painful or swollen joints (arthritis), unexplained fevers, photosensitiviy, skin rashes, and renal abnormalities [1-5].

Currently, there is no cure for lupus [6]. Nevertheless, lupus can be effectively treated with medications [7-11]. Lupus is characterized by periods of illness, called flares, and periods of wellness, or remission. Understanding how to prevent flares and how to treat them when they do occur helps people with lupus maintain better overall health; however, ongoing renal disease often remains an important issue [12].

Women present with lupus more often than men [12, 13]. Lupus is more common in African American women than in Caucasian women, and is also more common in women of Hispanic, Asian, and Native American background. African American and Hispanic women are also more likely to develop severe disease, involving several organs [14-15]. Lupus is common in several members of the same family [16]. In recent years, compelling evidence has been gathered that supports a role for epigenetic alterations in the pathogenesis of SLE [17]. Different populations of SLE patients are characterized by a global loss of DNA methylation [17]. The demethylation has been associated with defects in ERK pathway signaling, and consequent DNMT 1 downregulation [17]. Hypomethylation of gene promoters has been described, which permits 1) transcriptional activation and resultant functional changes within affected cells, and also 2) hypomethylation of the ribosomal RNA gene cluster [17]. Among the identified targets undergoing demethylation are genes involved in autoreactivity (ITGAL), osmotic lysis and apoptosis (PRF1, MMP14 and LCN2), antigen presentation (CSF3R), inflammation(MMP 14), B- and T-cell interaction (CD70 and CD40LG) and cytokine pathways (CSF3R, IL-4, IL-6 and IFNGR2) [17]. DNA methylation inhibitors are also known to induce autoreactivity in vitro and cause a lupus-like disease in vivo. Further, altered patterns of histone modifications have been described in SLE. For example, CD4 positive lymphocytes undergo global histone H3 and H4 deacetylation and consequent skewing of gene expression [17]. Although multiple lines of evidence highlight the contribution of epigenetic alterations to the pathogenesis of lupus in genetically predisposed individuals, many questions remain to be answered. Attaining a deeper understanding of this subject will create possibilities in the emerging area of epigenetic treatments. It is difficult to estimate how many people in the United States have the disease, because its symptoms vary widely and to date no obligatory governmental reporting system exists. However, in other countries, extended studies are yielding some pertinent epidemiologic data [18]. In one recent study in the Lugo region of northwestern Spain, performed between January 1987 and December 2006, 150 residents were diagnosed as having SLE according to the 1982 American College of Rheumatology (ACR) criteria for the classification of SLE. Women outnumbered men (127 [84.7%] vs. 23 [15.3%]) [18]. The mean age at the time of disease diagnosis was 46.1 ± 19.6 years. The mean follow-up from the time of disease diagnosis was 7.8 ± 4.5 years. The age- and sex-adjusted annual incidence rate over the 20-year study period was 3.6 (95% confidence interval [CI], 3.0-4.2) per 100,000 population aged 15 years and older [18]. The overall annual incidence rate over the 20-year study period in women (5.9/100,000 population aged $\geq$15 yr; 95% CI, 4.9-7.0) was higher than in men (1.1/100,000 population aged $\geq$15 yr; 95% CI, 0.7-1.7) ($p < 0.001$) [18]. By December 31, 2006, the overall age-adjusted SLE prevalence in the Lugo region for patients who fulfilled at least 4 of 1982 ACRC criteria was 17.5 per 100,000 population aged 15 years and older (95% CI, 12.6-24.1). Prevalence in women (29.2/100,000 population aged $\geq$15 yr; 95% CI, 20.0-40.7) was higher than in men (5.8/100,000 population aged $\geq$15 yr; 95% CI, 2.0-12.0).The most frequent clinical manifestation was arthritis [18]. As reported in population-based studies on SLE patients of European descent, renal disease was observed in only 27.3% of the patients. The rate of flares was 0.084/year. A younger age and the presence of nephritis at the time of disease diagnosis were significantly associated with the development of flares during the follow-up of Lugo patients. Compared with the general population, the probability of survival in patients with SLE was significantly reduced ($p = 0.04$). In conclusion, the Lugo study establishes a baseline estimate of the incidence and clinical spectrum of SLE in northwestern Spain. According to the results, the incidence of SLE in northwestern Spain is slightly greater than that reported in most European regions. Patients with SLE from northwestern Spain have a later age of onset and a lower frequency of nephritis than in the African-American population; however, the data show a reduced probability of survival in Spanish patients with SLE [18]. Most studies have shown that about 1 in 20 people with lupus will have a close relative (mother, aunt, sister, brother; less often father or uncle) with lupus. Occasionally the baby of a mother with lupus will be born with a special form of lupus called neonatal lupus syndrome, due to the passage of certain antibodies (anti-Ro and/or anti-La) from the mother to the baby during pregnancy. The neonatal form of lupus only lasts a few months, as the baby destroys the antibodies from the mother and does not generate more antibodies itself. Neonatal lupus does not predispose to future development of lupus in the child.

Lupus Incidence and Prevalence

Lupus can be difficult to diagnose because the symptoms resemble those of other conditions. A second important factor relative to diagnosis is the lack of extensive epidemiological studies regarding the incidence and the prevalence of the disease [19, 20]. Many studies are based on PubMed or other internet search engine data because the lack of obligatorily reporting of this disease, and cases of diagnosis where ACR criteria are not followed. A large study showed that autoimmune disease incidence and prevalence data found in the literature varied considerably between the 24 diseases reviewed [21]. The largest number of prevalence studies were conducted on multiple sclerosis (MS), rheumatoid arthritis(RA), and systemic lupus erythematosus (SLE) (>/= 23), followed by insulin-dependent diabetes (IDDM), myasthenia gravis, primary biliary cirrhosis, and scleroderma (>/= 7). The authors estimated in 1997 that 8,511,845 persons in the United States, or approximately 1 in 31 Americans, were afflicted with one of these autoimmune diseases [21]. The diseases with the highest prevalence rates were Graves disease/hyperthyroidism, IDDM, pernicious anemia, rheumatoid arthritis, thyroiditis, and vitiligo, comprising an estimated 7,939, 280 people or 93% of the total number estimated. Glomerulonephritis, MS, and SLE added an estimated 323,232 people. The other reviewed diseases were rare, affecting less than 5.14/100,000 persons. Most of the reviewed diseases were more common in women [21]. From the incidence data, we estimated that 237,203 Americans would develop an autoimmune disease in 1996 and that approximately 1,186,015 new cases of these autoimmune diseases would occur in the United States every 5 years. Women were at 2.7 times greater risk than men to acquire an autoimmune disease [21]. After reviewing the medical literature for incidence and prevalence rates of 24 autoimmune diseases, the authors concluded that many autoimmune diseases are infrequently studied by epidemiologists. As a result, the total burden of these diseases may be an underestimated [21].

One of the most common manifestations of lupus is the classic solar-induced rash [22]; the rash may be recognized by many physicians. However, one study has noted that other symptoms, including fatigue, may not be recognized unless occurring in a constellation; appropriate blood tests may help to confirm the diagnosis [23]. If the results of this small study were extrapolated to a larger scale, it could mean that up to 1 in 500 adult women (not 1 in 3,500) is affected with lupus. Such a figure probably represents an overestimate, but systemic lupus erythematosus (SLE or lupus) is a multisystem disease which can affect people of all ages and has been found worldwide. In our review, we aim to address the incidence of the disease (how many people will develop the disease) and the prevalence of the disease (how many people have the disease at a particular time). In other words, these estimates address "who gets the disease". "Why they get the disease" is more difficult to address, but will be also be briefly discussed. Until a few years ago, there was very little information on how prevalent lupus is in the UK [24]. It was generally considered a rare disease, most general practitioners only having one or two patients in their care. However, studies done in the late 1980s and early 1990s have shown that lupus is more common than was realized, particularly in women [24]. Results from the largest UK study in Birmingham showed that in a population of 1.2 million, there were 242 adult people known to have lupus and 33 new cases of lupus diagnosed in one year (ie, 1991; children were not studied) [24]. From these figures, the prevalence and incidence rates for lupus, corrected for the age of the population, were calculated. The prevalence was 28 per 100,000, that is, about one person in 3,500 had lupus [24]. The incidence (new cases per year) was 3.8 per 100,000, that is about one person in 26,300 developed the disease that year. Previous results from the smaller cities of Nottingham and Leicester were very similar. Many studies have shown that women are about 10 times more likely to have or to develop lupus than men [24]. In Birmingham, the figures showed that lupus occurred in almost exactly one in 2,500 adult women; which shows that lupus is not a rare disease in women. It is, however, rare in men; lupus occurred in approximately 1 in 25,000 adult men. Although the disease can start at any age, the first signs of the disease in women usually appear during the reproductive years (after the onset of menstrual periods and before the menopause) [24]. The disease is most commonly diagnosed in women between the ages of 20 and 40, and it appears to be milder than in those patients in whom the disease starts after menopause. There is no particular age pattern in men with lupus. It is also well recognized that people from different ethnic and racial backgrounds are at different risks of developing lupus. People of Afro-Caribbean origin are particularly likely to develop the disease, even when they are born and live in North America or the UK. Surprisingly, people of West African origin (from which the Afro-Caribbean populations were descended) are at low risk of developing lupus. Studies have suggested that up to 1 in 250 women in Jamaica develop lupus. In Birmingham, 1 in 500 women of Afro-Caribbean background have lupus, compared with about 1 in 1000 women from India and Pakistan, and about 1 in 2,500 white European Caucasians [24]. Other studies have shown that people of Chinese and Polynesian backgrounds are also at increased risk of developing lupus, compared with white Caucasians. These observations on the different risks of developing lupus in different populations have suggested that genetic factors play an important role in the development of the disease [24]. Of course, these findings do not rule out a role for environmental factors, which may be shared by people from differing genetic backgrounds. No single known gene puts people at risk of developing lupus (unlike hemophilia and cystic fibrosis). It seems most likely that between 20 and 80 genes contribute to the risk of lupus, and that these genes combine with environmental factors to determine whether the disease develops and when. The "environmental" factors include exposure to UV light (sun exposure), selected infections, possible chemicals in the environment, factors related to stress (not well-identified) and female hormonal activity (for example, estrogen-containing contraceptives, or pregnancy). These factors combine to influence the immune system such that immune abnormalities result, and the disease develops (or recurs) [24]. Multiple studies have tried to link genetical susceptibility to lupus to 1) genes downstream of TNFAIP3 and 2) to genetic variants in complement Factor H and Factor H-related genes [25, 26]. In studies of identical twins—genetically identical persons—when one twin has lupus, the other twin has a 24-percent chance of developing it [27]. The Gullah population of the Sea Islands of South Carolina is a unique group of African Americans who, due to geographic and cultural factors, remained isolated with minimal genetic admixture until the 1950s [28]. Because of the unique homogeneous nature of the Gullah, a large prevalence of SLE has been noted in this population, demonstrating genetic clustering when compared with other groups of people affected by lupus [28].

Causes of Lupus

Lupus is a complex disease, and its precise cause is unknown. As previously noted, while a person's genes may increase the chance that he or she will develop lupus, an environmental trigger is likely also needed to incite the initial illness or a flare [29]. Examples of environmental triggers may include: ultraviolet (UV) light, an infection, exhaustion, a physical injury, emotional stress(such as a divorce, illness, death in the family, or other life complication), surgery, pregnancy, or giving birth [30-35]. Hormones(especially the sex hormone estrogen) play a role in lupus. Men and women both produce estrogen, but estrogen production is much greater in females. Many women have more lupus symptoms before menstrual periods and/or during pregnancy, when estrogen production is high [30-37]. Thus, estrogen may somehow regulate the severity of lupus. However, this finding does not necessarily indicate that estrogen or any other hormone triggers lupus [30-37].

As noted, these findings suggest that genetics play an important role in the pathogenesis of lupus; however, the findings also confirm the central role of environmental triggers. Some of the environmental factors scientists have recently studied include sunlight, stress, hormones, cigarette smoke, medications, and infectious agents such as viruses [21,30-35]. Recent research has confirmed that one virus, Epstein-Barr virus (EBV), which causes mononucleosis, is a likely trigger of lupus in genetically susceptible people. As previously noted, scientists believe there is no single gene that predisposes people to lupus [30-35].

Diagnosing Lupus

Diagnosing lupus can be difficult. No single test can determine whether a person has lupus, but multiple laboratory tests may help a physician confirm the diagnosis of lupus, or rule out other causes for a patient's symptoms. In 1982, the Diagnostic and Therapeutic Criteria Committee of the American College of Rheumatology (ACR) published revised criteria for the classification of SLE (see Table 1) [36]. During the ensuing decades, several investigators have described the presence of antiphospholipid antibodies in patients with SLE. In addition, the primary antiphospholipid syndrome (Hughes syndrome) has been described in these patients, and it has been suggested that the 1982 ACR revised criteria be re-evaluated in light of these discoveries [37].

Autoantibodies in Lupus

The most useful serologic tests identify selected autoantibodies often present in the blood of people with lupus, such as antinuclear antibodies (ANAs). Most people with lupus test positive for ANAs; however, there are other causes of a positive ANA besides lupus, including infections and other autoimmune diseases; occasional positive results are found in healthy people [36]. Thus, ANA testing provides another clue for the physician in establishing a diagnosis. In addition, there are blood tests for autoantibodies that are more specific to lupus; however, not all people with lupus test positive for these antibodies, and not all people with these antibodies have lupus. These antibodies include antibodies to the small RNA-associated proteins Ro/SSA, La/SSB, Sm, U1RNP, Ku, anti-ribosomal P, monocyte chemotactic protein-1 (MCP-1), vascular cell adhesion molecule (VCAM) intercellular adhesion molecule (ICAM/CD54), and autoantibodies to RNA helicase A (RHA) among many [38-44]. Thus, the pathogenic significance and diagnostic value of lupus autoantibodies in the patients and in their relatives remains under investigation [38-44]. Some physicians may order a test for anticardiolipin (or antiphospholipid) antibody [45]. The presence of this antibody may indicate increased risk for blood clotting, as well as increased risk for miscarriage in pregnant women with lupus [45,46].

Lupus Blood Tests

We shall review five major tests that may be conducted on patient serum.

A. Antinuclear Antibody (ANA)

ANA stands for anti-nuclear antibody. This test detects a group of antibodies directed against components of the cell nucleus, including DNA and ribonucleoproteins (RNPs) [36-44]. Individual ANAs include anti-DNA antibodies, and anti-ENA antibodies (see below). Thus, the composite ANA test is used as a screening test for these autoantibodies, which may then be identified individually by other tests. The ANA test is positive in 95% of people with lupus, and only about 5% of healthy people. It can also be positive in people with related autoimmune conditions (sometimes called connective tissue diseases) such as dermatomyositis, polymyositis, and systemic sclerosis (scleroderma) [36-44]. It is sometimes positive in people with other types of diseases, such as chronic infections or selected malignancies.

B. DNA Antibodies

DNA antibody testing represents the gold standard serum test for lupus. For unknown reasons, the presence of antibodies against double-stranded DNA represents the hallmark of the disease. The finding is very specific, and rarely found in any other condition. Strongly positive anti-DNA antibody tests provide almost total confirmation of the diagnosis. In addition, the titer of the antibodies provides a rough guide to disease activity; this finding is thus utilized by physicians to monitor the clinical course of the disease [36-44].

C. Extractable Nuclear Antigens (ENAs)

The title "extractable nuclear antigens" applies to a battery of antiantibodies which are found in lupus variants, as well as in Sjögren's syndrome and mixed connective tissue disease [47].

D. Antiphospholipid Antibodies

These tests are associated with the important clinical issue of hypercoagulation [45,46]. Patients with high levels of antiphospholipid antibodies have an increased tendency to clotting in both the veins and arteries; in pregnant women with these antibodies there is a risk of thrombosis within the placenta and umbilical cord, leading to miscarriage [45-50].

E. Complement

The complement system represents a group of proteins in the blood which are involved in the immune response. In active lupus, the levels of complement (usually measured as "C3" and "C4") are low; thus, levels of these proteins may provide an estimate of disease activity [48-49]. Serum C3 and C4 levels have been used as biomarkers for lupus renal flares [50]. Further, recent studies have shown that complement anti-C1q antibodies levels have a higher correlation with flares of lupus nephritis than other serum markers [51].

Blood Testing

In addition to the specific blood tests described above, the physician usually requests a complete blood count (CBC) and serum chemistry studies. The blood count in lupus may show a low white cell count, a low red cell count and a low platelet count. Serum chemistry tests are also important, especially the blood creatinine and urea nitrogen measurements, which are classically elevated in renal disease. Elevated blood C-reactive protein (CRP) may also reflect lupus disease activity [52].

Urine Testing

Urine testing is vital in lupus patients; some lupus clinics teach all patients how to test their own urine. The most simple test utilizes a "dip-stick" to check for elevated urine protein, often the earliest clue to the presence of kidney disease. Following a positive dip stick test, more precise urine tests are performed on a "MSU" (mid-stream urine) - a sample of urine sent to the laboratory for microscopic analysis [53]. Under the microscope, the presence of white cells, red cells or clumps of cells - "casts" - is recorded - all possible signs of kidney disease. In addition,, urine sent to the laboratory may be tested for bacterial infection [53]. In one study, the authors 1) determined the sensitivity and the specificity of the qualitative urine dipstick test to detect 0.50 g or greater of a correlated quantitative 24-hour urine protein (24-hUP), 2) addressed overall agreement of the dipstick test results and the magnitude of the 24-hUP, and 3) examined the correlation between the spot urine protein creatinine index (S-UPCI) and the 24-hour UPCI with that of the 24-hUP. The authors found that a $\geq$ 2+ dipstick test is relatively sensitive to detect significant proteinuria, but it is poorly correlated with quantitative 24-hUP. Further, the authors concluded that the S-UPCI and the 24-hUP can be used interchangeably for follow-up in lupus nephritis patients with proteinuria of less than 2 g/d [54]. Finally, urine MCP-1 represents another biomarker of renal lupus in the absence of cytokines, interferon-γ and growth factors [55].

Other Tests

The lupus patient may require specialized tests to look for more widespread organ involvement. These may include echocardiograms, brain scans, and kidney scans; if evidence exists of renal involvement, possibly a renal biopsy.

Lupus and Affects on Different Organs

In Table 2, we summarized the affects of multiple lupus variants on multiple organ systems.

Lupus and the Gastrointestinal System

Lupus may demonstrate multiple manifestations within the gastrointestinal tract [55-58]. First, arteritis of the large intestine may cause diarrhea, lower abdominal pain and result in ulceration of the intestine. Excessive fluid build-up in the peritoneal cavity (ascites) has been described in lupus, and this may be caused by nephritis or other organ involvement. Chronic diarrhea may be seen as a side effect of lupus medications. Pancreatitis and splenomegaly may also be encountered [56-58]. Dysphagia may also occur, possibly due to arteritis in the esophagus resulting in painful or difficult swallowing; this symptom is usually limited to solid foods [55-58]. Gastroesophageal reflux (GER) disease may also occur with lupus. GER represents a condition in which food and/or liquid travels backwards from the stomach into the esophagus. It is common in lupus patients due to medications such as 1) corticosteroids, and 2) nonsteroidal anti-inflammatory drugs (NSAIDs) affecting the intestine [56-58]. Gastroparesis can also occur; it represents a condition that reduces the stomach's ability to empty contents in the absence of any blockage. Symptoms include bloating, abdominal distention, nausea, vomiting and unintentional weight loss. Gastroparesis can be caused by lupus itself, or by therapeutic medications. Enlargement of the liver (hepatomegaly) may also be encountered in lupus patients [55-58]. Hepatomegaly may cause a feeling of fullness under the right ribcage, and tenderness on examination. Inflammation of the liver (hepatitis) may also be encountered in lupus, again caused by either the disease itself or by therapeutic medications. Symptoms of hepatitis include dark urine, loss of appetite, nausea, vomiting, abdominal distension, pale or clay colored stools, fatigue, malaise and generalized itching. Nausea and vomiting can also be caused by an arteritis in the stomach or small intestine [56-58], or by a "pseudo-obstruction" (motility issue most likely caused by arteritis) of the intestine. Finally, pancreatitis represents inflammation of the pancreas. Pancreatitis in lupus may cause severe abdominal pain in the upper, middle or upper left part of the abdomen that may radiate to the back; nausea, vomiting, fever, chills, a swollen or tender abdomen, and a rapid heartbeat. Chronic pancreatitis may cause anemia, an inability to digest food, diabetes and jaundice [55-58].

Lupus and the Central Nervous System

Physicians are now recognizing the importance of subtle forms of brain involvement in lupus, as well as more clinically evident problems [59-61]. Brain disease in lupus may present with mild depression, memory loss, or more severe problems such as seizures. In general, there are two primary causes of brain disease in lupus. The first is the disease itself, which may cause alterations in the brain activity. The second is a clotting disorder presenting in some lupus patients, specifically the antiphospholipid or Hughes syndrome [62]. It is important for the physician to distinguish between these two major causes, as their respective treatments are distinctly different. Depression is an integral symptom of lupus in some patients; indeed, therapy of lupus itself often relieves the depression [59-61]. In more severe cases, management of depression in lupus may depend on treating the lupus itself combined with additional antidepressant therapy. One of the significant psychiatric advances of the last decade has been the introduction of milder antidepressants, with less severe side effects as those encountered with many earlier medications. Headaches are common in lupus. In some patients a history of headache going back to their early teens is feature of the disease [59-61]. The headaches may be a part of the lupus itself, or may be associated with antiphospholipid syndrome. The headaches may present with a migraine character, including visual disturbances and severe pain. In any lupus patient with headaches, a systematic workup should be performed including examination of blood pressure, sinuses, blood and if indicated, a brain scan (either MRI or CT) [59-61]. Sometimes, lupus may initially present in a dramatic way, with a seizure or a series of epileptic fits. Such a presentation may also represent an important feature of the antiphospholipid syndrome [62]. Fits or seizures are one of the non-specific ways the brain reacts to severe illness. Once the lupus is treated, further fits are the exception rather than the rule. Other movement disorders may also be encountered in lupus. Occasionally, patients develop chorea (Saint Vitus' dance) with jerky hand or head movements. The chorea is simply a manifestation of abnormal brain function and once again, is often associated with Hughes syndrome [62]. Spinal cord complications are a rare, acute and dangerous complication of lupus, which may lead to permanent paralysis. It is now recognized that immediate treatment with both steroids and anticoagulants may prevent any potential spinal cord injury. A variety of psychiatric and behavioral disorders have been described in SLE, ranging from mild personality disorders to severe psychotic behavior [59-62]. Some lupus patients are incorrectly diagnosed with schizophrenia at the initial presentation of their illness. Interestingly, treatment of the lupus in these patients results in total improvement in the psychiatric features. The rapid resolution is one of the most important observations gleaned from recent lupus research, as it provides possible insights into other mental diseases. Patients with the antiphospholipid syndrome may suffer memory impairment, from subtle to severe memory loss [62]. Physicians treating lupus patients are now confirming this important aspect of the disease. Clearly, any patient who presents with this feature of the disease requires a full neurologic examination, possibly including a MRI scan, as well as testing for the antiphospholipid syndrome.

In regard to therapy, it is first important to realize that neurologic involvement in lupus is common [62]. Second, in the vast majority of patients there is complete resolution of neurologic problems over time, provided they are addressed properly. If the neurologic symptoms present dramatically, ie, with fits or severe neuropsychiatric disease, the treatment (as with most active forms of lupus) should be with steroids and immunosuppressive drugs. The doses of steroids used are less than previously utilized (for example, 60mg daily in the majority of the worst cases); rarely is a higher dose required. An alternative way of giving steroids is by “pulse” injections on an intermittent basis [59-61]. The puse method is becoming more popular, as it is a simple and more rapidly effective way of administrating steroids, especially in emergencies. As previously noted, a distinct form of brain involvement in lupus is associated with the antiphospholipid or Hughes syndrome [62]. In this complication, the neurologic etiopathogenesis is secondary to microthrombi in neural blood vessels. In patients where the antiphospholipid syndrome is suspected, brain scans are usually performed. The brain scans may show localized areas where blood supply has been inadequate. The treatment in these patients requires thinning of the blood, either with aspirin or, in more severe cases with anticoagulants such as warfarin (Coumadin) [62]. For less dramatic brain involvement, the decision to treat is more problematic. Many patients are not treated, who should be treated. In some patients, depression is a major problem and requires conventional anti-depressive treatment. The more modern medications for depression are superior to older medications, causing far less side effects. The opinion of a psychiatrist may be sought to address whether medical psychiatric treatment is appropriate, especially given the dangers of drug interactions. In summary, the vast majority of patients who experience lupus brain involvement may be treated successfully and return to normal daily activities [59-61]. Anxiety and depression are common symptoms felt by lupus patients.

Finally, other neurologic sequelae may present in lupus patients. Central nervous system vasculitis represents inflammation of the blood vessels of the brain. It is characterized by high fevers, psychosis, seizures, and meningitis-like neck stiffness, leading to stupor and coma if not quickly and aggressively treated [63,64]. Cognitive dysfunction may occur in lupus, and may include memory loss, loss of concentration, confusion and difficulty expressing thoughts. Cognitive dysfunction may present as an intermittent or constant clinical problem; it is sometimes referred to as "lupus brain fog". Also, up to 30% of people with lupus have a simultaneous fibromyalgia, evidenced by tender points and increased pain in the soft tissues. Patients with a fibromyalgia may also experience cognitive dysfunction, difficulty sleeping, and lack of stamina. As previously noted, lupus headaches may present with a migraine character [59-61]; these headaches are more common in lupus patients with antiphospholipid syndrome or Raynaud's phenomenon. These severe headaches are often treated similar to other migraines; although corticosteroids are also usually helpful, distinguishing it from other types of migraines. Intracranial hypertension (pseudotumor cerebri) is a rare complication of lupus and can also be caused by the medications used to treat lupus. The most common symptoms are severe non-specific headaches, transient altered vision, and tinnitus [59-61]. Other symptoms may include a stiff neck, back pain, double vision, pain behind the eyes, and exercise intolerance. Diagnosis is achieved via 1) a complete eye examination, 2) tests to rule out other causes of increased intercranial pressure and 3) a high opening pressure on lumbar puncture (spinal tap). Peripheral neuropathy is a symptom most commonly associated with diabetes; however, peripheral neuropathy may also be encountered in lupus. Peripheral nerves, in contradistinction to cranial nerves, represent nerves located in the arms, legs and torso. When these nerves do not communicate properly with the spinal cord, a peripheral neuropathy results. A peripheral neuropathy may cause pain, numbness, tingling, burning or itching. Some 10-25% of lupus patients may have one or more seizures as part of their disease [59-61]. Finally, patients with antiphospholipid syndrome are at risk for stroke [62].

Lupus and the Kidney

In lupus patients, the kidney is often seriously affected by the disease. Lupus nephritis represents disease inflammation of the kidney, characterized by damage to these organs and progressive loss of kidney function [66-71]. Symptoms and signs of lupus nephritis include 1) blood and/or protein in the urine, 2) elevated blood pressure, 3) abnormal blood serum studies and 4) swelling of the ankles, hands and face. Lupus nephritis may develop into a life-threatening complication of the disease [65-71]. Lupus nephritis ascites is defined as excessive fluid build up within the peritoneal cavity, secondary to kidney inflammation and failure. Estimates vary depending on the type of clinic and the patient population studied, but it is usually estimated that approximately half of all lupus patients will have clinical evidence of kidney inflammation within their clinical course [66-71]. In mild cases of lupus, the nephritis percentage will be lower. Fortunately, severe kidney disease requiring kidney dialysis or transplantation is rare in lupus. Kidney involvement in lupus rarely causes discomfort or pain (as distinct, for example, from kidney stones or renal infections) [66-71]. The most common clinical renal problem is excessive protein (albumin) leakage into the urine. The excess protein loss may be mild and detected only via testing, or severe and result in lowering of the blood protein (ie, a low plasma albumin level) [66-71]. If the blood albumin concentration is lowered, ankle swelling, fluid retention and truncal edema may result. Further, when the kidney is inflamed, blood pressure frequently rises; blood pressure measurement is thus important in any physical examination of lupus patients [66-71]. When the kidney is more severely damaged, its normal filtering process is impaired; toxic metabolites such as urea and creatinine (normally present in the blood in small amounts) build up, leading to weight loss, nausea and general malaise [66-70]. Simple outpatient urine testing involves the use of a urine dipstick. Modern urine dipsticks test for a variety of substances in the urine, including glucose, albumin protein, blood and so on. The test involves dipping the dipstick in the urine, and comparing resultant color changes to a interpretation chart. If the lupus patient is losing excess protein in the urine (proteinuria) then the amount of protein loss may need to be quantified [66-71]. Often, this is accomplished by evaluating the ratio of albumin to creatinine in a sample of urine (ie, the albumin: creatinine ratio), which is technically easier than measuring the total protein in all patient urine over a 24 hour period [66-71]. The patient urine may also be sent to the laboratory for detection of infectious agents, and for further detailed microscopic examination. The three primary blood tests affected by kidney function include 1) the urea (ie, blood urea nitrogen or BUN), 2) creatinine and 3) albumin [66-71]. The creatinine may be further utilized to calculate the estimated glomerular filtration rate (eGFR), which permits grading of the severity of kidney disease; stage 1 represents the mildest disease, and stage 5 the most severe. Overall, if the filtering function of the kidney is impaired, then serum BUN and creatinine levels rise and the eGFR falls. The serum albumin falls if significant, pathologic leakage of albumin into the urine is present. In addition to these tests, other blood tests give important information regarding the lupus patient. These include the serum sodium, potassium, calcium and phosphate levels, as well as the hemoglobin [66-71].

A kidney ultrasound may also be performed, to confirm that two kidneys are present and to document their size. Sometimes other tests may be undertaken such as an radiologic isotope renogram, which can measure the extent that each kidney contributes to overall renal function [66-71]. If clinically indicated, the precise degree of disease activity may be ascertained via a kidney biopsy. Renal biopsy is now a routine procedure in hospitals throughout the world. For best results, it is often conducted with ultrasound guidance. Following local anesthesia, a needle is inserted into the kidney and a small core biopsy is obtained. The patient is usually kept in the hospital overnight, as there is a small risk of bleeding following the biopsy. The procedure has a high safety margin, and does not adversely affect kidney function.

Classically, the first pathologic signs of lupus renal involvement involve lymphohistiocytic infiltrates surrounding the glomeruli. A more advanced histologic stage is direct inflammation and damage within the glomeruli. Severe histologic stages involve extensive involvement and scarring of the glomeruli [66-71]. There are international conventions about staging the damage within the kidney biopsy; pathologists are thus able to determine the chances of response to treatment from their reading of the biopsy. Current clinical consensus mandates that if histologic kidney inflammation exists, a therapeutic regimen of 1) steroids and 2) an additional immunosuppressive agent is warranted [66-71]. For active or severe lupus renal disease, the most widely used additional immunosuppressive is cyclophosphamide (given intermittently by injection). In the past, cyclophosphamide was given as a tablet; however, this route of administration produced more side effects and most clinics have now converted to intermittent injection "pulses" [72].

Doses vary from clinic to clinic; however, a recent trend has been to utilize lower doses, with the benefit of fewer side effects. A second, milder and widely used lupus immunosuppressive is azathioprine, given as tablet and usually at a dose of about 2mg/kg body weight. A third tablet immunosuppressive that is becoming more widely used is mycophenolate mofetil [72].

Studies are underway to see if it might supersede cyclophosphamide, which would be advantageous as it does not cause as many serious side effects. It would further be useful if a patient does not tolerate azathioprine. All immunosuppressives can affect the blood cell count; thus, regular complete blood counts are mandatory for patients taking these medications. Other immunosuppressive drugs such as cyclosporine A are increasingly utilized in lupus therapy, but the current primary mainstays of treatment remain cyclophosphamide and azathioprine [73].

Finally, if the kidney damage reaches a stage where toxic blood metabolites are increasing, then dialysis is vital. Dialysis is one of the major advances in twentieth century medicine; either haemodialysis or peritoneal dialyses have assisted thousands of patients with lupus renal failure [74].

One of the surprises in the early days of lupus renal transplantation was the finding that lupus consistently did not damage the transplanted kidney [75]. The reasons for the finding are not known; however, the finding could be related to the strong immunosuppression utilized with transplantation, and possibly to other factors. Patients with lupus who undergo renal transplantation have largely successful clinical outcomes [75].

Lupus and the Heart and Lungs

The main symptoms and signs of heart or lung involvement are pleuritic pain (specifically, pain experienced on deep inhalation), shortness of breath, cough and ankle swelling. In addition, because the drugs used to treat lupus patients suppress the immune system, chest infections are increased in these patients [76-79]. Pleuritic pain is common in lupus – estimates vary that between 30% and 60% of patients develop this problem during their clinical course. More severe presentations of lupus may cause pleural effusions; specifically, these effusions are collections of fluid, often usually starting at the base of the lungs and occasionally covering a large proportion of the lung surface. Pleural effusion fluid may constrict the lungs, causing shortness of breath. Pleuritic pain may be confirmed via the clinical history and examination, and pleural effusions confirmed on a chest x-ray [76-79]. Pleural effusions usually respond rapidly to a short course of steroids. A number of pathologic conditions may affect the anatomic structure of the lungs themselves, although no structural alterations are as specific for lupus as interstitial fibrosis. Confirmation of this abnormality is achieved via chest x-rays and CT (or MRI) scanning. Some lupus patients are more susceptible to blood clots, which in turn elicit a pulmonary embolus; a pulmonary embolus may present acutely, or chronically with coughing up of blood [76-79].

Classically, pulmonary embolus pain is at the center front of the chest, and may be misinterpreted by the patient (or the physician) as a heart attack. Clinical examination, chest x-rays and an echocardiogram may help to make the distinction [76-79]. A small number of lupus patients develop heart valvular disease [76-79]. There is a strong association with the presence of anti-phospholipid antibodies and leaky heart valves; these valve abnormalities may result in shortness of breath, and should be treated with the assistance of a cardiologist. Rarely, lupus patients require heart valve surgery. Although the actual number of lupus patients suffering from myocardial infarctions (MIs) is small, there is an increased risk of occurrence, especially in women between the ages of thirty five and forty five. The reasons for this increased risk are not entirely clear; however, some traditional MI risk factors such as high blood pressure are increased in lupus patients [76-79].

Significantly, anti-phospholipid antibody effects can be minimized by the use of aspirin or warfarin. Pleuritic pain may often be successfully treated with low to moderate doses of steroids [76-79]. Increased emphasis is being placed on determining the risk factors for the development of MIs in lupus patients, including abnormalities in clotting factors and possible abnormal cholesterol levels. Smoking cessation is also a vital factor in the long-term management of these problems.

Pregnancy and Contraception for Women with Lupus

Although pregnancy in women with lupus is considered high risk, most women with lupus carry their babies safely to the end of their pregnancy. Some babies have been born with neonatal lupus [80-84]. Overall, women with lupus have a higher rate of miscarriage and premature birth relative to the general population. In addition, women who have antiphospholipid antibodies are at a greater risk of miscarriage in the second trimester because of increased risk of blood clots in the placenta or umbilical cord [80-84]. Lupus patients with a history of kidney disease have a higher risk of pre-eclampsia. Pregnancy counseling and planning before pregnancy are important for lupus patients. Ideally, a woman should have no signs or symptoms of lupus and be taking no medications for at least 6 months before she becomes pregnant.

Some women may experience a mild to moderate flare during or after their pregnancy; others do not. Pregnant women with lupus, especially those taking corticosteroids, also are more likely to develop high blood pressure, diabetes, hyperglycemia and renal complications; thus, regular prenatal care and good nutrition during pregnancy are essential. It is also advisable to have access to a neonatal intensive care unit at the time of delivery, in case the baby requires special medical attention [80-84]. For women with lupus who do not wish to become pregnant or who are taking drugs that could be harmful to an unborn baby, reliable birth control is important. Previously, oral contraceptives were not an option for women with lupus because doctors feared the hormones in the pill would cause a flare of the disease [85]. However, a large NIH-supported study termed Safety of Estrogens in Lupus Erythematosus National Assessment (SELENA) found that severe flares were no more common among women with lupus taking oral contraceptives than those taking a placebo (inactive pill). As a result of this study published in 2005, physicians are increasingly prescribing oral contraceptives to women with inactive or stable lupus [85].

Current Research in Lupus

Lupus is the focus of intense research, as scientists try to determine precisely what causes the disease and how it can best be treated. Some of the central research questions include: 1) Why are women more likely than men to have the disease? 2) Why are there more cases of lupus in selected racial and ethnic groups, and why are cases in these groups often more severe than in Caucasian patients? 3) What specific derangements occur in the immune system, and why do they occur? 4) How can we therapeutically correct the way the immune system functions? 5) What treatment approaches will work best to ameliorate lupus symptoms? 6) How can we cure lupus?. To help address these questions, scientists are developing new and improved ways to study the disease. They are performing laboratory studies that compare aspects of the immune systems of lupus patients with those of healthy people. They also utilize mouse models with disorders resembling lupus, to better understand the abnormalities of the immune system that occur in lupus and to identify possible new therapies. In the US, the National Institute of Arthritis and Musculoskeletal and Skin Diseases (NIAMS) within the U.S. Department of Health and Human Services National Institutes of Health (NIH), funds many lupus researchers. A tissue bank collection from children affected by neonatal lupus and their mothers is also available.

Genetics in Lupus

Identifying genes that 1) play a role in the development of lupus, or 2) affect lupus severity is an active area of research. NIAMS intramural and extramural investigators have established that a polymorphism in the STAT4 gene (which is associated with lupus susceptibility) is preferentially associated with lupus disease severe symptoms, including renal malfunction [86]. The STAT4 finding may allow physicians to determine which patients are at risk of severe disease, and may lead to the development of new treatments for these patients. Scientists have also identified a gene that may confer susceptibility to lupus. They have shown that having an alternative form of the gene Ly108 may impair the body's ability to keep self-destructive B cells under control [87]. The Ly108 gene is part of a gene family (SLAM) that has been linked to a lupus-like disease in mice [87].

Biomarkers

Biomarkers represent another significant area of lupus research. Biomarkers are defined as molecules that reflect a specific biological or pathological process, a consequence of a process, or a response to a therapeutic intervention. Patients with SLE and metabolic syndrome had significantly raised serum uric acid, C-reactive protein (CRP), lipid hydroperoxides, and protein oxidation, in contradistinction to patients with SLE without metabolic syndrome. Lipid hydroperoxides were correlated with CRP, whereas protein oxidation was associated with waist circumference and uric acid. There was a positive association between serum Complement C3 and C4 and glucose, as well as between C3 and CRP [88]. Researchers have identified anti-double-stranded DNA antibodies and Complement C3a (both of which can be identified utilizing blood tests) as biomarkers for flares, in that they can predict that a flare will occur. They also showed that moderate doses of prednisone can prevent flares in people possessing these biomarkers [89].

The Disease Process

Because lupus presentations differ between patients and the disease is characterized by autoimmunity in variable organ systems, the initial presentation in a given patient can be difficult to detect. Many symptoms may increase and decrease over time, often delaying the diagnosis and initiation of therapy. Many researchers have reported that autoantibodies are important in the diagnosis and classification of SLE; however, whether these autoantibodies specifically correlate with changes in disease activity in individual patients is controversial [51]. One group of researchers reported the association between changes in SLE global disease activity and renal activity, vis-a-vis changes in multiple autoantibodies and cell adhesion molecules [51]. The researchers utilized stored sera, collected during clinic visits from each of 49 SLE patients (91% female, 59% African-American, 31% Caucasian, 10% other ethnicity, 38% under 30 years, 41% between 30-44 years, and 21% 45-63 years); the sera were then were analyzed [51]. Specific patient clinic visits were further selected to include one visit with proteinuria and one or two without proteinuria for each patient. Global disease activity was measured by the Physician's Global Assessment (PGA), and SLEDAI (SLE Disease Activity Index modified to exclude anti-dsDNA and complement); renal activity assessed via urine protein (by urine dipstick) and renal activity score [51]. Sera were assayed for anti-Complement C1q, anti-chromatin, anti-dsDNA, anti-ribosomal P protein, monocyte chemotactic protein-1 (MCP-1), vascular cell adhesion molecule (VCAM) intercellular adhesion molecule (ICAM/CD54) and overall complement [51]. Associations between changes in disease activity and changes in biomarker levels were assessed [90]. In terms of global disease activity, anti-C1q had the highest association with the PGA ($p = 0.09$) and was strongly associated with modified SLEDAI ($p = 0.009$). In terms of renal activity, anti-C1q had the highest association with proteinuria ($p = 0.079$), and was strongly associated with the renal activity score ($p = 0.006$) [51]. The authors concluded that anti-C1q demonstrated the best performance of the potential biomarkers, being significantly associated with the modified SLEDAI and with the renal activity score. This study indicated the potential superior utility of anti-C1q over anti-dsDNA and other measures to track lupus renal activity [51].

Lupus and the Skin, Hair and Mucosae

In Table 3, we outline multiple mucocutaneous manifestations of lupus erythematosus. The classic, presenting skin finding in lupus is the malar butterfly rash. The malar rash is a red rash (and occasionally a mild blush) that occurs across the bridge of the nose and on the cheeks, resulting in a distinctive butterfly shape appearance. Butterfly rashes tend to come and go, depending on how active the underlying lupus is; it does not leave scars as it heals, but may leave pigmentary alterations [90-101]. Discoid lupus is a type of lupus that tends to be confined to the skin, with other organs in the body not involved. Discoid lupus occurs in patches. The patches tend to be well defined, thickened and scaly; they are slightly red in color and may itch. As the patches heal, they tend to leave scars; in dark skin the skin pigment may be lost, forming residual white areas. If discoid lupus occurs on the scalp, the hair will often be lost, leaving permanent bald areas [90-101]. Subacute cutaneous lupus erythematosus (SCLE) presents as a distinctive rash, that usually occurs in sun exposed areas of the body. It begins as scaly patches which increase in size to form circular areas, which then gradually heal without leaving scars [90-101]. SCLE clinically often presents in a range between the systemic form and the discoid form; specifically, patients with subacute cutaneous lupus often have some of the blood abnormalities found in systemic lupus and frequently experience joint pains, but they do not classically develop the serious complications that can occur in SLE [90-101]. A panniculitis represents inflammation of the fat below the skin, resulting in tender red subcutaneous lumps; these heal slowly over time and can cause residual dimpling of the skin. Lupus patients may manifest a panniculitis, presenting as either lupus panniculitis or lupus profundus. Lupus may affect the blood vessels in the skin, causing a vasculitis [90-101]. Vasculitis may cause painful red macules, often present on the legs and arms. A lupus vasculitis may also occur in other areas of the body; for example, it may occur in the kidney, and if present, may represent a serious complication necessitating prompt treatment. In addition, blood flow through skin blood vessels may become sluggish in lupus patients with the antiphospholipid antibody syndrome (APS/Hughes Syndrome) [90-101]. In these patients, the skin may take on a mottled or net-like appearance known as livedo reticularis. Livedo reticularis often presents on the legs and arms. Patient scalp hair may be affected in lupus. The hair often thin, and can become patchy when lupus is active. It will often regrow if the disease is brought under control. However, as previously noted, in discoid lupus disease scars may leave permanent bald areas. Also, sometimes medication therapy may make the hair thin in lupus patients. Medication hair thinning occurs in some people undergoing steroid treatment, and in most people when cytotoxic drugs such as cyclophosphamide are used. In both cases, the hair should regrow when the drug is discontinued [90-101]. Approximately 60% of people with lupus will be sensitive to sunlight. Sunlight may cause 1) exacerbation of skin rashes, 2) a generalized burning of the skin and 3) increased activity of lupus in other organs within the body. The lupus band test is classically found when performing direct and/or indirect immunofluorescence for lupus patients. The lupus band represents linear deposits of immunoglobulins at the DEJ, combined with a thickened basement membrane in lesional skin of LE patients [96-99]. A number of treatments are available for the skin in lupus. These can be divided into topical, injection and oral treatments. Topical treatments tend to consist of steroid creams and ointments. These can contain mild steroids such as hydrocortisone, or stronger steroids such as betamethasone [102-104]. These topical therapies may sometimes be adequate to control mild lupus rashes; however, they should not be used for extended periods, particularly on the face. In discoid lupus, particularly troublesome skin areas can be injected with long acting steroids under the skin to promote healing. Over time, most people will require oral treatment to control their skin problems. The antimalarials such as chloroquine, hydroxychloroquine, mepacrine and mycophenolate mofetil are all very useful in controlling skin rashes [102-104]. They tend to work slowly, and need to be taken for a number of months before any effect is seen. Other oral treatments include steroids, which may also be given intravenously if the skin lesions are very severe. Oral and intravenous steroids obviously have a number of side effects; thus, these options are usually reserved for skin problems that have not responded to topical treatments and antimalarial agents [102-104]. Occasionally, skin rashes cannot be controlled with the above treatments or they recur on steroid dose reduction. In these people, other medications such as azathioprine or cyclosporin can be used. These drugs are often reserved for noncutaneous problems in lupus such as kidney disease; however, they may be given for the skin alone in difficult cases. One important way that those with lupus can help themselves is to avoid sun exposure [102-104]. Thus, patients should be encouraged to cover up their skin with long sleeves and trousers in the sunlight, and wear a hat if exposed to the sun for extended periods. The use of UV screening film on windows may also be helpful for those who are particularly sun sensitive. Also, sun block cream with a minimum sun protection factor (SPF) of 25, should be applied to exposed areas of skin, although many patients will require higher SPF level protection.

Lupus and the Sun

As previously noted, lupus lesions may be exacerbated after exposure to sunlight. The resultant rashes are titled photosensitive rashes, and represent classic clinical lesions of lupus. In addition, patients with these rashes may develop migraine headaches, nausea or joint pains. The joints may become tender to touch and swollen. Other clinical aspects of lupus may also be exacerbated after sun exposure, including fever, pleuritic pain (chest pain on inhalation), kidney disease and neurologic problems. Patients with severe light sensitivity may further be adversely affected by fluorescent and halogen lighting, energy-saving bulbs or any very bright light. Precautionary measures may be warranted, including amber window film or blinds, which screen out blue spectrum light. Certain types of sunblock are also available on prescription for lupus patients [105-107]. Sunblocks which screen out visible light as well are available by prescription, or over the counter. Clinically, it is always best to be on the lowest possible dose of steroids; thus, avoiding UV light and wearing sunblock is important even for patients on steroids. Hydroxychloroquine (Plaquenil) seems to be particularly helpful for preventing rashes, arthritis and pleuritic pain; however, this theapy is also not a replacement for sunlight avoidance. Other agents (such as azathioprine, methotrexate and cyclophosphamide) which are often used for more serious disease or to minimize steroid dosages may also reduce the risks of sunlight induced flares. Sunblock should be sun protection factor (SPF) 25 or greater, and effective against both UVA and UVB light. It should be applied in the morning and reapplied during the day (at least once or twice), as it tends to get rubbed off or sweated away [105-107]. Sunblock should be used even on cloudy days by light-sensitive people because UV light can penetrate the cloud layer.

Lupus and the Musculoskeletal System

Joint and muscle pain represent two of the most common symptoms of lupus. Vertebral fractures may also occur in patients with lupus [108-112]. In lupus, the joint tissue may become inflamed, causing pain and swelling. The joints most frequently involved are located in the hands, wrists and knees, although any joint may be involved [108-112]. The arthritis is often intermittent, and affects different joints at different times. The ligaments and tendons around the joints can also become inflamed and tender. If the inflammation is not brought under control with medication and continues for a long period of time, the tendons and ligaments can weaken. Once this happens, the tendons and ligaments can no longer support the joint properly. The affected joint becomes lax, or unstable, and can appear to be deformed. The hand joints are most frequently affected by these deformities [108-112]. The joint bones themselves are not affected by lupus arthritis, and at least initially the deformities can be painlessly corrected by pushing the joint back into position. Painkillers such as paracetamol may control the joint pain. If this is not adequate, then the addition of nonsteroidal anti-inflammatory drugs (NSAIDs) may be indicated. If only one or two troublesome joints are present, an injection of steroids into the affected joints may be recommended; this is often an effective way of obtaining maximum benefit from the steroids, with a minimal risk of side effects. If there are more joints affected, steroids may be administered into nearby muscles or intravenously. Intramuscular and intravenous steroids may result in rapid and dramatic reduction in pain and inflammation of affected joints [108-112]. However, the improvement is often of short duration, and the treatment usually needs to be supplemented by oral medication. The most common oral medications utilized are antimalarials, and specifically hydroxychloroquine is frequently employed. These medications are effective in reducing joint pain and inflammation over a long period of time, but can take up to three months to become maximally effective. Oral steroids are also effective in controlling joint pain, and are commonly used. Sometimes joint pain and inflammation can be particularly problematic and stronger agents such as azathioprine, methotrexate and cyclosporine may be prescribed [108-112]. Surgery may be helpful for some people. Hand surgeons can correct some of the hand deformities with operations on the tendons and ligaments. Orthopedic surgeons can replace some of the larger joints, for example knees and hips, if they are badly damaged. Surgery is a significant stress in lupus patients; thus, the disease needs to be well controlled to make the procedure as safe as possible and to increase the likelihood of satisfactory results. Lupus may also affect the muscles. The most common cause of muscle pain is related to arthritis in nearby joints; treating the joints helps to address the muscle pain. An infrequent but serious cause of muscle pain in lupus is direct inflammation of the muscles, or myositis. In myositis, muscle weakness is often morea of a problem than pain; the weakness may be a serious problem if it occurs in muscles that control breathing and swallowing. A less serious, but more common muscle problem is a condition called fibromyalgia. Fibromyalgia can occur in people both with and without lupus. It causes persistent pain in most muscles, but tends to be centred on the shoulders and hips. It causes sleep disturbances; tender spots in the muscles can develop. The causes of fibromyalgia are unknown; it does not progress to muscle or joint destruction although it can cause considerable discomfort [108-112]. Although a serious problem, myositis usually responds well to treatment with steroids. Other drugs are frequently prescribed and used in combination with steroids to improve or maintain the myositis; these medications include azathioprine and cyclosporin. In severe cases, cyclophosphamide and gamma globulins may be prescribed. Table 4 outlines a summary of different organ systems affected by lupus.

Podiatric Care in Lupus

Lupus may also cause joint and muscle pains in the feet. Resultant abnormal walking patterns can lead to misshapen feet, and deformities such as bunions and hammertoes [113-114]. Toe deformities can then increase the risk of friction and pressure inside the shoes, causing calluses and corns. Corns and callus occur frequently in older patients, those with problems walking, or those who wear badly fitting shoes. Lupus and the drugs used to treat lupus can aggravate the problem of hard or dry skin. Specific skin problems associated with lupus may occur on the feet, but are uncommon [113-114]. Verrucae may sometimes be a nuisance to people who are taking immunosuppressants. Lupus patients may also have nail problems. In some lupus patients, nail growth may be slow. The slow growth may lead to weak, thin nails, pitting in the nail plate and loose nails. In other patients, periungual inflammation or Raynaud's phenomenon may lead to thickened or ridged nails. Nail problems are generally cosmetic in lupus, although involuted or ingrown toenails are common [113-114]. These can be very sensitive; it is important to obtain professional help to prevent ingrown toenails from becoming infected. About 20-30% of lupus patients develop Raynaud's phenomenon (spasms in the blood vessels, causing cold or white fingers or toes). Chilblains are also frequent, often in association with Raynaud's phenomenon. Chilblains may become painful and represent an abnormal reaction to cold, usually on toes and fingers [113-114]. They can resolve leaving cracks in the skin, which then expose it to infection. It is important to keep the feet warm, but not to warm them up too quickly if they are cold. Vasculitis occasionally causes painful toes and feet, and may lead to infections. Vasculitis may cause small red lines in the cuticles or nail folds, or small red nodules on the legs; from time to time, painful red nodules can form on the legs. Occasionally, these red nodules may also ulcerate. Steroid therapy may make the skin thin, and more prone to damage and infection.

Nails must be cut carefully; it is often easier and safer to file them rather than cut them, particularly if they are thick or uneven. The patient's feet should be washed and examined daily for any damage or problems. Any dry skin should be kept moist with a good moisturizing cream, to prevent cracks from occurring [113-114]. It is vital to wear well-fitting, supportive footwear.

Ideally, shoes should also have a soft cushioned sole, a pliable yielding upper and fasten firmly around the instep. There should be no high-pressure areas on the shoes which rub the skin. Also, the feet must be kept warm. Two thin pairs of socks are warmer than one thick pair; in cold weather, thermal insoles should be put into shoes and bed socks worn at night. Lupus patients should visit a podiatrist on at least one occasion for foot care advice [113-114].

Lupus and the Mucosae

One of the most common features of lupus is oral ulcers [115]. Bullous SLE represents a rare but serious disease, in which patients have antibodies against their own skin and/or oral mucosa. Lesions associated with this condition consist of grouped blisters, typically presenting on the head and neck; blisters may also present on the arms and legs [116]. Systemic corticosteroids and immunosuppressives represent the classic treatment for this disease [116].

Herpes simplex (fever blisters) may appear as a side effect of immunosuppressive therapy [117]. These lesions appear as small groups of painful, fluid filled blisters that usually resolve without medical treatment within 2-4 weeks [117]. Oral and intranasal ulcers may also occur in some lupus patients [118].

These ulcers may cause soreness, difficulty chewing, and visible sores in the mouth [118]. Oral candidiasis may occur usually a side effect of immunosuppressive therapy. Oral candidiasis appears as whitish red, flaky plaques that can affect any area of the mouth; plaques often affect the esophagus. Patients may feel a burning sensation, or have difficulty swallowing. Oral anti-fungals are utilized for therapy. If the mouth is particularly sore, a soft toothbrush and gentle brushing of teeth, flossing and smoking cessation should be recommended.

Depending on the type of lesion, steroid paste may also be utilized, coupled with antimalarial tablets such as hydroxychloroquine. In many cases, an antifungal nystatin mouthwash may be warranted. Approximately a third of lupus patients have some sort of eye problem related to their disease. Fortunately, in most people only the surface of the eye is affected [119]. Corneal dryness does not significantly affect the vision, and is readily treated with eye drops. Much less commonly, the disease may involve the interior of the eye or the visual pathways within the brain.

These complications may reduce vision and usually require systemic treatment, either by oral or intravenous routes. A retinopathy due to antimalarial medications should also be excluded in patients receiving this treatment [120]. Lupus may cause "scleritis", which may be very painful and is usually visible as a bright red patch on part or all of the external, white sclera of the eye [119,120]. Treatment may require steroids or other immunosuppressive medications once infection has been ruled out.

Other medications used to treat lupus can themselves contribute to eye problems. Steroids, particularly if used at high doses over a long period, increase the risk of developing cataracts at an earlier age than other people not receiving these drugs [121]. Also, patients receiving steroids are at increased risk of optic nerve damage from glaucoma [121]. Regular eye examinations with an optician will generally pick up on such problems at an early stage, and treatment for these conditions can then be sought from an ophthalmologist.

As previously noted, antimalarial medications may cause a retinopathy, particularly chloroquine [119]. Antimalarial medication retinopathy is currently not frequently encountered, due to 1) lower dosages and 2) a preference for hydroxychloroquine over chloroquine than in the past. However, if a patient notices a deterioration in reading vision or in perception of color, her or she should undergo an eye examination. Notably, the most common reasons for changes in vision in lupus patients are age related changes in focusing or cataracts, rather than side effects from hydroxychloroquine therapy [119-121].

Mixed Connective Tissue Disease, or Overlap Syndrome

Overlap syndrome is an entity that satisfies the criteria of at least two connective tissue diseases (CTD). These conditions include scleroderma/systemic sclerosis (SSc), dermatomyositis or polymyositis, Sjogren's syndrome, rheumatoid arthritis and systemic lupus erythematosus. A combined syndrome affects the clinical features, diagnosis and treatment of the disorder.

The classic features of an overlap syndrome include severe Raynaud's phenomenon and joint pains, often with puffy, swollen "sausage" fingers [122]. One recent study explored features of scleroderma overlap syndrome [122].

The authors studied the medical records of 165 consecutive SSc patients, and reviewed scleroderma overlap syndrome cases in depth. Specifically, an internet PubMed search was conducted for the period 1977 to 2009 using the key words "overlap syndrome", "systemic sclerosis", "connective tissue disease" and "biological agents." The authors found that forty of the original 165 patients satisfied inclusion criteria for scleroderma overlap syndrome.

The incidences of additional connective tissue diseases present in 1) the original group and 2) in the overlap syndrome group (respectively) were as follows: dermatomyositis or polymyositis 11.5% and 47.5%, Sjogren's syndrome 10.3% and 42.5%, rheumatoid arthritis 3.6% and 15.4%, and systemic lupus erythematosus 1.2% and 5.0%. Coexistence of SSc and another CTD aggravated the clinical course of the disease, especially vis-a-vis lung, kidney, digestive tract, vascular and articular involvement.

In the overlap group, coexisting non-rheumatic complications were similar to non-overlap SSc complications. An additional rheumatic or non-rheumatic disease did affect treatment choice [122]. A little less than 1 in 10 patients with lupus are affected with an additional autoimmune disorder such as Graves' disease, psoriasis, Hashimoto's thyroiditis, sarcoidosis, erythema nodosum, or other conditions [123].

Differential Diagnoses of Lupus

Other conditions are occasionally incorrectly diagnosed as lupus; these disorders include many vasculitic disorders. The differential diagnosis disorders include Wegener's granulomatosis, Takayasu arteritis, giant cell (temporal) arteritis, Behçet's disease, rheumatoid arthritis, sarcoidosis, Cogan syndrome, Kawasaki disease and ankylosing spondylitis. Of interest, recent reports have also established associations between 1) inflammatory abdominal aortic aneurysms and lymphoplasmacytic thoracic aortitis and 2) multiple sclerosis [124-127]. In Tables 5 and 6, we summarize some diagnostic tools to assist in differentiating between lupus and differential entities, as well as a summary of primary symptoms and signs encountered in lupus patients.

Coping with Lupus among Family and Friends

The lupus patient may have to bear the burden of the illness largely alone, either because partners 1) do not appreciate a real and deserving condition, or 2) do not understand the chronic nature of lupus.

Please refer to Table 1 for a summary of multiple organizations providing excellent supportive material for lupus patients and their families and friends. In general, the following recommendations should be considered: 1) pursue education about lupus; 2) counterbalance fatigue by resting and by pacing daily activities; 3) try to resolve stress, depression, pain or anger, and avoid other triggering factors such as sun exposure or fluorescent lights; 4) be open and honest with family and friends regarding lupus unpredictability, especially in regard to neurological and or behavioral alterations; and 5) try to pursue new interests and skills if desired, and ask for help as needed from family, friends and health professionals.

Treatment

Multiple researched treatments are available for lupus patients; several therapies are based on large clinical trials, or on other studies [73-75, 102-104, 108-112, 120, 125,126, 127].

NSAIDs

For lupus patients with joint pain, chest pain or fever, nonsteroidal anti-inflammatory drugs (NSAIDs), are often prescribed; some, such as ibuprofen and naproxen, are available over the counter. Common side effects of NSAIDs include stomach irritation, heartburn, diarrhea, and fluid retention. Some lupus patients may also develop liver, kidney, or neurological complications; thus, it is important to maintain access to a physician while taking these medications [73-75, 102-104, 108-112, 120, 125,126, 127].

Antimalarials

Antimalarials are another class of drug frequently used in lupus therapy. These medications, such as hydroxycloroquine, were originally used to treat malaria and are now utilized to treat lupus [73-75, 102-104, 108-112, 120, 125-128].

Antimalarials may be used alone, or in combination with other drugs; they are generally used to address fatigue, joint pain, skin rashes, and inflammation of the lungs. Clinical studies have also found that continuous treatment with antimalarials may prevent flares from recurring. Side effects of antimalarials may include stomach irritation, and rarely damage to the retina of the eye [73-75, 102-104, 108-112, 120, 125,126, 127,128].

Corticosteroids

The mainstay of lupus treatment involves the use of corticosteroid hormones, including prednisone, hydrocortisone, methylprednisolone and dexamethasone [129-133]. Corticosteroids are related to cortisol, which is a natural anti-inflammatory hormone. They work by rapidly suppressing inflammation. Corticosteroids can be given orally, via topical creams, by injection or by intravenous (IV) infusion. Corticosteroid side effects generally cease when drug administration is stopped. It is clinically dangerous to suddenly cease corticosteroid therapy.

Sometimes, a large amount of therapeutic corticosteroid is administered by IV infusion over a brief period of time (ie, hours or days), constituting "bolus" or "pulse" therapy. Long-term side effects of corticosteroids include stretch marks on the skin, weakened or damaged bones (osteoporosis and osteonecrosis), high blood pressure, damage to the arteries, diabetes mellitus, infections, and cataracts [129-133]

Lupus patients undergoing corticosteroid therapy should discuss adding supplemental calcium, vitamin D or other agents (to reduce osteoporosis risk) with their physician.

Immunosuppressives

For patients whose renal or central nervous systems are affected by lupus, immunosuppressive therapy may be considered. Immunosuppressives, including cyclophosphamide and mycophenolate mofetil, restrain the overactive immune system in lupus by blocking the production of immune cells. These drugs may be given orally, or via IV infusion [73-75, 102-104, 108-112, 120, 125-133].

Side effects may include nausea, vomiting, hair loss, urinary bladder problems, decreased fertility, and increased risks of cancer and infection. The risk of side effects increases with the length of treatment. As with other treatments for lupus, there is also a risk of disease relapse after the immunosuppressives have been stopped.

Table 1. The 1982 Revised criteria for classification of systemic lupus erythematosus

Criteria	Definition
1. Malar rash (skin)	Fixed erythema, flat or raised, over the malar eminences, tending to spare the nasolabial folds.
2. Discoid rash (skin)	Erythematous raised patches with adherent keratotic scaling and follicular plugging; atrophic scarring may occur in older lesions.
3. Photosensitivity	Skin rash as a result of unusual reaction to sunlight, by patient history or physician observation.
4. Oral ulcers	Oral or nasopharyngeal ulceration, usually painless, observed by a physician.
5. Arthritis	Nonerosive arthritis involving 2 or more peripheral joints, characterized by tenderness, swelling, or effusion.
6. Serositis	a) Pleuritis--convincing history of pleuritic pain or rubbing heard by a physician or evidence of pleural effusion. *OR* b) Pericarditis--documented by ECG or rub or evidence of pericardial effusion.
7. Renal abnormalities	a) Persistent proteinuria greater than 0.5 grams per day or grater than 3+ if quantitation not performed. *OR* b) Cellular casts--may be red cell, hemoglobin, granular, tubular, or mixed.
8. Neurologic alterations	a) Seizures--in the absence of offending drugs or known metabolic derangements; e.g., uremia, ketoacidosis, or electrolyte imbalance *OR* b) Psychosis--in the absence of offending drugs or known metabolic derangements, e.g., uremia, ketoacidosis, or electrolyte imbalance.
9. Hematologic disorders	a) Hemolytic anemia--with reticulocytosis *OR* b) Leukopenia--less than 4,000/mm<>3<> total on 2 or more occasions. *OR* c) Lyphopenia--less than 1,500/mm<>3<> on 2 or more occasions. *OR* d) Thrombocytopenia--less than 100,000/mm<>3<> in the absence of offending drugs.
10. Immunologic disorder	a) Positive LE cell preparation. *OR* b) Anti-DNA: antibody to native DNA in abnormal titer. *OR* c) Anti- Anti-Smith (Sm): presence of antibody to Sm nuclear antigen. *OR* d) False positive serologic test for syphilis known to be positive for at least 6 months and confirmed by *Treponema pallidum* immobilization or fluorescent treponemal antibody absorption test.
11. Antinuclear antibody (ANA)	An abnormal titer of antinuclear antibody by immunofluorescence (direct or indirect)or an equivalent assay at any point in time and in the absence of drugs known to be associated with "drug-induced lupus" syndrome

Modified from www.rheumatology.org.

Table 2. Types of lupus

Type	Definition	Organs affected
Systemic lupus erythematosus (SLE).	SLE is the form of the disease that most people are referring to when they say "lupus." The word "systemic" means the disease can affect many parts of the body. The symptoms of SLE may be mild or serious. Although SLE usually first affects people between the ages of 15 and 45 years, it can occur in childhood or later in life as well.	- Skin and mucosal: phtosensitivity, baldness, skin rashes, butterfly rashes. Mucoasal erosions, raynouds syndrome. - Gastrointestinal: poor appetite diarrhea, vomiting, gastroesophageal reflux disease, gastroparesis hepatomegaly, lupus hepatitis, nausea & pancreatitis. - Eyes: Retinal exudates, blindness, conjuctivitis, Sjongres syndrome. - Kidney: renal failure, proteinuria, edema, hypertension. - Reproductive system: Menorrhagia, amenohrrea, prematurity, stillbirths. - Lymphatic:Lymph and spleen enlargement. -Lining membranes: Pericarditis, pleurisy, endocarditis. - Blood: Deplete platelets, presence of multiple autoantibodies. - Central nervous system: Depression, seizures, paralysis, neuropathies, psychiatric disorders, migraines, headaches. - Musculoeskeletal: Arthralgias, arthritis and myalgias.
Discoid lupus erythematosus (DLE).	DLE is a chronic skin disorder in which a red, raised rash appears on the face, scalp, or elsewhere. The raised areas may become thick and scaly and may cause scarring. The rash may last for days or years and may recur. A small percentage of people with discoid lupus have or develop SLE later.	Mainly skin and the histology shows in general, vacuolar alteration of the basal cell layer, thickening of the basement membrane, follicular plugging, hyperkeratosis, atrophy of the epidermis, incontinence of pigment, and inflammatory cell infiltrate (usually lymphocytic) in a perivascular, periappendiceal, and subepidermal location.
Subacute cutaneous lupus erythematosus (SCLE)	SCLE refers to skin lesions that appear on parts of the body exposed to sun. The lesions do not cause scarring but they may result in dyspigmentation. Patients with SCLE frequently fulfill 4 or more of the criteria used to classify SLE. Serologic abnormalities are common. Therapy with sunscreens, topical corticosteroids, and antimalarial agents is usually effective.	SCLE is a nonscarring, non–atrophy-producing, photosensitive dermatosis. SCLE may occur in patients with (SLE), Sjögren syndrome, or deficiency of the second component of complement (C2d), or it may be drug induced. Some patients also have the lesions of (DLE), and some may develop small vessel vasculitis.

Type	Definition	Organs affected
Drug-induced lupus (DIL)	DIL is a form of lupus caused by medications. Many different drugs can cause drug-induced lupus. They include some antiseizure medications, high blood pressure medications, antibiotics and antifungals, thyroid medications, and oral contraceptive pills. Symptoms are similar to those of SLE (arthritis, rash, fever, and chest pain), and they typically go away completely when the drug is stopped. The kidneys and brain are rarely involved.	There are multiple known medications to cause DIL but there are three that report the highest number of cases: hydralazine, procainamide, and isoniazid. While the criteria for diagnosing DIL has not been thoroughly established, symptoms of DIL typically present as myalgia and arthralgia. Generally, the symptoms recede after discontinuing use of the drugs. Others drug that have moderate to low risk of producing DIL are: Isoniazid, minocycline, pyrazinamide, quinidine, D-penicillamine), carbamazepine, oxcarbazepine, phenytoin and propafenone.
Neonatal lupus (NL)	NL is a rare disease that can occur in newborn babies of women with SLE, Sjögren's syndrome, or no disease at all. It has been suspect that neonatal lupus is caused in part by autoantibodies in the mother's blood called anti-Ro (SSA) and anti-La (SSB). At birth, the babies have a skin rash, liver problems, and low blood counts. These symptoms gradually go away over several months. In rare instances, babies with neonatal lupus may have congenital heart block, a serious heart problem in which the formation of fibrous tissue in the baby's heart interferes with the electrical impulses that affect heart rhythm.	Neonatal lupus is rare, and most infants of mothers with SLE are entirely healthy. All women who are pregnant and known to have anti-Ro (SSA) or anti-La (SSB) antibodies should be monitored by echocardiograms (a test that monitors the heart and surrounding blood vessels) during the 16th and 30th weeks of pregnancy. It is important for women with SLE or other related autoimmune disorders to be under a doctor's care during pregnancy. Doctors can now identify mothers at highest risk for complications, allowing for prompt treatment of the infant at or before birth. SLE can also flare during pregnancy, and prompt treatment can keep the mother healthier longer.

Table 3. Cutaneous manifestations of lupus erythematosus

SLE	SCLE (8%)	DLE (70%)	Rare
Butterfly rash and or	Annular-polycyclic type	Discoid lesions (sores) tend to be red and raised and become scaly	Bullous LE
Macular exanthema, mucosal ulcers.	Papulo-squamous type	Discoid rash. This rash is coin-shaped or oval in shape, like a disk and it is seen on areas of the skin that are exposed to sunlight.	LE tumidus
Generalized or acrolocalized vasculitis	Xerophthalmia	Atrophic plaque with hypo and or hyperpigmentation	LE profundus
Photosensitivity	Psoriasiform plaques	Palmar-plantar erosive discoid LE	Photosensitivity
Livedo reticularis	Characteristically the lesions appear in sun-exposed areas such as the vee of the neckline or the forearms, but not the face.	Predominantly affects the cheeks, nose and ears	Chilblain LE
Non-scarring alopecia	Palatal erosions	Follicular plugging with adherent scale.	Urticarial vasculitis
Raynaud's phenomenon	Nodular form		LE hypertrophic/verrucous
Periungual telangiectasia			Lupus pernio
Red patches across the cheeks			Lupus eythematosus-lichen planus (LE-LP)

Table 4. Summary of different organ systems affected by lupus

Organ system	Kidneys	Lungs:	Central nervous system:	Blood vessels	Heart
Type of compromise	Inflammation of the kidneys (nephritis) can impair their ability to get rid of waste products and other toxins from the body effectively. There is usually no pain associated with kidney involvement, although some patients may notice dark urine and swelling around their eyes, legs, ankles, or fingers. Most often, the only indication of kidney disease is an abnormal urine or blood test. Because the kidneys are so important to overall health, lupus affecting the kidneys generally requires intensive drug treatment to prevent permanent damage.	Some people with lupus develop pleuritis, an inflammation of the lining of the chest cavity that causes chest pain, particularly with breathing. Patients with lupus also may get pneumonia.	In some patients, lupus affects the brain or central nervous system. This can cause headaches, dizziness, depression, memory disturbances, vision problems, seizures, stroke, or changes in behavior.	Blood vessels may become inflamed (vasculitis), affecting the way blood circulates through the body. The inflammation may be mild and may not require treatment or may be severe and require immediate attention. People with lupus are also at increased risk for atherosclerosis (hardening of the arteries).	In some people with lupus, inflammation can occur in the heart itself (myocarditis and endocarditis) or the membrane that surrounds it (pericarditis), causing chest pains or other symptoms. Endocarditis can damage the heart valves, causing the valve surface to thicken and develop growths, which can cause heart murmurs. However, this usually doesn't affect the valves' function.

Table 5. Diagnostic Tools for Lupus

Medical history: Focus in the skin rashes, butterfly rash over the cheeks and nose, migraine, nausea (feeling sick) or joint pains. The joints may even become tender to the touch and swollen. This is one of the most common and certainly one of the most prominent features of lupus. Patients often describe it as an "unnatural fatigue". Its causes are not well understood. Often it precedes the diagnosis by months or years and only when treatment has been successfully started does the patient realize how major a feature it had been. The majority of lupus patients suffer at some stage from joint and muscle pains. In many patients this presents as "pain all over". In acute flares of lupus the symptoms are often described as being "flu-like". Unlike other rheumatic diseases such as rheumatoid arthritis, there is often very little to see in the way of joint swelling. It is not just the joints that are affected but the tendons and muscles as well. In the majority of cases the joint inflammation does not progress to permanent damage.
Complete physical examination:, focus in skin rashes, loss of hair, edema and erythema of the joints, chest pain at the end of taking a deep breath, shortness of breath, cough and ankle swelling,
Laboratory tests:
1. Complete blood count (CBC): The complete blood count or CBC test is used as a broad screening test to check for such disorders as anemia, infection, and many other diseases.
2 .Erythrocyte sedimentation rate (ESR) also called a sedimentation rate or Biernacki Reaction, is the rate at which red blood cells sediment in a period of 1 hour.
3. Urinalysis
4. Blood chemistries.
Complement levels: A low level of complement could mean the substance is being used up because of an immune response in the body, such as that which occurs during a flare of lupus.
5. ANA Test
6. Other autoantibody tests (anti-DNA, anti-Sm, anti-RNP, anti-Ro [SSA], anti-La [SSB])
7. Anticardiolipin antibody test
Skin biopsy: take a 4 microns punch and embed in formalin 10% and other of similar size embed in Michel's medium for direct immunofluorescence.
Kidney biopsy: Any consideration of the benefits of kidney biopsy must include knowledge of the risks of the procedure. With improved imaging and the use of semi-automated biopsy guns, complications are uncommon. However, bleeding remains of foremost concern. Major complications, those requiring blood transfusion or invasive intervention, have been reported in 0–6.4% of biopsies. Predictors of complications have included low haematocrit and high creatinine. Patients with SLE may have an additional risk of bleeding due to concurrent corticosteroid use or platelet dysfunction, though this has not been studied. *Suggested indications for performance of a kidney biopsy in lupus nephritis*: 1) Acute renal failure indicated by a rising creatinine, 2) Urine protein >500mg per 24h or urine protein: creatinine ratio >0.5g protein/g creatinine. 3) Haematuria in the presence of any level of proteinuria. 4) Presence of red and/or white cell casts (cellular casts).5) Failure to respond adequately to therapy or relapse after therapy.

Table 6. Common symptoms of lupus

Painful or swollen joints (arthritis), and muscle pain.
Unexplained fever: Fever is usually a feature of a flare of the disease. Fever is unusual when the disease is in a quiet phase: therefore in an adult or a child known to have lupus who develops fever the possibility that a separate diagnosis such over infection might be present always needs consideration.
Skin rashes: Red rashes, most commonly on the face, especially in the cheeks. Rashes may also occur in the ears, upper arms, shoulders, chest, and hands and other areas exposed to the sun. A wide variety of skin rashes occur in lupus. Traditionally these are sun-sensitive ("photosensitive") but this is not always the case. The commonest rashes are on the cheeks (the "butterfly" rash across the nose and cheeks), however other rashes can occur on the elbows, on the palms and soles and on the V-neck area. The rashes vary from pinkish discoloration through to blisters and purpura. Most rashes in lupus have a tendency to come and go. Pale or purple fingers or toes from cold or stress (Raynaud's phenomenon) could also be present. Unusual loss of hair.
Chest pain upon deep breathing, or changing positions. These may caused by pericarditis, tamponade, and constriction. These complications can produce reduced cardiac pumping, lung congestion, and organ failure. Doctors can usually diagnose pericarditis by taking a careful medical history, performing a physical examination, and doing an ECG Sometimes an echocardiogram can be helpful in making the diagnosis. Tamponade occurs when fluid accumulating in the pericardial sac prevents the heart from filling completely. When this happens, the blood pressure drops and the lungs become congested, and the patient experiences weakness, dizziness and lightheadedness, and extreme shortness of breath. If treatment is not given, death can occur.
• Photosensitivity (sunlight skin rashes often first develop or worsen after sun exposure).
• Edema in the legs and or ankles and or around the eyes.
• Mouth, nose and or other mucosa ulcers with pain.
• Swollen of several glands and or swollen lymph glands.
• Extreme fatigue.
• Anemia.
• Headaches, dizziness, depression, confusion, or seizures
• Pale or purple fingers and toes from cold and stress.

BLyS-Specific Inhibitors

Belimumab, a B-lymphocyte stimulator (BLyS) protein inhibitor, was approved by the U.S. Food and Drug Administration (FDA) in March 2011 for patients with lupus who are receiving other standard therapies, including those listed above [73-75, 102-104, 108-112, 120, 125-133]. Given by IV infusion, it may reduce the number of abnormal, pathologic B cells in lupus. Common side effects include nausea, diarrhea, and fever. Patients may also experience reactions at the infusion site, for which antihistamines can be given in advance. Less commonly, serious infections may result.

Other Lupus Therapies

In some patients, methotrexate or other hormonal therapies such as dehydroepiandrosterone and intravenous gamma globulins may be useful for controlling lupus when other treatments have failed [73-75, 102-104, 108-112, 120, 125,126, 127-133]. In addition to medications to address the lupus itself, it may be necessary to take additional medications to treat problems related to lupus such as high cholesterol, high blood pressure, or infections.

Alternative and Complementary Therapies

Because of the cost of the medications used to treat lupus and the potential for serious side effects, many patients seek other ways of treating the disease. Some alternative approaches include special diets, nutritional supplements, fish oils, ointments and creams, chiropractic treatments and homeopathy [134]. Although these methods may not be harmful and may be associated with symptomatic or psychosocial benefit, no research to date conclusively demonstrates that they ameliorate the disease process itself, or prevent organ damage. An open dialogue between the patient and physician regarding the relative values of complementary and alternative therapies will allow the patient to make an informed choice about these treatment options [134].

References

[1] O'Neill S, Cervera R. Systemic lupus erythematosus. *Best Pract. Res. Clin. Rheumatol.* 2010;24:841-555.

[2] Aringer M, Hiepe F. [Systemic lupus erythematosus]. *Z. Rheumatol.* 2011;70:313-323.

[3] Feng X, Zou Y, Pan W, Wang X, Wu M, Zhang M, Tao J, Zhang Y, Tan K, Li J, Chen Z, Ding X, Qian X, Da Z, Wang M, Sun L. Prognostic indicators of hospitalized patients with systemic lupus erythematosus: a large retrospective multicenter study in China. *J. Rheumatol.* 2011;38:1289-1295.

[4] Costenbader KH, Desai A, Alarcón GS, Hiraki LT, Shaykevich T, Brookhart MA, Massarotti E, Lu B, Solomon DH, Winkelmayer WC. Trends in the incidence, demographics, and outcomes of end-stage renal disease due to lupus nephritis in the US from 1995 to 2006. *Arthritis Rheum.* 2011;63:1681-1688.

[5] Dubois' Lupus Erythematosus. Daniel J. Wallace, (Editor), Bevra Hannahs Hahn (Editor). Seventh edition. Publishers Lippincott Williams and Wilkins 2006.

[6] Wofsky D. Trials and tribulations in systemic lupus erythematosus. *Bull. NYU Hosp. Jt Dis.* 2010;68:175-178.

[7] Lateef A, Petri M. Biologics in the treatment of systemic lupus erythematosus. *Curr. Opin. Rheumatol.* 2010;22:504-509.

[8] Espinosa G, Cervera R. Belimumab, a BLyS-specific inhibitor for the treatment of systemic lupus erythematosus. *Drugs Today.* (Barc). 2010;46:891-899.

[9] De Souza A, Ali-Shaw T, Strober BE, Franks AG Jr.Successful treatment of subacute lupus erythematosus with ustekinumab. *Arch. Dermatol.* 2011;147:896-898.

[10] Daikeler T, Tyndall A. [Stem cell treatment of autoimmune disease]. *Dtsch Med. Wochenschr.* 2011;136:1684-1686.

[11] Lash AA. Systemic lupus erythematosus. Part 2: Diagnosis, treatment modalities, and nursing management. *Medsurg. Nurs.* 1993;2:375-385.

[12] Pullen RL Jr, Cannon JD, Rushing JD. Managing organ-threatening systemic lupus erythematosus. *Medsurg. Nurs.* 2003;12:368-379.

[13] Pons-Estel GJ, Alarcón GS, Scofield L, Reinlib L, Cooper GS. Understanding the epidemiology and progression of systemic lupus erythematosus. *Semin. Arthritis Rheum.* 2010;39:257-268.

[14] Kliukvina NG. Systemic lupus erythematosus in men: difficulties of diagnosis and specific features of clinical picture. *Ter. Arkh.* 2011;83:47-50.

[15] Sanchez ML, McGwin G Jr, Durán S, Fernández M, Reveille JD, Vilá LM, Alarcón GS; LUMINA Study Group. Factors predictive of overall health over the course of the disease in patients with systemic lupus erythematosus from the LUMINA cohort (LXII): use of the SF-6D. *Clin. Exp. Rheumatol.* 2009;27:67-71.

[16] Rhew EY, Manzi SM, Dyer AR, Kao AH, Danchenko N, Barinas-Mitchell E, Sutton-Tyrrell K, McPherson DD, Pearce W, Edmundowicz D, Kondos GT, Ramsey-Goldman R. Differences in subclinical cardiovascular disease between African American and Caucasian women with systemic lupus erythematosus. *Transl. Res.* 2009;153:51-59.

[17] Pan Y, Sawalha AH. Epigenetic regulation and the pathogenesis of systemic lupus erythematosus. *Transl. Res.* 2009;153:4-10.

[18] Javierre BM, Richardson B. A new epigenetic challenge: systemic lupus erythematosus. *Adv. Exp. Med. Biol.* 2011;711:117-136.

[19] Alonso MD, Llorca J, Martinez-Vazquez F, Miranda-Filloy JA, Diaz de Teran T, Dierssen T, Vazquez-Rodriguez TR, Gomez-Acebo I, Blanco R, Gonzalez-Gay MA. Systemic lupus erythematosus in Northwestern Spain: A 20-Year Epidemiologic study. *Medicine.* (Baltimore). 2011 Aug 18. [Epub ahead of print] PMID: 21857367.

[20] Pineles D, Valente A, Warren B, Peterson MG, Lehman TJ, Moorthy LN. Worldwide incidence and prevalence of pediatric onset systemic lupus erythematosus. *Lupus.* 2011 Jul 18. [Epub ahead of print].

[21] Danchenko N, Satia JA, Anthony MS. Epidemiology of systemic lupus erythematosus: a comparison of worldwide disease burden. *Lupus.* 2006;15:308-318.

[22] Jacobson DL, Gange SJ, Rose NR, Graham NM. Epidemiology and estimated population burden of selected autoimmune diseases in the United States. *Clin. Immunol. Immunopathol.* 1997;84:223-243.

[23] Patel LM, Lambert PJ, Gagna CE, Maghari A, Lambert WC. Cutaneous signs of systemic disease. *Clin. Dermatol.* 2011; 29:511-522.

[24] Johnson AE, Gordon C, Hobbs FD, Bacon PA. Undiagnosed systemic lupus erythematosus in the community. *Lancet.* 1996;347:367-369.

[25] Johnson AE, Gordon C, Palmer RG, Bacon PA. The prevalence and incidence of systemic lupus erythematosus in Birmingham, England. Relationship to ethnicity and country of birth. *Arthritis Rheum.* 1995;38:551-558.

[26] Adrianto I, Wen F, Templeton A, Wiley G, King JB, Lessard CJ, Bates JS, Hu Y, Kelly JA, Kaufman KM, Guthridge JM, Alarcón-Riquelme ME; BIOLUPUS and GENLES Networks, Anaya JM, Bae SC, Bang SY, Boackle SA, Brown EE, Petri MA, Gallant C, Ramsey-Goldman R, Reveille JD, Vila LM, Criswell LA, Edberg JC, Freedman BI, Gregersen PK, Gilkeson GS, Jacob CO, James JA, Kamen DL, Kimberly RP, Martin J, Merrill JT, Niewold TB, Park SY, Pons-Estel BA, Scofield RH, Stevens AM, Tsao BP, Vyse TJ, Langefeld CD, Harley JB, Moser KL, Webb CF, Humphrey MB, Montgomery CG, Gaffney PM. Association of a functional variant downstream of TNFAIP3 with systemic lupus erythematosus. *Nat. Genet.* 2011;43:253-258.

[27] Zhao J, Wu H, Khosravi M, Cui H, Qian X, Kelly JA, Kaufman KM, Langefeld CD, Williams AH, Comeau ME, Ziegler JT, Marion MC, Adler A, Glenn SB, Alarcón-Riquelme ME; BIOLUPUS Network; GENLES Network, Pons-Estel BA, Harley JB, Bae SC, Bang SY, Cho SK, Jacob CO, Vyse TJ, Niewold TB, Gaffney PM, Moser KL, Kimberly RP, Edberg JC, Brown EE, Alarcon GS, Petri MA, Ramsey-Goldman R, Vilá LM, Reveille JD, James JA, Gilkeson GS, Kamen DL, Freedman BI, Anaya JM, Merrill JT, Criswell LA, Scofield RH, Stevens AM, Guthridge JM, Chang DM, Song YW, Park JA, Lee EY, Boackle SA, Grossman JM, Hahn BH, Goodship TH, Cantor RM, Yu CY, Shen N, Tsao BP. Association of genetic variants in complement factor H and factor H-related genes with systemic lupus erythematosus susceptibility. *PLoS Genet.* 2011 May;7(5):e1002079.

[28] Rasmussen A, Sevier S, Kelly JA, Glenn SB, Aberle T, Cooney CM, Grether A, James E, Ning J, Tesiram J, Morrisey J, Powe T, Drexel M, Daniel W, Namjou B, Ojwang JO, Nguyen KL, Cavett JW, Te JL, James JA, Scofield RH, Moser K, Gilkeson GS, Kamen DL, Carson CW, Quintero-del-Rio AI, del Carmen Ballesteros M, Punaro MG, Karp DR, Wallace DJ, Weisman M, Merrill JT, Rivera R, Petri MA, Albert DA, Espinoza LR, Utset TO, Shaver TS, Arthur E, Anaya JM, Bruner GR, Harley JB. The lupus family registry and repository. *Rheumatology.* (Oxford). 2011;50:47-59.

[29] Crow MK. Collaboration, genetic associations, and lupus erythematosus. *N. Engl. J. Med.* 2008;358:956-961.

[30] Kamen DL, Barron M, Parker TM, Shaftman SR, Bruner GR, Aberle T, James JA, Scofield RH, Harley JB, Gilkeson GS. Autoantibody prevalence and lupus characteristics in a unique African American population. *Arthritis Rheum.* 2008;58:1237-1247.

[31] D'Cruz DP, Khamashta MA, Hughes GR. Systemic lupus erythematosus. *Lancet.* 2007;369:587-596.

[32] James JA, Harley JB, Scofield RH. Epstein-Barr virus and systemic lupus erythematosus. *Curr. Opin. Rheumatol.* 2006;18:462-467.

[33] James JA, Harley JB, Scofield RH. Role of viruses in systemic lupus erythematosus and Sjögren syndrome. *Curr. Opin. Rheumatol.* 2001;13:370-376.

[34] Pavlovic M, Kats A, Cavallo M, Shoenfeld Y. Clinical and molecular evidence for association of SLE with parvovirus B19. *Lupus.* 2010;19:783-792.

[35] Getts MT, Miller SD. 99th Dahlem conference on infection, inflammation and chronic inflammatory disorders: triggering of autoimmune diseases by infections. Clin Exp Immunol. 2010;160:15-21.

[36] Adhami E. Calculating the etiology of systemic lupus erythematosus. *Med. Hypotheses.* 2004;62:237-246.

[37] Hess EV, Farhey Y. Environmental relationships, epidemiology, and genetics of systemic lupus erythematosus. *Curr. Opin. Rheumatol.* 1995;7:371-375.

[38] Tan EM, Cohen AS, Fries JF, Masi AT, McShane DJ, Rothfield NF, Schaller JG, Talal N, Winchester RJ: The 1982 revised criteria for the classification of systemic lupus erythematosus. *Arthritis Rheum.* 1982;25:1271-1277.

[39] Hochberg MC. Updating the American College of Rheumatology revised criteria for the classification of systemic lupus erythematosus [letter]. *Arthritis Rheum.* 1997;40:1725.

[40] Tomer Y, Buskila D, Shoenfeld Y. Pathogenic significance and diagnostic value of lupus autoantibodies. *Int. Arch. Allergy Immunol.* 1993;100:293-306.

[41] Wang CL, Ooi L, Wang F. Prevalence and clinical significance of antibodies to ribonucleoproteins in systemic lupus erythematosus in Malaysia. *Br. J. Rheumatol.* 1996;35:129-32.

[42] Harley JB Scofield RH. Systemic lupus erythematosus: RNA-protein autoantigens, models of disease heterogeneity, and theories of etiology. *Clinical Rheumatology.* 1991;10:367-368.

[43] Huang SC, Pan Z, Kurien BT, James JA, Harley JB, Scofield RH. Immunization with vesicular stomatitis virus nucleocapsid protein induces autoantibodies to the 60 kD Ro ribonucleoprotein particle. *J. Investig. Med.* 1995;43:151-158.

[44] Autoantibodies to RNA helicase A: a new serologic marker of early lupus. Yamasaki Y, Narain S, Yoshida H, Hernandez L, Barker T, Hahn PC, Sobel ES, Segal MS, Richards HB, Chan EK, Reeves WH, Satoh M. *Arthritis Rheum.* 2007;56:596-604.

[45] Anti-Ro and anti-nRNP response in unaffected family members of SLE patients. Heinlen LD, McClain MT, Kim X, Quintero DR, James JA, Harley JB, Scofield RH. *Lupus.* 2003;12:335-337.

[46] Arbuckle MR, McClain MT, Rubertone MV, Scofield RH, Dennis GJ, James JA, Harley JB. Development of autoantibodies before the clinical onset of systemic lupus Erythematosus. *N. Engl. J. Med.* 2003;349:1526-1533.

[47] Plowman EK, Okun MS. Antiphospholipid syndrome and other lupus-related movement disorders. Handb Clin Neurol. 2011;100:237-245.

[48] Silvariño R, Sant F, Espinosa G, Pons-Estel G, Solé M, Cervera R, Arrizabalaga P. Nephropathy associated with antiphospholipid antibodies in patients with systemic lupus erythematosus. *Lupus.* 2011;20:721-729.

[49] Somarelli JA, Mesa A, Rodriguez R, Avellan R, Martinez L, Zang YJ, Greidinger EL, Herrera RJ. Epitope mapping of the U1 small nuclear ribonucleoprotein particle in

patients with systemic lupus erythematosus and mixed connective tissue disease. *Lupus.* 2011;20:274-289.

[50] Julkunen H, Ekblom-Kullberg S, Miettinen A. Nonrenal and renal activity of systemic lupus erythematosus: a comparison of two anti-C1q and five anti-dsDNA assays and complement C3 and C4. *Rheumatol Int.* 2011 Jun 26. [Epub ahead of print].

[51] Sinico RA, Radice A. [The clinical immunology laboratory in diagnosis and monitoring of systemic lupus erythematosus and connective tissue diseases]. *G. Ital. Nefrol.* 2005;33:S21-26.

[52] Birmingham DJ, Irshaid F, Nagaraja HN, Zou X, Tsao BP, Wu H, Yu CY, Hebert LA, Rovin BH. The complex nature of serum C3 and C4 as biomarkers of lupus renal flare. *Lupus.* 2010;19:1272-1280.

[53] Akhter E, Burlingame R, Seaman A, Magder L, Petri M. Anti-C1q antibodies have higher correlation with flares of lupus nephritis than other serum markers. *Lupus.* 2011 Aug 3. [Epub ahead of print].PMID:21813587.

[54] Lozovoy M, Simão A, Hohmann MS, Simão TN, Barbosa DS, Morimoto HK, Reiche EM, Cecchini R, Dichi I. Inflammatory biomarkers and oxidative stress measurements in patients with systemic lupus erythematosus with or without metabolic syndrome. *Lupus.* 2011 Aug 25. [Epub ahead of print]. PMID: 21868433

[55] Chotayaporn T, Kasitanon N, Sukitawut W, Louthrenoo W. Comparison of proteinuria determination by urine dipstick, spot urine protein creatinine index, and urine protein 24 hours in lupus patients. *J. Clin. Rheumatol.* 2011;17:124-129.

[56] Barbado J, Vega L, González-Gallego R, Jimeno A, Ortiz De Lejarazu R, Bermejo-Martin JF. [MCP-1 in urine as biomarker of renal lupus in absence of cytokines, interferon-γ and growth factors]. *Reumatol. Clin.* 2010;6:296-298.

[57] Ebert EC, Hagspiel KD. Gastrointestinal and hepatic manifestations of systemic lupus erythematosus. J Clin Gastroenterol. 2011;45:436-441.

[58] Xanthouli P, Mühleisen H, Briem S, Weis D, Fiehn C. protein-losing enteropathy: a cause of hypoalbuminaemia in patients with systemic lupus erythematosus]. *Z. Rheumatol.* 2011;244:239-242.

[59] Tian XP, Zhang X. Gastrointestinal involvement in systemic lupus erythematosus: insight into pathogenesis, diagnosis and treatment. *World J. Gastroenterol.* 2010;16:2971-2977.

[60] Nowicka-Sauer K, Czuszynska Z, Smolenska Z, Siebert J. Neuropsychological assessment in systemic lupus erythematosus patients: clinical usefulness of first-choice diagnostic tests in detecting cognitive impairment and preliminary diagnosis of neuropsychiatric lupus. *Clin. Exp. Rheumatol.* 2011;29:299-306.

[61] Hanly JG, Urowitz MB, Jackson D, Bae SC, Gordon C, Wallace DJ, Clarke A, Bernatsky S, Vasudevan A, Isenberg D, Rahman A, Sanchez-Guerrero J, Romero-Diaz J, Merrill JT, Fortin PR, Gladman DD, Bruce IN, Steinsson K, Khamashta M, Alarcón GS, Fessler B, Petri M, Manzi S, Nived O, Sturfelt G, Ramsey-Goldman R, Dooley MA, Aranow C, Van Vollenhoven R, Ramos-Casals M, Zoma A, Kalunian K, Farewell V; Systemic Lupus International Collaborating Clinics (SLICC). SF-36 summary and subscale scores are reliable outcomes of neuropsychiatric events in systemic lupus erythematosus. *Ann. Rheum. Dis.* 2011;70:961-967.

[62] Padovan M, Castellino G, Bortoluzzi A, Caniatti L, Trotta F, Govoni M. Factors and comorbidities associated with central nervous system involvement in systemic lupus

erythematosus: a retrospective cross-sectional case-control study from a single center. *Rheumatol. Int.* 2010 Jul 31. [Epub ahead of print].

[63] Hughes GR. Hughes syndrome (the antiphospholipid syndrome): a disease of our time. *Inflammopharmacology.* 2011;19:69-73.

[64] Giannitti C, Cerase A, Miracco C, Fioravanti A. Cerebral haemorrhage in a patient with systemic lupus erythematosus and vasculitis treated with intravenous immunoglobulins for a long-time and in absence of other risk factors. *Clin. Ter.* 2011;162:125-127.

[65] Bihl GR, Petri M, Fine DM. Kidney biopsy in lupus nephritis: look before you leap. *Nephrol. Dial. Transplant.* 2006;21:1749-1752.

[66] Edelbauer M, Ho J. Molecular evaluation of renal biopsies: a search for predictive and prognostic markers in lupus nephritis. *Expert Rev. Mol. Diagn.* 2011;11:561-565.

[67] Costenbader KH, Desai A, Alarcón GS, Hiraki LT, Shaykevich T, Brookhart MA, Massarotti E, Lu B, Solomon DH, Winkelmayer WC. Trends in the incidence, demographics, and outcomes of end-stage renal disease due to lupus nephritis in the US from 1995 to 2006. *Arthritis Rheum.* 2011;63:1681-1688.

[68] Ardoin S, Birmingham DJ, Hebert PL, Yu CY, Rovin BH, Hebert LA. An approach to validating criteria for proteinuric flare in systemic lupus erythematosus glomerulonephritis. *Arthritis Rheum.* 2011;63:2031-2037.

[69] Liu Y, Yang HF, Wang LX. [Pathological classification and clinical characteristics of lupus nephritis: a report of 49 cases]. *Nan Fang Yi Ke Da Xue Xue Bao.* 2010;30: 1915-1917.

[70] Austin HA III, Boumpas DT, Vaughan EM, Balow JE. Predicting renal outcomes in severe lupus nephritis: contributions of clinical and histologic data. *Kidney Int.* 1994;45:544–550.

[71] Weening JJ, D'Agati VD, Schwartz MM, Seshan SV, Alpers CE, Appel GB, et al, on behalf of the International Society of Nephrology and Renal Pathology Society Working Group on the Classification of Lupus Nephritis. The classification of glomerulonephritis in systemic lupus erythematosus revisited. *Kidney Int.* 2004;65: 521–530.

[72] Andrade-Ortega L, Irazoque-Palazuelos F, López-Villanueva R, Barragán-Navarro Y, Bourget-Pietrasanta F, Díaz-Ceballos Mde L, Hernández-Paz R, Urenda-Quezada A, Rivas-Ruiz R. [Efficacy of rituximab versus cyclophosphamide in lupus patients with severe manifestations. A randomized and multicenter study]. *Reumatol. Clin.* 2010;6:250-255.

[73] El-Sehemy MS, Al-Saaran AM, Baddour NM, Adam AG, Moez PE. Comparative clinical prospective therapeutic study between cyclophosphamide, cyclosporine and azathioprine in the treatment of lupus nephritis. *Egypt J. Immunol.* 2006;13:39-52.

[74] Liang CC, Huang CC, Wang IK, Chang CT, Chen KH, Weng CH, Lin JL, Hung CC, Yang CW, Yen TH. Impact of renal survival on the course and outcome of systemic lupus erythematosus patients treated with chronic peritoneal dialysis. *Ther. Apher. Dial.* 2010;14:35-42.

[75] Tang H, Poynton MR, Hurdle JF, Baird BC, Koford JK, Goldfarb-Rumyantzev AS. Predicting three-year kidney graft survival in recipients with systemic lupus erythematosus. *ASAIO J.* 2011;57:300-309.

[76] Duman D, Masatlioğlu S, Demirtunç R, Karadağ B. Increased pulmonary artery stiffness and its relation to right ventricular function in patients with systemic lupus erythematosus].*Turk Kardiyol. Dern. Ars.* 2008;36:82-89.

[77] Yeh TT, Yang YH, Lin YT, Lu CS, Chiang BL. Cardiopulmonary involvement in pediatric systemic lupus erythematosus: a twenty-year retrospective analysis. *J. Microbiol. Immunol. Infect.* 2007;40:525-531.

[78] Beresford MW, Cleary AG, Sills JA, Couriel J, Davidson JE. Cardio-pulmonary involvement in juvenile systemic lupus erythematosus. *Lupus.* 2005;14:152-158.

[79] Mulić S, Selesković H, Krizić M, Kusljugić Z, Baraković F, Smajić E, Kapidzić-Basić N, Kasumagić S, Hajdarović A, Krizić N, Sabitović D. [Pericarditis and exudative pleuritis in patients with systemic lupus erythematosus before and after therapy]. *Med. Arh.* 2004;58:13-15.

[80] Kwok LW, Tam LS, Zhu T, Leung YY, Li E. Predictors of maternal and fetal outcomes in pregnancies of patients with systemic lupus erythematosus. *Lupus.* 2011;20:829-836.

[81] Liu J, Zhao Y, Song Y, Zhang W, Bian X, Yang J, Liu D, Zeng X, Zhang F. Pregnancy in women with systemic lupus erythematosus: a retrospective study of 111 pregnancies in Chinese women. *J. Matern. Fetal Neonatal Med.* 2011 Apr 19. [Epub ahead of print].

[82] Rajewski M, Skrzypczak J. Frequency of antiphospholipid antibodies and antiphospholipid syndrome in women with recurrent miscarriages. *Ginekol. Pol.* 2011 ;82:32-38.

[83] Li L, Dong GF, Han FZ, Cui Y, Shi YZ, Zhang X. [Neonatal lupus erythematosus: a report of 7 cases and review of 87 cases of China]. *Zhonghua Er Ke Za Zhi.* 2011;49:146-150.

[84] Giancotti A, Spagnuolo A, D'ambrosio V, Pasquali G, Muto B, De Gado F. Pregnancy in lupus patients: our experience. *Minerva Ginecol.* 2010;62:551-558.

[85] Isenberg DA, Allen E, Farewell V, D'Cruz D, Alarcón GS, Aranow C, Bruce IN, Dooley MA, Fortin PR, Ginzler EM, Gladman DD, Hanly JG, Inanc M, Kalunian K, Khamashta M, Merrill JT, Nived O, Petri M, Ramsey-Goldman R, Sturfelt G, Urowitz M, Wallace DJ, Gordon C, Rahman A. An assessment of disease flare in patients with systemic lupus erythematosus: a comparison of BILAG 2004 and the flare version of SELENA. *Ann. Rheum. Dis.* 2011;70:54-59.

[86] Kawasaki A, Ito I, Hikami K, Ohashi J, Hayashi T, Goto D, Matsumoto I, Ito S, Tsutsumi A, Koga M, Arinami T, Graham RR, Hom G, Takasaki Y, Hashimoto H, Behrens TW, Sumida T, Tsuchiya N. Role of STAT4 polymorphisms in systemic lupus erythematosus in a Japanese population: a case-control association study of the STAT1-STAT4 region. *Arthritis Res. Ther.* 2008;10:R113.

[87] Kumar KR, Li L, Yan M, Bhaskarabhatla M, Mobley AB, Nguyen C, Mooney JM, Schatzle JD, Wakeland EK, Mohan C. Regulation of B cell tolerance by the lupus susceptibility gene Ly108. *Science.* 2006;312:1665-1669.

[88] Lozovoy M, Simão A, Hohmann MS, Simão TN, Barbosa DS, Morimoto HK, Reiche EM, Cecchini R, Dichi I. Inflammatory biomarkers and oxidative stress measurements in patients with systemic lupus erythematosus with or without metabolic syndrome. *Lupus.* 2011 Aug 25. [Epub ahead of print].

[89] Tseng CE, Buyon JP, Kim M, Belmont HM, Mackay M, Diamond B, Marder G, Rosenthal P, Haines K, Ilie V, Abramson SB. The effect of moderate-dose corticosteroids in preventing severe flares in patients with serologically active, but

clinically stable, systemic lupus erythematosus: findings of a prospective, randomized, double-blind, placebo-controlled trial. *Arthritis Rheum.* 2006;54:3623-3632.
[90] Kuhn A, Ruland V, Bonsmann G. Skin manifestations in lupus erythematosus: clinical aspects and therapy. *Z. Rheumatol.* 2011;70:213-226.
[91] Rosato E, Molinaro I, Pisarri S, Salsano F. Digital ulcers as an initial manifestation of systemic lupus erythematosus. *Intern. Med.* 2011;50:767-769.
[92] Lehmann P. Sun exposed skin disease. Clin Dermatol. 2011;29:180-188.
[93] Lipozencic J, Ljubojevic S. Perioral dermatitis. *Clin. Dermatol.* 2011;29:157-161.
[94] Reich A, Marcinow K, Bialynicki-Birula R.The lupus band test in systemic lupus erythematosus patients. *Ther. Clin. Risk Manag.* 2011;24;27-32.
[95] Cervera R, Tektonidou MG, Espinosa G, Cabral AR, González EB, Erkan D, Vadya S, Adrogué HE, Solomon M, Zandman-Goddard G, Shoenfeld Y. Task Force on Catastrophic Antiphospholipid Syndrome (APS) and Non-criteria APS Manifestations (II): thrombocytopenia and skin manifestations. *Lupus.* 2011;20:174-181.
[96] Burnham TK, Neblett TR, Fine G. The application of the fluorescent antibody technic to the investigation of lupus erythematosus and various dermatoses. *J. Invest. Dermatol.* 1963;41:451–456.
[97] Abreu-Velez AM, Smith JG Jr, Howard MS. Activation of the signaling cascade in response to T lymphocyte receptor stimulation and prostanoids in a case of cutaneous lupus. *North Am. J. Med. Sci.* 2011;3:251-254.
[98] Abreu Velez AM, Smith JG Jr, Howard MS. Cutaneous lupus erythematosus with autoantibodies colocalizing with glial fibrillary acidic protein. *N. Dermatol. Online.* 2011; 2:8-11.
[99] Abreu Velez AM, Smith JG Jr, Howard MS. Vimentin compartamentalization in discoid lupus. *North Am. J. Med. Sci.* 2010; 2:106-110.
[100] Abreu Velez AM, Girard JG, Howard MS. Antigen presenting cells in a patient with hair loss of and systemic lupus erythematosus. *North Am. J. Med. Sci.* 2009;1:205-210.
[101] Abreu-Velez AM, Loebl AM, Howard MS. Autoreactivity to sweat and sebaceous glands and skin homing T cells in lupus profundus. *Clin. Immunol.* 2009;132:420-424.
[102] Gammon B, Hansen C, Costner MI. Efficacy of mycophenolate mofetil in antimalarial-resistant cutaneous lupus erythematosus. *J. Am. Acad. Dermatol.* 2011 Jun 2. [Epub ahead of print].
[103] Petri M. Use of hydroxychloroquine to prevent thrombosis in systemic lupus erythematosus and in antiphospholipid antibody-positive patients. *Curr. Rheumatol. Rep.* 2011;13:77-80.
[104] Kuhn A, Ochsendorf F, Bonsmann G. Treatment of cutaneous lupus erythematosus. *Lupus.* 2010;19:1125-1136.
[105] Kuhn A, Gensch K, Haust M, Meuth AM, Boyer F, Dupuy P, Lehmann P, Metze D, Ruzicka T. Photoprotective effects of a broad-spectrum sunscreen in ultraviolet-induced cutaneous lupus erythematosus: a randomized, vehicle-controlled, double-blind study. *J. Am. Acad. Dermatol.* 2011;64:37-48.
[106] Hua-Li Z, Shi-Chao X, De-Shen T, Dong L, Hua-Feng L. Seasonal distribution of active systemic lupus erythematosus and its correlation with meteorological factors. *Clinics.* (Sao Paulo). 2011;66:1009-1013.
[107] Kuhn A, Gensch K, Haust M, Meuth AM, Boyer F, Dupuy P, Lehmann P, Metze D, Ruzicka T. Photoprotective effects of a broad-spectrum sunscreen in ultraviolet-induced

cutaneous lupus erythematosus: a randomized, vehicle-controlled, double-blind study. *J. Am. Acad. Dermatol.* 2011;64:37-48.

[108] Garciá-Carrasco M, Mendoza-Pinto C, Riebeling C, Sandoval-Cruz M, Nava A, Etchegaray-Morales I, Jiménez-Hernández M, Montiel-Jarquín A, López-Colombo A, Cervera R. Influence of prevalent vertebral fractures on the quality of life of patients with systemic lupus erythematosus. *Isr. Med. Assoc. J.* 2011;13:333-337.

[109] Wiland P. Musculoskeletal symptoms in systemic lupus erythematosus and their differential diagnosis with rheumatoid arthritis]. *Ann. Acad. Med. Stetin.* 2010;56:40-44

[110] Cronin ME. Musculoskeletal manifestations of systemic lupus erythematosus. *Rheum. Dis. Clin. North Am.* 1988;14:99-116.

[111] Grossman JM. Lupus arthritis. *Best Pract. Res. Clin. Rheumatol.* 2009;23:495-506.

[112] Klippel JH, Gerber LH, Pollak L, Decker JL. Avascular necrosis in systemic lupus erythematosus. Silent symmetric osteonecroses. *Am. J. Med.* 1979;67:83-87.

[113] McCarthy DJ, Lagana FJ. Podiatric pathology of lupus erythematosus. *J. Am. Podiatr. Med. Assoc.* 1989;79:281-290.

[114] Lagana FJ, McCarthy DJ. Podiatric implications of lupus erythematosus. *J. Am. Podiatr. Med. Assoc.* 1988;78:577-583.

[115] Talacko AA, Gordon AK, Aldred MJ. The patient with recurrent oral ulceration. *Aust. Dent. J.* 2010;55:14-22.

[116] Mekouar F, Hammi S, Elomri N, Ghafir D. Bullous systemic lupus erythematosus. *Intern. Med.* 2011;50:1445.

[117] Strohmeyer G, Kalbfleisch H, Mennel HD. [Fever of unknown origin with arthralgia and exanthema, herpes labialis, encephalopathy with myoclonus, acute kidney failure]. *Internist.* (Berl). 1981;22:568-5677.

[118] Muñoz-Corcuera M, Esparza-Gómez G, González-Moles MA, Bascones-Martínez A. Oral ulcers: clinical aspects. A tool for dermatologists. Part II. Chronic ulcers. *Clin. Exp. Dermatol.* 2009;34:456-461.

[119] Read RW. Clinical mini-review: systemic lupus erythematosus and the eye. *Ocul. Immunol. Inflamm.* 2004;12:87-99.

[120] Chiffoleau A, Guillet A, Zanlonghi X, Jolliet P. [Antimalarial's retinopaty remains a current threat]. *Presse Med.* 2009;38:662-663.

[121] Brydak-Godowska J. Ocular changes and general condition in lupus erythematosus (SLE)--own observation]. *Klin. Oczna.* 2007;109:11-14.

[122] Balbir-Gurman A, Braun-Moscovici Y. Scleroderma overlap syndrome. *Isr. Med. Assoc. J.* 2011;13:14-20.

[123] Jørgensen KT, Pedersen BV, Nielsen NM, Jacobsen S, Frisch M. Childbirths and risk of female predominant and other autoimmune diseases in a population-based Danish cohort. *J. Autoimmun.* 2011 Aug 1. [Epub ahead of print].

[124] Miller DV, Maleszewksi JJ. The pathology of large-vessel vasculitides. *Clin. Exp. Rheumatol.* 2011 Jan-Feb;29 (1 Suppl 64):S92-8.

[125] Strand V, Chu AD. Measuring outcomes in systemic lupus erythematosus clinical trials. *Expert Rev. Pharmacoecon. Outcomes Res.* 2011;11:455-468.

[126] Merrill J, Buyon J, Furie R, Latinis K, Gordon C, Hsieh HJ, Brunetta P. Assessment of flares in lupus patients enrolled in a phase II/III study of rituximab (EXPLORER). *Lupus.* 2011;20:709-16.

[127] Mitka M. Treatment for lupus, first in 50 years, offers modest benefits, hope to patients. *JAMA*. 2011;305:1754-1755.

[128] Bertsias G, Ioannidis JP, Boletis J, Bombardieri S, Cervera R, Dostal C, et al. EULAR recommendations for the management of systemic lupus erythematosus. Report of a Task Force of the EULAR Standing Committee for International Clinical Studies Including Therapeutics. *Ann. Rheum. Dis*. 2008;67:195-205.

[129] Crosbie D, Black C, McIntyre L, Royle PL, Thomas S. Dehydroepiandrosterone for systemic lupus erythematosus. *Cochrane Database Syst. Rev*. 200717;CD005114.

[130] Sabahi R, Anolik JH. B-cell-targeted therapy for systemic lupus erythematosus. *Drugs*. 2006;66:1933-1948.

[131] Sanz I, Yasothan U, Kirkpatrick P. Belimumab. *Nat. Rev. Drug Discov*. 2011;10: 335-336.

[132] Ledford H. After half-century's wait, approval paves path for new lupus drugs. *Nat. Med.* 2011;17:400.

[133] Thompson CA. First new lupus drug approved in half-century. *Am. J. Health Syst. Pharm*. 2011;68:646.

[134] Haija AJ, Schulz SW. The role and effect of complementary and alternative medicine in systemic lupus erythematosus. *Rheum. Dis. Clin. North Am.* 2011;37:47-62.

In: Lupus: Symptoms, Treatment and Potential Complications ISBN: 978-1-62081-078-1
Editors: T. D. Marquez and D. U. Neto

Chapter II

Autoantibody-Producing B Cells and B Cell Therapy in Systemic Lupus Erythematosus - Possible New Targets of Novel Subsets of RP105-Negative B Cells

Syuichi Koarada*
Division of Rheumatology, Faculty of Medicine, Saga University, Nabeshima, Saga, Japan

Abstract

A recent study has significantly improved the prognosis of systemic lupus erythematosus (SLE), a prototypic systemic autoimmune disease with multiple organ disorders. However, corticosteroids and immunosuppressive agents are still used in medical care. There are a significant proportion of patients with refractory disease and complications by the conventional drugs. In fact, few novel drugs have been approved for SLE during the past decades. Many studies suggest that the center in pathophysiology of SLE is autoreactive B cells producing autoantibodies. Therefore, B cell may be one of the most promising targets in therapies of SLE. Moreover, B cells would function as antigen-presenting cells, providers of pro-inflammatory cytokines, and activators of T cells other than function of effector cells that produce immunoglobulins in immune system. It is also evident that large population of abnormal B cells exists in active SLE. RP105 (CD180), one of the toll-like receptor associated molecules, is expressed on mature B cells. Previously, we found significantly increased population of RP105-negative B cells in SLE. Interestingly, phenotype of RP105(-) B cell subsets in SLE patients is greatly different from normal subjects and, importantly, RP105(-) B cells produce autoantibodies including anti-dsDNA antibodies. RP105(-) B cells are assigned as the B cell subsets in

* Corresponding author: S.Koarada, koarada@cc.saga-u.ac.jp 81-(952) 34-2367(O), 81-(952) 34-2017(Fax).

final stages of differentiation and may be one of the central B cells dysregulated in SLE. This review provides basic information of B cell biology and RP105(-) B cells in SLE and illustrates new insights of novel and alternative concept of B cell targeting therapies in SLE.

Introduction

SLE and RP105(CD180)

Systemic lupus erythematosus (SLE) is an autoimmune disease that is characterized by polyclonal B cell activation and hypergammaglobulinemia [1, 2, 3, 4]. The autoimmune inflammation affects multiple organ systems, including kidney, central and peripheral nervous system, joints, blood, lungs, cardiovascular system, and skin. Although various B cell subsets play important roles in pathogenesis of SLE, especially, autoantibody-producing B cells against nuclear proteins and DNA are key players in immune system and tissue damages in SLE [5]. Toll-like receptors (TLRs) are sensors that belong to innate immunity and recognize various pathogens such as lipopolysaccharides (LPS), lipopeptides, CpG-DNA, and so on (Figure 1). RP105 (CD180), one of the members of TLRs, is expressed on cell surface of normal mature B cells [6]. RP105 consists of extracellular leucine-rich repeats (LRRs) and a short cytoplasmic portion (Figure 2) [7]. The extracellular LRRs are associated with a molecule called MD-1 and form the surface receptor complex, RP105/MD-1. RP105/MD1 works in concert with TLR4, controlling B cell recognition and signaling of LPS, that is a membrane constituent of Gram-negative bacteria [8].

It has been shown that B cells from RP105-deficient mice are hyporesponsive to TLR4 and TLR2 stimulation [9, 10]. In mice, RP105 is considered to regulate the growth and death of B cells. RP105 interacts with TLR4 and negatively regulates TLR4 signaling [11]. These results suggest that loss of RP105 may induce the dysregulation of TLRs' signals and sustain hyperreactivity, hyperactivation and autoreactivity, and then may finally result in autoimmunity.

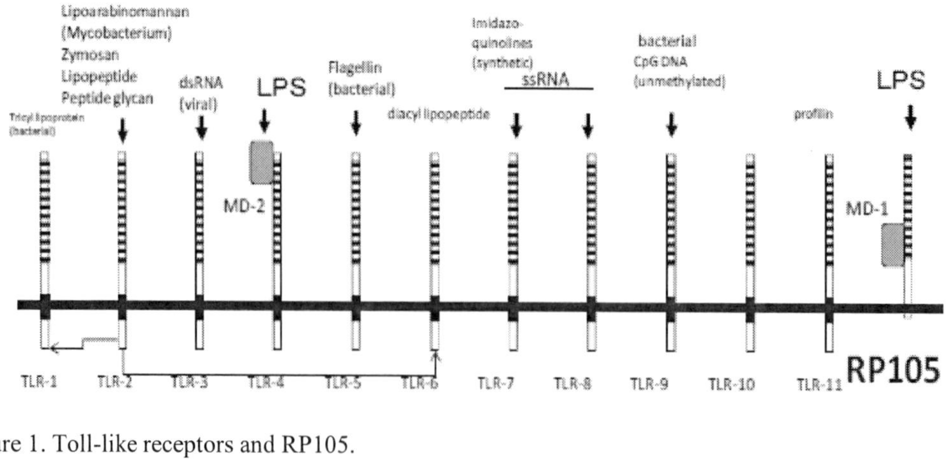

Figure 1. Toll-like receptors and RP105.

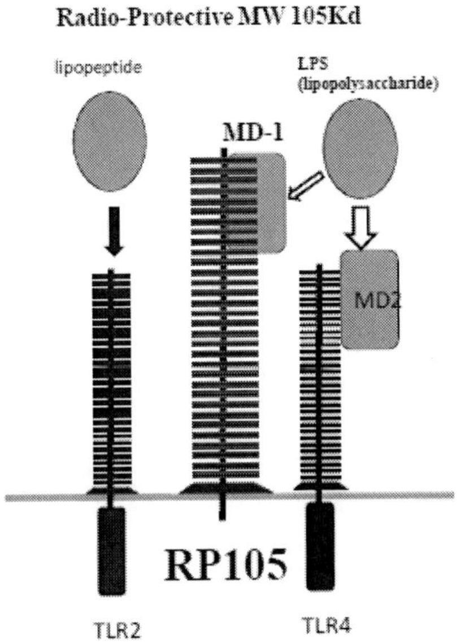

Figure 2. Structure of RP105 (CD180).

However, in human, there had been very little information on RP105. Therefore, we have investigated RP105 in human SLE, because SLE patients evidently have hyperactivated B cells in peripheral blood. In the peripheral blood of active patients with SLE, there are many B cells lacking RP105 expression on the cell surface. These cells are called as RP105-negative B cells [RP105(-) B cells]. In our previous reports, the numbers of RP105(-) B cells were arguably increased [12]. Most importantly, RP105(-) B cells produce autoantibodies, including IgG class anti-dsDNA (double stranded DNA) and ssDNA (single stranded DNA) antibodies in vitro [13]. A great demand for new therapies with high efficacy remains because some patients treated with conventional drugs, corticosteroids and immunosuppressive agents, still have refractory diseases and/or show various complications with drug toxicity. B cell therapy is presently the central strategy in the novel treatment with SLE. Moreover, the narrower target of B cells, especially focused on the autoreactive B cell itself, may be much more fascinating, considering its roles in the pathophysiology of SLE. However, to date, the effective therapies of targeting autoantibody-producing B cells have not been established yet. For treatment of SLE, some B cell therapies have shown effective response. If possible, a strategy of targeting RP105(-) autoantibody-producing B cells may be a possible treatment for SLE. In this review we discuss general information on the RP105 biology, its clinical significance and B cell therapy, in SLE.

Section 1. B Cell Biology in SLE

Autoantibodies in Human SLE

In SLE patients, various autoantibodies against ssDNA, dsDNA, histones, and phospholipids, have been identified and established their clinical significance. Among these autoantibodies, especially, anti-dsDNA and anti-Sm antibodies are specific for SLE.

Autoantibodies produced by autoreactive B cells form immune-complexes that deposit in organs causing tissue damage and dysfunction. Anti-dsDNA antibodies directly show pathogenic roles in lupus nephritis [14].

Autoantibodies in Lupus-Prone Mice

The central roles of autoantibodies in pathogenesis of SLE have been definitely established in murine lupus models, for example, New Zealand Black (NZB) and White (NZW) mice and MRL/lpr mice. Parental strains, NZB and NZW mice, do not have the phenotype of SLE.

On the other hand, (NZB/NZW)F1 mice, the first filial generation, develop autoimmunity and show diffuse proliferative lupus nephritis. MRL/lpr mice have a severe spontaneous autoimmune syndrome with massive generalized lymphadenopathy, arthritis, vasculitis, skin lesions and lupus nephritis. The mice are characterized by a mutation in the fas gene and have excessive proliferation of T cells and production of anti-DNA autoantibodies.

B Cell Development and Differentiation; Various B Cell Subsets

The population of B cells is one of the main parts of the immune system. Especially, in humoral response of adaptive immunity, the formation and development of B cells is essential.

In the bone marrow, pro-B cells, the earliest B-lineage cells, are derived from pluripotential hematopoietic cells. After rearrangement of heavy-chain immunoglobulin genes, pro-B cells differentiate into pre-B cells. At the next stage of immature B cells, light-chains and heavy-chains assemble and then immunoglobulin M (IgM) molecules express on cell surface. Importantly, in this stage, autoreactive B cells, having strong reactivity with self-antigens, are censored by the mechanism including apoptosis, clonal deletion and anergy. The remaining immature B cells without self-reactivity can survive and leave the bone marrow. Immature B cells migrate into the peripheral and then differentiate into mature B cells. The mature B cells express IgD and IgM on the surface.

In the peripheral, B cells encounter various antigens. The antigen-activated B cells migrate into T cell zones, because humoral response generally requires assistance of CD4+ T cells. B cells are activated, proliferated, and differentiated there via T cell-B cell interaction.

Some B cells encountered by antigens move to lymphoid follicle and form the germinal center. Somatic hypermutation of genes of immunoglobulin variable domain, affinity maturation, and class-switch of immunoglobulin from IgM to other isotypes are taken place there. B cells that do not bind antigens result in apoptosis and die. B cells, having high affinity binding to antigens, survive the selection. These surviving B cells become either memory B cells or plasma cells after leaving the germinal center. Finally, B cells migrate to the bone marrow and differentiate into plasma cells. Plasma cells are the terminally differentiated cells of B cell lineage and function as effector cells that produce circulating immunoglobulin. On the other hand, memory B cells reside in the lymphoid organ and can quickly respond the same antigen later.

Late B Cell Differentiation; Plasmablasts and Plasma Cells

Late B cells, including plasmablasts and plasma cells, play critical roles in humoral immunity [15]. However, in human, precise phenotypes of these B cells have not been fully understood yet. RP105(-) B cells are assigned as human late B cells. Therefore, the phenotypic analysis of RP105(-) B cells is helpful to understand differentiation and dysregulation of late B cells in human SLE [16].

Interestingly, RP105(-) B cells are not single cell population. They are divided into at least 5 subsets and each subset may represent the final step of differentiation of B cells towards plasma cells (Figure 3), subset 1; activated B cells, subset 2; pre-plasmablasts, subset 3; (early-)plasmablasts, subset 4; pre-plasma cells, and subset 5; circulating plasma cells. These may be novel classification of human B cell subsets that were first identified by using three markers of CD19, RP105 and CD138, using flow cytometry (Figure 4).

The analysis of phenotype also presents that these subsets exist even in healthy subjects. The phenotypes of normal RP105(-) B cells are similar to those from SLE patients. However, several antigens are differently expressed in levels between SLE patients and normal subjects.

In general, plasma cells are divided into two classified cells, long- and short-lived plasma cells. In SLE, long-lived plasma cells are responsible for the production of anti-RNA and anti-cardiolipin antibodies.

On the other hand, anti-DNA antibodies are mainly produced by plasmablasts and short-lived plasma cells [17]. To clarify the relationship between RP105(-) B cell subsets and long- and short-lived plasma cells is also challengeable.

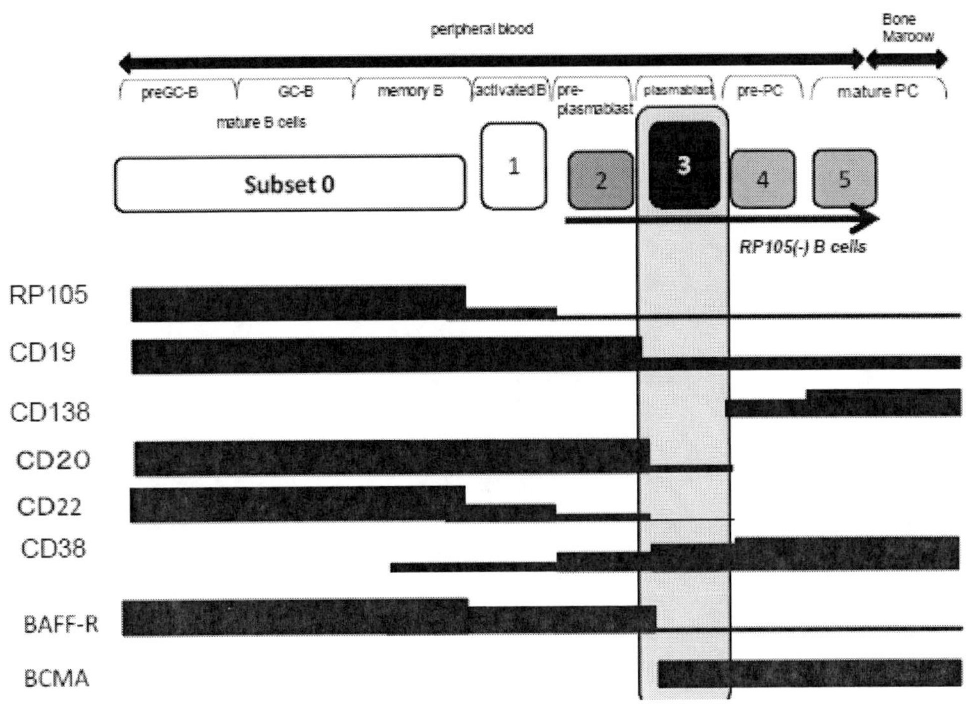

Figure 3. Antigen expression of RP105(-)B cell subsets.

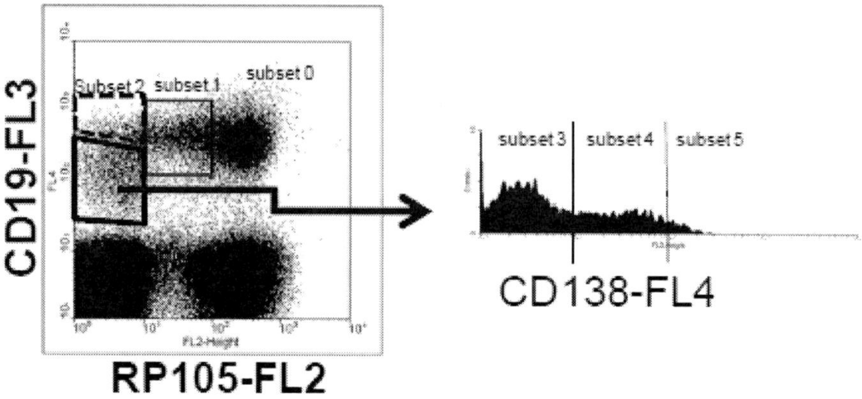

Figure 4. Five subpopulations of RP105(-) B cells.

Surface Antigens on B Cells

According to the stages of B cell development, expression of surface makers is characterized. CD19, CD20, CD22 and CD138 molecules are important to define the developing stage of B cell (Figure 5).

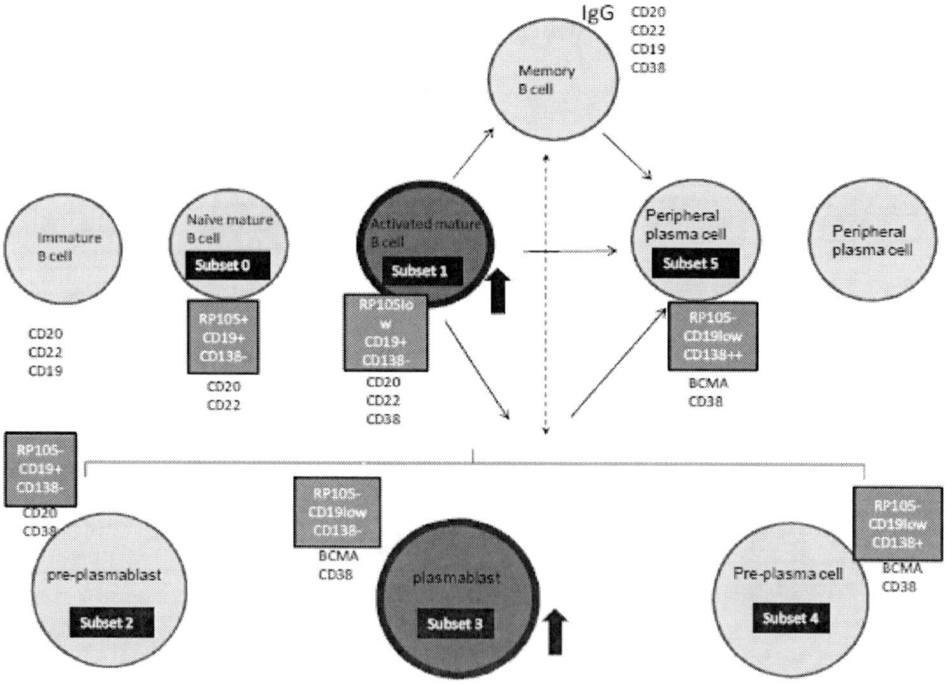

Figure 5. RP105(-)B cell subsets in SLE.

CD19

CD19, a cell surface molecule that assembles with the antigen receptor of B cells, is expressed throughout B cell development. CD19 transduces a critical signal that regulates B cell development, activation, and differentiation. Human activated B cells and plasmablasts/plasma cells express CD19. However, the levels are lower on plasmablasts and plasma cells compared to activated B cells [18].

In our study of phenotype of RP105(-) B cell subsets (Figure 6), CD19 expression is lower, especially, in subset 3, 4, and 5 among RP105(-) B cell subsets. However, CD19 expression is constantly found in all subsets.

CD20

CD20, an activated-glycosylated phosphoprotein, is expressed on the surface of all but earliest and latest stages of B cell development, beginning at the pro-B cells and progressively increasing in expression levels until mature B cells. However, stem cells and normal plasma cells lack CD20 expression. CD20 knockout mice do not show deficit of B cells. The function of CD20 is not known [19].

In RP105(-) B cell subsets, subset 0 and 1 B cells are positive for CD20, but the expression levels on subset 2 is reduced by half (Figure 6). Subset 3, 4, and 5 B cells lost CD20 expression. Therefore, rituximab, anti-CD20 monoclonal antibody, targeting B cells does not cover these late B cells lacking CD20 expression.

CD22

CD22 is a 135kDa B cell-specific transmembrane sialoglycoprotein. Pre-B cells express cytoplasmic CD22 expression at low levels. The levels of surface CD22 expression are low in immature B cells and higher levels in mature B cells (IgM+IgD+) [20]. However, CD22 has disappeared in plasma cells and memory B cells [21].

The expression of CD22 antigen on RP105(-) B cells is gradually disappeared during differentiation of late B cells (Figure 6). Subset 0 expresses high levels of CD20 but the expression is lower even in subset 1. CD22 disappeared earlier than CD20 in the development of RP105(-) B cell subsets.

CD138

CD138, one of the members of syndecan family, is a transmembrane proteoglycan. In the hematopoietic system, CD138 is mainly expressed on late stages of B cell differentiation [22]. It is expressed at high levels in plasma cells among B cell lineage. Therefore, the molecule is generally used as a plasma cell marker. In SLE patients we investigated the molecule in RP105(-) B cells (Figure 4 and 5) and defined them as late B cells. Subset 1, 2, and 3 of RP105(-) B cells are negative for CD138 (Figure 6). Therefore, due to lacking CD138, subset 3 B cells may be assigned as (early-)plasmablasts not as plasma cells. Subset 4 B cells may be assigned as pre-plasma cells due to intermediate CD138 expression. B cells of subset 5 are CD138 bright plasma cells in peripheral blood.

Interaction between B Cells and T Cells

The signals between B cells and T cells are essential to activation, proliferation and differentiation of B cells. CD28/B7 families and CD40/CD40L are considered as critical costimulatory molecules. Therefore, they can be targets for B cell therapy (Figure 7).

CD40/CD40L

CD40 is expressed on surface of B cells and binds to CD40L on activated helper T cells (Figure 7). Interaction between B cells and T cells via antigen binding and CD40/CD40L activates and proliferates B cells, and results in differentiation from B cells into plasma cells. Interaction of CD40-CD40L plays a significant role in the production of autoantibodies and tissue injury in lupus nephritis.

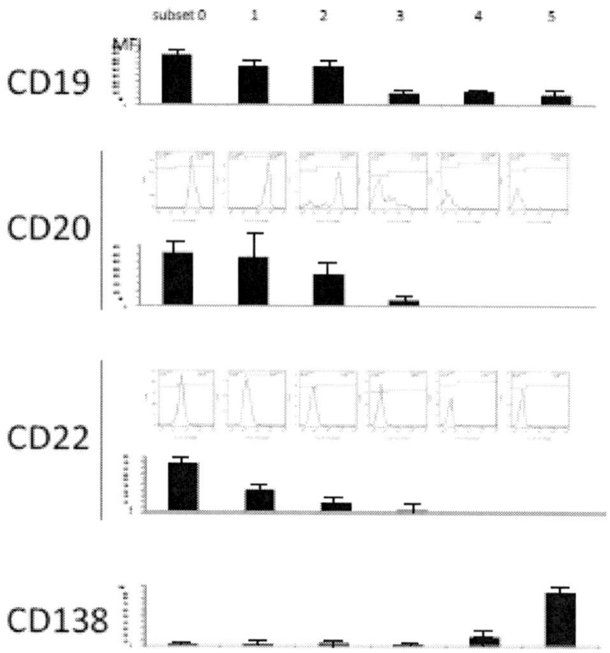

Figure 6. B cell-T cell interaction.

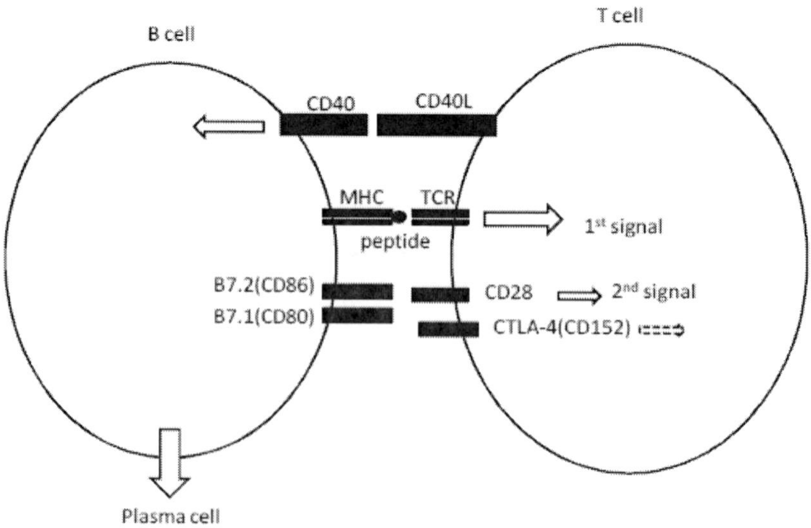

Figure 7. BAFF/APRIL and three BBRs.

B7.1 (CD80), B7.2 (CD86) / CD28, CTLA-4 (CD152)

B7.1 (CD80) and B7.2 (CD86), also called B7 molecules, are members of immunoglobulin superfamily and costimulatory molecules that enhance interaction with T cells as the second signal and activate T cells. These molecules, expressed on surface of activated B cells, bind to CD28 on naïve T cells. Activation by TLR ligands upregulates expression of CD80 in antigen presenting cells (APCs). On the other hand, CD86 expression on APCs is constitutive. CD86 expression is increased in peripheral blood B cells from SLE patients [23]. The percentage of CD86+ cells is significantly higher in B cells from SLE patients compared to normal subjects. The percentage of CD80+ cells are increased in the subset of large activated B cells of SLE patients. Comparison of the small resting B cell subset does not show a significant difference in CD80 expression between them.

RP105(-) B cells express higher levels of CD86 but not CD80 compared to RP105(+) B cells. More precisely, from subset 0 to subset 2 B cells, CD86 expression is very low, but CD86 were positive on subset 3 4, and 5 cells. CD80 were low or negative in all RP105(-) B cell subsets. CD86+ RP105(-) B cell subsets may function as APCs.

CD28, expressed on T cells, provides costimulatory signals, which are essential for T cell activation. CD28 binds to CD80 and CD86. CD28 molecule is constitutively expressed on naive T cells. Stimulation via CD28 and T cell receptor (TCR) can provide a proper stimulatory signal to T cells for the production of various cytokines such as interleukin (IL)-2 and IL-6. Without interaction CD28 and B7, association of TCR on a naive T cell with major histocompatibility complex (MHC)-antigen peptide complex on APC makes T cells anergic.

CTLA-4 (CD152) is a member of the immunoglobulin superfamily. CTLA-4 is expressed on surface of activated helper T cells and has an inhibitory signal to regulate response of activated T cells [24, 25]. CTLA-4 is structurally similar to CD28 molecule, and both molecules, CD28 and CTLA-4, bind to CD80 and CD86 on APCs. In SLE patients, the splice variant soluble CTLA-4 (sCTLA-4) is also found to be aberrantly production. sCTLA-4 is found in the serum of patients with active SLE.

Antigen Presentation; As Antigen-Presenting Cells, Providers of Pro-Inflammatory Cytokines, and T Cell Activators

B cells regulate T cells, dendritic cells and even the population of B cells itself. Normal B cells express MHC class II molecules, costimulatory molecules such as CD80 and CD86 and present antigens to T cells efficiently. In autoimmune diseases, out-of-regulated autoreactive B cells may strongly stimulate autoreactive T cells by antigen presentation. B cells play important roles in pathophysiology of autoimmunity as stimulators that present autoantigens. Therefore, the regulation of function of antigen presentation and activation is one of the possible targets of B cell therapies.

Interestingly, in RP105(-) B cells, only subset 3, 4 and 5 B cells from SLE patients express significantly higher levels of HLA-DR (MHC class II) compared to normal subjects. Bronchoalveolar lavage fluid from a dermatomyositis (DM) patient with interstitial pneumonitis contained a large number of RP105(-) B cells [26]. Increased RP105(-) B cells are also observed in peripheral blood of DM. However, RP105(-) B cells are accumulated much more in the local area with inflammation. Large proportion of circulating RP105(-) B cells exists in Sjögren's syndrome (SS) patients [27, 28]. Salivary glands in SS patients have lymphoid follicles of which germinal centers consist of RP105(-) B cells. A larger proportion of B cells infiltrating the area other than lymphoid follicles are also negative for RP105. Collectively, from above observations, RP105(-) B cells may be directly associated with the inflammation and tissue damage of the local organs such as lungs, salivary glands and so on.

Cytokines for B Cells; Activation and Cell Survival

Cytokines such as B-cell activating factor (BAFF), a proliferation-inducing ligand (APRIL), IL-4, IL-7, tissue growth factor (TGF)-beta, and interferons (IFNs) are important to activate and survival of B cells.

BAFF/APRIL and Three BBRS

BAFF, also known as B-lymphocyte stimulator (BLyS), zTNF4, TALL-1, THANK, and APRIL, is essential factors for B cell immunity [29, 30, 31, 32]. BAFF is one of the tumor necrosis factor (TNF) ligand family and required for B cell growth, survival via inhibition of apoptosis, and immunoglobulin production from transitional and mature B cells [31, 33, 34]. APRIL also induces B-cell activation [35]. In general, BAFF exists as homotrimers on cell surface and is also in soluble form. Moreover, circulating BAFF is more abundant in NZB/W F1 and MRL/lpr mice during the onset and progression of SLE.

As shown in Figure 8, BAFF binds to three different BAFF-binding receptors (BBRs) of the TNF receptor family: B-cell maturation antigen (BCMA), BAFF receptor (BAFF-R) and transmembrane activator and cyclophilin ligand interactor (TACI) [36, 37, 38]. APRIL has homology with BAFF and bind to only TACI and BCMA, among BBRs, and then influences humoral responses, class-switching of immunoglobulin, and activity of B1 cells. Although knowledge of distinct function among three BBRs is still lacking [39, 40], expression on normal B cells in human has been already reported [41, 42, 43, 44, 45].

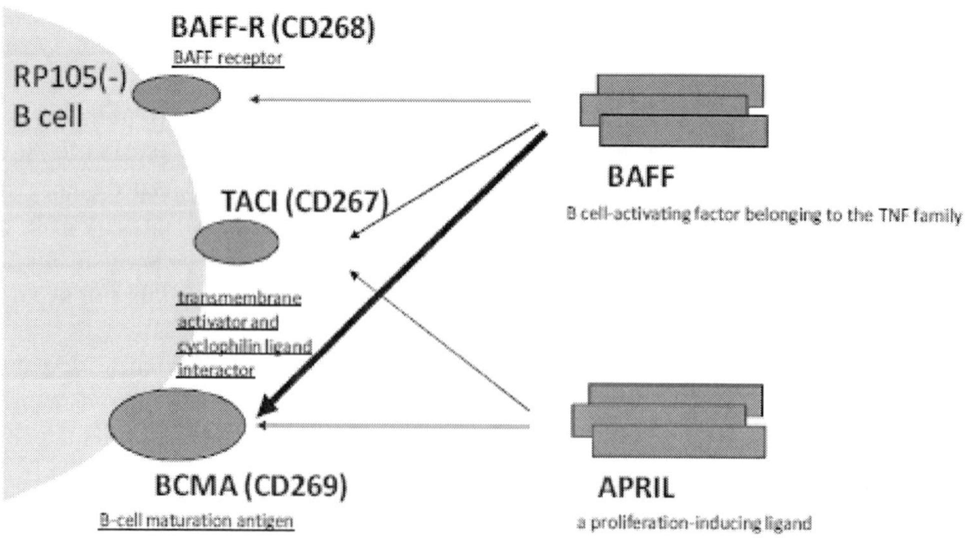

Figure 8. B cell surface markers on RP105(-) B cells subsets.

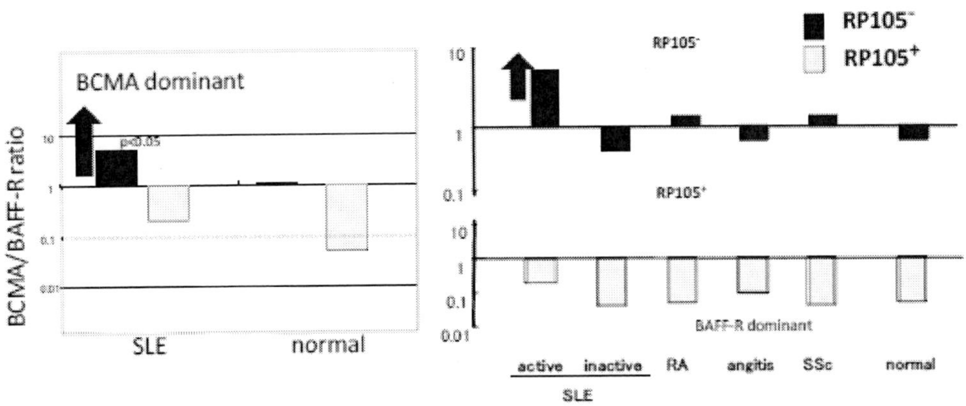

Figure 9. BAFF-R and BCMA expression on RP105(-) B cells.

In the process of differentiation of mature B cells into plasma cells, BAFF-R expression is decreased. On the other hand, BCMA expression is increased and TACI expression remains unchanged. However, there had been no information on BBR's expression in B cells derived from SLE patients. Therefore, we investigated their expression on B cells. RP105(-) B cells. In SLE, RP105(-) B cells express higher levels of BCMA than normal subjects, and are possibly regulated by BAFF/APRIL (Figure 9).

Interestingly, we found preferential expression of BCMA on RP105(-) B cells compared with RP105(+) B cells. However, BAFF-R expression on RP105(-) B cells is significantly lower. The ratios of BCMA/BAFF-R on RP105(-) B cells are increased in SLE patients compared to normal subjects. Therefore, RP105(-) B cells from SLE patients more preferentially express BCMA compared to BAFF-R than normal subjects. Stimulation of trimers of CD40L is so strong that it decreases the numbers of surviving both RP105(-) and RP105(+) B cells. RP105(+) B cells are not rescued from sCD40L-induced cell death by BAFF and/or APRIL. In contrast, either BAFF or APRIL can maintain the living RP105(-) B cells due to avoidance of apoptosis. Strongly activated RP105(-) B cells reduced BAFF-R and increased BCMA levels. Collectively, the pathway of BCMA-BAFF/APRIL may be primary surviving function in late B cells from SLE.

IL-7

IL-7 is another cytokine produced by bone marrow stromal cells and can act as a growth factor for B cell precursors, pro-B cells. However, IL-7 has little effect on the stages of later B cells.

IFNs (Interferons)

IFN-alpha has anti-viral function and promotes maturation of myeloid dendritic cells. IFNs play critical roles in immunity and autoimmunity. IFNs take part in T cell activation and survival, and follicular helper T cell differentiation [46]. Importantly, they produce BAFF [47]. IFN- α stimulates CD4+ T cells that enhance activation of antigen-specific B cells with antibody production, and increase levels of TLR7 in B cells. IFN-α promotes the differentiation of activated B cells into plasmablasts, and then, finally, plasmablasts differentiate into antibody-secreting plasma cells by IL-6 [48].

Recent evidence suggests that Type I IFNs are involved in pathogenesis of SLE. In lupus-prone mice, IFNs accelerate the break of B cell tolerance to nucleic acids. Moreover, immune complexes with nucleic acids activate TLRs and then it result in production of IFNs and pro-inflammatory cytokines [49]. Sometimes, in medical practice, treatment with recombinant IFNs in patients with hepatitis or neoplastic diseases induces SLE. However, a genetic predisposition is also essential for IFN-alpha induced autoimmunity. The result from mice explains the reason why not all patients develop SLE due to IFN therapy. Elevated serum IFNs and IFN-stimulated gene expression are also found in SLE patients. IFNs are correlated with disease activity and involvements of renal and central nervous system.

In our preliminary study, when strong stimulation of sCD40L-trimers induces B cell apoptosis, RP105(-) B cells survive by exogenous IFNs in vitro.

Abnormal B Cells in Lupus-Prone Mice

(NZB × NZW) F1, NZM2410, BXSB, and MRL/lpr mouse strains show a fatal lupus-like syndrome. These mice spontaneously develop signs and symptoms of SLE. To a greater or lesser extent, the mice present lymphoid hyperplasia, B cell hyperactivation, autoantibody production and immune complexes, complement consumption, and lupus nephritis [50].

Germinal centers (GC) may be important sites of immune dysregulation in autoimmune diseases. Spontaneously, GCs are formed in many strains of lupus-prone mice. The spontaneous GC formation is found in the spleens of several autoimmune mouse strains that develop a lupus-like disease. GC B cells are predominantly composed of PNA+, B220+, and GL7+ B cells. In MRL/lpr lupus strain, CD138(int) B cells with intermediate CD138 expression, produce autoantibodies, including anti-Sm antibodies, and accumulate in peripheral blood. The cells are strongly related to autoimmunity [15]. The stage of CD138(int) B cells is a checkpoint for regulation of autoreactive B cells. Accumulation of peripheral CD138(int) B cells is related to breaking checkpoint of tolerance. Increased numbers of autoreactive CD138(int) B cells are associates with production of autoantibodies against nuclear antigens such as Sm. Moreover, in CD138(int) B cells, there are two subsets, autoreactive and normal CD138(int) B cells. The differential phenotype between autoreactive and normal CD138(int) B cells is defined. Autoreactive CD138(int) B cells have remarkably activated phenotype with expressing higher levels of CD80, larger size and increased granularity compared to normal CD138(int) B cells. Therefore, activated phenotype in CD138(int) B cells is one of the hallmarks of autoreactivity.

B-1 cells show different phenotype from conventional B cells (B-2 cells). B-1 cells are self-reconstituting and long-lived. They produce low-affinity but cross reactive IgM antibodies [51, 52]. While NZB, (NZBxNZW)F1 and motheaten mice have B-1 cells that produce anti-erythrocyte and anti-DNA antibodies, B-1 cells in other lupus-prone mice do not correlate with autoimmunity [53, 54].

Abnormal B Cells in Human SLE

As stated above, the pathogenesis of SLE is still unknown, however, B cell overactivity, especially in autoreactive B cells that produce pathogenic autoantibodies is the center in immune cell dysregulation of SLE. Therefore, emergence of autoreactive B cells is a hallmark of human and murine SLE. Altered B cell subsets, immature transitional B cells, memory B cells, plasmablasts and plasma cells in peripheral blood are found in patients with SLE.

B-1 cell in human has CD5 (Ly-1 in mice), the T cell surface marker. In human SLE, pathogenic role of B-1 cells is more questionable. Suzuki N et al. reported that both of B-1 and B-2 cells produce anti-dsDNA autoantibodies in SLE patients [55].

Analysis in detail of B cells from SLE patients revealed that there are primary disturbances in the different peripheral B cell subsets. Among abnormal B cell subpopulations in SLE patients, RP105(-) B cells are remarkable. Therefore, B cell subpopulations other than RP105(-) B cells were also reported. CD27(high) CD38(+) CD19(dim) Ig(low) CD20(-) CD138+ plasma cells [56] and CD27(high) plasma cells [57], a plasma cell precursor subset (CD20(-)CD19(+/low)CD27(+/++) CD38(++)) [58] are found in peripheral blood in active patients. However, these cells may be identical with RP105(-) B cell subsets. Other interesting subpopulations, type I transitional (T1) B cells [59] and VH4.34 B cells [60] were also reported. Extraordinary numbers of circulating B cells with pregerminal center phenotype (IgD(+)CD38(+)centerin(+)) are found in SLE patients [58].

Although virtually all mature B cells from normal subjects express RP105, the number of RP105(-) B cells is increased in active SLE patients. The disease activity of SLE is closely associated with the number of cells. In serial analysis, the percentages of RP105(-) B cells decrease as the disease turned inactive. The levels of IgG, one of the B cell functions, are correlated with the percentage of cells. Circulating RP105(-) B cells disappeared in inactive state of the disease after conventional treatment with corticosteroids. RP105(-) B cells are more sensitive to corticosteroid-induced apoptosis than RP105(+) B cells.

The diagnosis of ANA-negative SLE may be difficult sometimes due to lack of hallmarks of obvious serological autoimmune disorders. Very interestingly, increased RP105(-) B cells were found in the peripheral blood from ANA-negative SLE [61]. When SLE patients show no serological abnormality, the cytological screening of detection of RP105(-) B cells may be helpful in possible diagnosis of SLE.

In human SLE, pathogenic subsets of B cells have not fully identified yet. RP105(-) B cells are late B cells and consist of at least 5 subsets. Therefore, we investigated the percentages of each circulating RP105(-) B cell subset. The populations of subset 1 and 3 B cells are larger than other subsets, although all subsets in SLE patients are significantly increased compared to normal subjects. Moreover, the phenotype of each normal RP105(-) B cell subset seems similar to those from SLE patients. However, the expression levels of several antigens are different between them like autoreactive and normal CD138(int) B cells in lupus-prone mice. Although in subset 3, 4 and 5, levels of CD38 and HLA-DR of SLE patients are significantly higher, levels CD95 were lower compared to normal subjects.

Phenotype of RP105(-) B cells show strikingly similar to CD138(int) B cells; larger cell size and increased granularity, cytoplasmic Ig and IgM expression. CD19(low)RP105(-)CD138(int) B cells may be the human counterparts of CD138(int) B cells in MRL/lpr mice. RP105(-) B cells also have highly activated phenotypes. Because the similar observations have been found in human SLE , we could lead to the hypothesis that most of the RP105(-) B cells in SLE might be autoreactive. These results suggest the existence of common mechanisms, with breaking checkpoints of autoreactivity, in dysregulation of B cells in human and murine autoimmune diseases. To reconstruct these checkpoints may be possible targets of treatment of SLE.

TLRs

RP105 belongs to TLR families. Therefore, the relationship TLRs and SLE is interesting. TLRs control acquired immune response as well as innate immunity. TLR7 and TLR9 on B cells and plasmacytoid dendritic cells (pDC) recognize self-nucleic acids [62]. The signaling via TLRs is also an important step in the pathogenesis of SLE [63]. It was reported that the inhibitors of TLR7 and 9 signaling could be effective corticosteroid-sparing drugs [62].

Section 2. Therapies of Targeting B Cells in SLE

B cell therapies include targeting surface antigens [blinatumomab (CD19), rituximab (CD20) and epratuzumab (CD22)], maturation and growth factors of B cells [belimumab, briobacept, and atacicept (BAFF/APRIL)], costimulatory molecules [abatacept (CTLA-4 and B7 molecules)], and B cell tolerogen [abetimus]. There are also other targets including TLRs, plasma cells and plasmablasts, IFNs and BCMA. In this article we review these B cell therapies and present a novel strategy targeting RP105(-) B cells in SLE.

Anti-Surface Antigens

Anti-CD19

Blinatumomab, Anti-CD19

Blinatumomab is an antibody targeting the CD19 antigen. Anti-CD19 immunotherapy could offer a new therapy in B cell depletion for the treatment of multiple autoimmune diseases [64] including RA and SLE.

Anti-CD20

Rituximab, Anti-CD20 (Rituxan, Mab Thera)

Rituximab is a mouse-human chimeric IgG1κ immunoglobulin that targets CD20 molecules on B cells. Although CD20 levels on B cells are high, there is not a soluble form. At the ligation of CD20, it is not shed from cell surface and is not internalized. Therefore, the molecule would be an ideal target to eliminate B cells.

In 1997, the drug was approved by Food and Drug Administration (FDA) of the US for treatment of low-grade B cell lymphoma [65]. After FDA approved rituximab for the treatment of lymphoma, many researchers have investigated its use in patients with autoimmune diseases including refractory SLE patients. In 2006, rituximab was approved for rheumatoid arthritis (RA) in the U. S.

Rituximab depletes B cells in peripheral blood rapidly and efficiently [66]. Mechanisms of the agents are cytotoxicity including complement-dependent cytotoxicity (CDC) and antibody dependent cellular cytotoxicity (ADCC) [67]. Rituximab can also directly induce apoptosis of B cells [68]. Therefore, rituximab has been a great expectation to treat SLE patients.

Noncontrolled Series

A preliminary noncontrolled series [69, 70, 71, 72, 73] and many case reports [74, 75] of patients with SLE treated with rituximab have shown that the disease improves after the treatment of rituximab.

Clinical Trials

Although there was great promise of preliminary studies, controlled phase III trials of rituximab were failed. EXPLORER; patients with moderately active non-renal SLE [76] and LUNAR; patients with class III or IV lupus nephritis [77] were conducted but they failed to demonstrate superiority of rituximab over placebo plus conventional therapy at the primary endpoints.

Ocrelizumab, Anti CD20 (Rg1594)

In addition to rituximab, another anti-CD20 targeted therapy existed. Ocrelizumab is a humanized anti-CD20 monoclonal antibody. Its targets are mature B cells and then may be an immunosuppressive drug candidate.

Clinical Trials

The development of clinical trial of phase III of ocrelizumab for SLE and RA has been discontinued due to serious opportunistic infections in March 2010 [78].

Ofatumumab, Anti-CD20 (Arzerra)

Ofatumumab (trade name Arzerra, also known as HuMax-CD20) is a human anti-CD20 monoclonal antibody. Although it was reported that ofatumumab is clinically effective in patients with active RA, there is no information of clinical trials for treatment of SLE.

Veltuzumab, Anti-CD20

Veltuzumab (hA20) is a humanized anti-CD20 monoclonal antibody having 90-95% human antibody sequences. Structure of veltuzumab is similar to rituximab and functions, including antibody-dependent cell-mediated cytotoxicity, apoptosis and growth inhibition, are similar between them. Additionally, veltuzumab is the first anti-CD20 antibody with a subcutaneous administration. Veltuzumab also shows an excellent safety and tolerability profile. Therefore, this drug may avoid infusion-related side effects and increase convenience for the patient via its subcutaneous route compared to other ani-CD20 therapies. Low-dose veltuzumab are well tolerated and durable objective responses in non-Hodgkin's lymphoma (NHL) [79]. Phase I/II clinical trials have been completed in patients with non-Hodgkin's lymphoma. The results show a high complete response rate in follicular lymphoma, even at low doses of 80-120 mg/m2 once weekly for 4 weeks.

In autoimmune diseases, patients with ITP can also respond to low doses of veltuzumab in a Phase I/II clinical trial.

Anti-CD22; Epratuzumab

Epratuzumab is a humanized anti-CD22 IgG1 monoclonal antibody. It has murine sequence comprising only 5-10% of molecule, to reduce immunogenicity [67, 68, 80]. It was developed for the treatment of NHL with good safety. In SLE patients, treatment with epratuzumab decreases the number of B cells by about 35-40% [81]. Although epratuzumab only partially deletes B cells, it modulates B cells via a negative signal by binding to cell surface CD22. The targets of the drug are preferentially naïve and transitional B cells in peripheral blood [82]. Epratuzumab induces moderate ADCC, with no direct apoptosis or CDC.

Open-Label Trial

An open-label trial [81] examines the safety of the drug in SLE patients. A single-center study with moderately active SLE suggested improved disease activity.

Clinical Trials

Epratuzumab has been evaluated in one phase II trial [81] and two phase III studies (SL0003/SL0004 and NCT00383513) [82]. These results suggest that treatment of SLE with epratuzumab is effective, well tolerated and significantly improves the quality of life (QOL) of SLE patients. SL0003 (severe patients)/SL0004 (moderate patients), randomized controlled phase III trials, resulted in better reductions in total BILAG scores, steroid sparing effect, and improving of QOL compared with placebo. Another phase III study (NCT00383513) investigates efficacy and safety of epratuzumab in long-term.

Anti-CD138 Therapy

See below in the section of "anti-plasma cells" for further details.

Blockade of Survival and Differentiation of B Cells

Blocking of the factors for survival, differentiation and their signaling is another therapeutic target for B cells. Deprivation of B cell survival factors has demonstrated clinical benefit in both oncologic and immunologic diseases as well as removal of pathogenic B cells by depletion of monoclonal antibodies, Especially, BAFF and APRIL may be ideal candidates in this strategy.

To achieve this, anti-BAFF antibodies and fusion proteins of BBRs are available agents. However, BAFF/APRIL and their receptors are the system of 2-ligands-and-3-receptors. The system is so complicated that many strategies have been presented.

Anti-BAFF

The BAFF is a potent survival factor for B cells. It binds three receptors (BBRs): TACI, BCMA, and BAFF-R (BR3). Belimumab was the first novel drug to be approved for SLE after over 50 years in the U. S. Industry analysts expect belimumab, to be a blockbuster, with annual sales of $2.2 billion by 2014 [83].

Belimumab, Anti-BAFF (Trade Name Benlysta, Lymphostat-B)

Belimumab is a fully human IgG1λ anti-BAFF monoclonal antibody that inhibits BAFF (BAFF or BLyS-specific inhibitor). Belimumab may bind primarily to circulating soluble BAFF, and then decrease the numbers of B cells and the levels of anti-dsDNA antibodies [84]. Belimumab is approved in the U.S. on March 9, 2011. It has been investigated for the effectiveness in other autoimmune diseases. The phase II clinical trial for RA shows preliminary results that are encouraging. However, belimumab only works in a subset of patients and is not effective against the deadliest forms of the disease. Additionally, it did not work in African Americans, who are disproportionately affected by SLE.

Clinical Trials

Two phase III trials, BLISS-76 (NCT00410384) and BLISS-52 (NCT00424476), in SLE have been concluded with the primary endpoints being met in both studies. The safety profile and efficacy of belimumab were proved in controlling SLE. Inhibition of soluble BAFF with belimumab provides a new option for the treatment of SLE [85]. Belimumab has shown significant benefits for patients with SLE in the Phase III trials. A phase II trial in rheumatoid arthritis has also been completed, with positive results.

Briobacept, BR3-Fc

Briobacept (BR3-Fc) is a homodimeric fusion glycoprotein with two cytokine receptor BAFF-Rs (human extracellular domain-containing fragment BR3, ligand-binding portion) linked to IgG1 (human Fc domain containing fragment). BR3-Fc (briobacept) blocks BAFF from binding to BAFF-R, thus inhibiting activation and promoting apoptosis of B cells.

Results in Animal Models

Although there is no information of clinical trial using briobacept, in NZB/WF1 mice, which develop a fatal lupus-like syndrome, briobacept attenuated the disease process [86].

Anti-BAFF/APRIL

Atacicept; TACI-Ig

Because both BAFF and APRIL bind to TACI, TACI-Ig inhibits two ligands. Atacicept (TACI:Fc5) is a recombinant fusion protein of TACI receptor and human IgG1. Clinically, it is interesting that broader effect of the drug inhibiting both BAFF and APRIL would result in better than other drugs targeting BAFF or APRIL alone.

Results in Animal Models

In NZB/WF1 mice, soluble TACI-Ig fusion protein inhibits the development of proteinuria and prolongs survival [87]. These results suggested the involvement of BAFF/APRIL and its receptors in the development of SLE. TACI-Ig may be a promising treatment of autoimmune disease also in humans.

Clinical Trials

Atacicept was well tolerated and demonstrated biologic activity. Atacicept showed dose-dependent reductions in immunoglobulin levels and in mature and total B cell numbers in peripheral blood of SLE [88]. A phase II/III trial of atacicept intends to compare to placebo in reducing the number of flares for people with SLE [89]. Estimated study completion date is October 2012.

Anti-BAFF-R (BR3) (CD268)

As a novel B cell therapy, anti-BR3 monoclonal antibodies used in preclinical studies are effective. Anti-BR3 antibodies block BAFF-dependent human B-cell proliferation in vitro and reduce murine B-cell populations in vivo [90]. Anti-BR3 antibodies decrease the numbers of B cells more effectively than anti-BAFF monoclonal antibodies, BR3-Fc and TACI-Fc [91]

A-623, AMG 623

A-623 (AMG 623) is a polypeptide fusion protein (peptibody) (peptide-Fc FP) that inhibits B cell survival and maturation by neutralizing BAFF. AMG-623 has begun clinical trials, and appears to be well tolerated by patients. However, its efficacy of treating SLE and improving disease activity remains undetermined. A-623 is currently in Phase II clinical trials [92].

Blockade of Costimulatory Molecules

The autoimmune response in SLE, especially autoantibody production, depends on T cells and is executed via cognate interactions between T cells and APCs. To perform a proper T cell activation, interactions of specific signals generated through TCR and the second signals, provided by the interaction of costimulatory molecules, are essential. Lacking of the second costimulatory signal results in the interruption of autoimmune response, leading to anergy, a state of immune unresponsiveness. Therefore, costimulatory molecules, B7/CD28, are promising targets for B cell therapy in SLE. CD40L (CD40 ligand)/CD40 are also targets of blocking costimulatory signals between T cells and B cells.

Anti-CD40L

Anti-human CD40L humanized monoclonal antibodies, ruplizumab, [hu5c8, BG-9588, Antova™ (Biogen, Cambridge, MA, USA)] and E6040/IDEC-131 (IDEC Pharmaceuticals, San Diego, CA, USA) have been developed. They were used in clinical trials for patients with SLE.

Ruplizumab, Anti-CD40L, Antova

An open-label, multiple-dose study of ruplizumab, anti-CD40L antibodies, was examined in SLE [93]. A short course of the treatment in patients with active lupus nephritis showed reduction disease activity and levels of anti-dsDNA antibodies and increase of C3 concentrations.

These findings suggest that blockade of CD40L–CD40 signal seems to be a promising strategy for treating human autoimmune diseases. Although initial data in the serology and renal function of the patients was encouraging, surprisingly, ruplizumab was not fruitful in human SLE. Short-term administration of ruplizumab in lupus nephritis was correlated with life-threatening prothrombotic events [94]. Thromboembolic events during anti-CD40L treatment led to a halt in all clinical trials. Blockade of CD40L–CD40 interaction may be a potentially effective therapy for SLE [95].

From other group reported that anti-CD40L autoantibody is associated with thrombocytopenia but not with thromboembolism in SLE [96]. However, naturally, the potential risk of thromboembolic events should be considered in this system.

IDEC-131, Anti-CD40L

In a study of IDEC-131, another humanized anti-CD40L antibody, treatment of SLE patients proceeded without apparent thromboembolic activity [97]. However, IDEC-131 treatment did not show effectiveness in SLE patients, despite being well tolerated. Moreover, in 2003, after a thromboembolic event in a Crohn's disease patient was reported, all IDEC-131 studies stopped [98].

Anti-CD28

In 2006, a phase I clinical study was operated for anti-CD28 superagonist monoclonal antibody TGN1412 in six human volunteers. TGN1412 rapidly caused a life-threatening cytokine storm and multiple organ failure in all six volunteers [99, 100].

Anti-CD28; Abatacept (CTLA-4-Ig)

CTLA-4 has higher binding affinity than CD28. It is a genetically engineered soluble form of the inhibitory molecule CTLA-4. Abatacept is a fusion protein of the extracellular domain of CTLA-4 and constant region of immunoglobulin. The agent blocks costimulatory molecules, CD28/CTLA-4 and B7.1/B7.2. Abatacept have been used in treatment of rheumatoid arthritis [101]. Abatacept induce the remission of refractory RA patients with methotrexate treatment.

Results in Animal Models

In lupus model mice, (NZB/W)F1, treatment with CTLA4-Ig reduces autoantibody production and prolongs survival. Even when treatment is delayed until the most advanced stage of clinical illness, it is still effective. These findings suggest a potential role for human CTLA-4-Ig in the treatment of SLE [102].

Clinical Trials

A phase IIb randomized, double-blind, placebo-controlled trial of SLE patients with polyarthritis, discoid lesions, or pleuritis and/or pericarditis was performed. The primary and secondary end points were not met in the study. However, some improvements by abatacept were found in patients with non-life-threatening manifestations of SLE [103].

B Cell Tolerogens

LJP394 Compound (Abetimus Sodium, Riquent)

LJP394 is a synthetic agent of four double-strand oligonucleotides attached to a platform of polyethylene glycol. The agent binds to anti-dsDNA antibodies and cress-links B cell receptors recognizing dsDNA, and then the anti-dsDNA antibody-producing B cells are in anergy or depleted [104, 105].

Animal Studies

Animal studies show that abetimus reduces the titers of anti-dsDNA antibodies as well as of anti-dsDNA antibody-secreting cells [105].

Clinical Trials

The phase III trials of abetimus failed without clinical benefit in SLE patients [105]. Although abetimus has been associated with reductions in circulating anti-dsDNA antibodies, two pivotal trials with large numbers of lupus nephritis patients failed to demonstrate efficacy in renal flare. A trial was also abruptly terminated in February 2009.

New Strategy for B Cell Therapies

Rituximab depletes nearly all circulating B cells, while the agent does not show effectiveness in controlled clinical trials of SLE patients. These results disappointed many patients and physicians. Anti-DNA antibodies are mainly produced by plasmablasts and short-lived plasma cells [17]. However, rituximab does not delete plasma cells. To delete later B cells, plasmablasts and plasma cells, by agents may be more rational than just CD20+ B cell targeted therapies. Moreover, belimumab is successful in SLE treatment, but the drug is not effective in all patients. It does not work in subsets of African Americans or with severe activity of SLE. Therefore, new strategies for B cell therapy are required.

Anti-RP105(-) B Cells

As mentioned above, RP105(-) B cells are assigned as plasmablasts and plasma cells and produce anti-dsDNA antibodies. Therefore, it is possible that these cells can be targets for treatment of SLE. Interestingly, RP105(-) B cells can divide further into at least five subgroups. If the narrower targets can be available, the toxicity would be lower and efficacy may be strengthened. We planned to investigate the antigens specific for RP105(-) B cells.

For this purpose, we try to identify the antigens specific for RP105(-) B cells using a DNA microarray. Differential expression of genes between RP105(-) and RP105(+) B cells was analyzed. The surface expression of possible antigens specific for RP105(-) B cells was confirmed using flow cytometry. BCMA is one of the identified antigens. These results also suggest that BCMA may be one of the targets for elimination of RP105(-) B cells to treat the SLE patients. The data of higher BCMA expression suggest that RP105(-) B cells from active SLE patients may have predisposition toward survival response in high levels of BAFF and/or APRIL in vivo via BCMA.

Anti-BCMA and Other Targets on RP105(-) B Cells

Most interestingly, of BBRs (three BAFF receptors), levels of BAFF-R are higher in pre-plasmablasts (subset 2) RP105(-) B cells, but BCMA expression was conversely higher in plasmablasts (subset 3), pre-plasma cells (subset 4), and circulating plasma cells (subset 5 RP105(-) B cells) (Figure 9).

Although BCMA is expressed on normal plasma cells, the levels of expression are increased in active SLE. BCMA may be a potential target for therapeutic intervention. The blocking of the signals between BAFF/APRIL and their receptors, especially via BCMA, may be effective. To target BCMA for plasmablasts and plasma cells, antibodies with ligand blocking activity and cytotoxicity of B cells are required.

Although there is no information on anti-BCMA therapy in SLE, antibody targeting of BCMA on malignant plasma cells in vitro has been reported recently [106].

Apart from BCMA, prevention of emerging or depletion of RP105(-) B cells may be other options for treatment of SLE. We have investigated various antigens specific for RP105(-) B cells using DNA microarray and a flow cytometry.

The study is presently ongoing and several candidates for specific antigens have been found. If RP105(-) B cell-specific antigens would be available and specific antibodies be established, they may provide novel strategies and tools of targeting B cells in SLE. Especially, antigens specific for subset 3 [RP105(-) plasmablasts], the most possible pathogenic subset, are hopeful to treatment.

RP105 belongs to TLR family. Therefore RP105 itself and other TLRs may be good candidates to modulate activity of SLE. Further examination will be required to establish targeting RP105(-) B cells therapy inhibiting autoimmunity. Our study in human SLE would provide a new insight of potential mechanism and intervention of autoreactive B cells in SLE.

Anti-IFN-I

Accumulating evidence shows that IFN-I links to the pathogenesis of SLE, and targeting of IFN-I may be useful to B cell therapy. IFN-I, IFN-producing cells, IFN-inducers and molecules of the IFN signaling pathway may work as potential therapeutic targets.

Results in Animal Models

Several anti-IFN-I therapies have already shown evidence of effects in animal models [107]

Clinical Trials

A phase I clinical trial suggests that neutralizing monoclonal antibodies against IFN-α can ameliorate disease activity [108].

Anti-Plasma Cells and Plasmablasts

Because CD138 is highly expressed on plasma cells, the molecules may function as a target for B cell therapy, especially targeting plasma cells. However, there has been no information on the therapy of SLE.

In mice, the anti-tumor effect of murine and human chimeric CD138-specific monoclonal antibody, nBT062, against multiple myeloma cells was reported [109]. The result may promote evaluation of nBT062 in clinical trials to treat patients with multiple myeloma.

In RP105(-) B cells, CD138 is expressed in subset 5 alone. Subset 4 B cells express CD138 only intermediately.

Especially, plasmablasts, subset 3 B cells, do not have any CD138. Therefore, it is possible that anti-CD138 antibodies would not deplete subset 3 cells, which are increased in active SLE and assigned as possible pathogenic B cells. Then, to discover each antigen specific for plasmablasts, pre-plasma cells, or circulating plasma cells is very interesting and essential for developing future medicine.

Anti-TLRs

Soluble decoy receptors and neutralizing antibodies may inhibit interaction between receptor and ligand of TLRs. Strategies of clinical and preclinical candidates inhibiting TLRs are available for the treatment of autoimmune diseases. Targeting of TLRs may be effective for the prevention and treatment of SLE. Several novel candidates are undergoing preclinical and clinical evaluation. The drugs inhibit TLR2, TLR4, TLR7 and TLR9. It is reported that TLR antagonists could lower steroid dosage and thus reduce side effects in lupus patients [62]. DV-1179 is an inhibitor of TLR7 and TLR9, DNA-based compound, developed by Dynavax. Phase I study of DV1179 examines the safety in 2011. After successful completion of the trial, a proof-of-mechanism study in lupus patients may be started. IMO-3100 is another DNA based TLR7/9 inhibitor. The drug is under Phase I trial by Idera Pharmaceuticals. Although many strategies targeting TLRs exist, there are little information on treatment of SLE presently.

Lastly, there is a large question whether RP105 itself, one of the TLR members, could be a target for SLE treatment. The strategy of restoration of RP105 expression on RP105(-) B cells may be interesting in future study.

Conclusion

The nonspecific conventional immunosuppressive therapies induce significant adverse effects and disability in autoimmune diseases. Therefore, novel therapies, with safer and more effective, specific for pathogenic cells or molecules are required. The evidence of the pathophysiological importance of B cells in SLE has shown a rationale to B cell therapy. Especially, anti-plasmablasts and plasma cells therapy may be more useful to treatment of SLE patients. The aims of our investigation may be not only the development of new drug, but also clarification of the role of B cells in pathogenesis of human SLE. Identification of new targets including antigens and subsets of B cells, should be required. RP105(-) B cells are representatives of B cells dysregulated in SLE patients. Studies of RP105(-) B cells provide new insights into alternative therapy of novel B cells therapy in SLE.

Reference

[1] Hahn, B. H. Antibodies to DNA. *N Engl. J. Med.* 1998;338:1359-68.

[2] Von Muhlen, C. A., Tan, E. M. Autoantibodies in the diagnosis of systemic rheumatic diseases. *Semin. Arthritis. Rheum.* 1995;24:323-58.

[3] Lipsky, P. E. Systemic lupus erythematosus: an autoimmune disease of B cell hyperactivity. *Nat. Immunol.* 2001;2:764-6.

[4] Pisetsky, D. S. Anti-DNA and autoantibodies. *Curr. Opin. Rheumatol.* 2000;12:364-8.

[5] Itchison, N. A., Wedderburn, L. R. B cells in autoimmunity. *Proc. Natl. Acad. Sci. US* 2000;97:8750-1.

[6] Miyake, K., Yamashita, Y., Hitoshi, Y. et al. Murine B cell proliferation and protection from apoptosis with an antibody against a 105-kD molecule: unresponsiveness of X-linked immunodeficient B cells. *J. Exp. Med.* 1994; 180:1217-24.

[7] Miyake, K., Yamashita, Y., Ogata, M., Sudo, T., Kimoto, M. RP105, a novel B cell surface molecule implicated in B cell activation, is a member of the leucine-rich repeat protein family. *J. Immunol.* 1995; 154: 3333-40.

[8] Miura, Y., Shimazu, R., Miyake, K., Akashi, S., Ogata, H., Yamashita, Y., Narisawa, Y., Kimoto, M. RP105 is associated with MD-1 and transmits an activation signal in human B cells. *Blood* 92: 2815–22.

[9] Ogata, H., Su, I., Miyake, K., Nagai, Y. et al. The Toll-like receptor protein RP105 regulates lipopolysaccharide signaling in B cells. *J. Exp. Med.* 2000;192:23–9.

[10] Nagai, Y., Kobayashi, T., Motoi, Y. et al. The radioprotective 105/MD-1 complex links TLR2 and TLR4/MD-2 in antibody response to microbial membranes. *J. Immunol.* 2005;174:7043–9.

[11] Divanovic, S., Trompette, A., Atabani, S. F. et al. Negative regulation of Toll-like receptor 4 signaling by the Toll-like receptor homolog RP105. *Nat. Immunol.* 2005;6:571-8.

[12] Koarada, S., Tada, Y., Ushiyama, O. et al. B cells lacking RP105, a novel B cell antigen, in systemic lupus erythematosus. *Arthritis. Rheum.* 1999; 42: 2593-600.

[13] Kikuchi, Y., Koarada, S., Tada, Y. et al. RP105-lacking B cells from lupus patients are responsible for the production of immunoglobulins and autoantibodies. *Arthritis. Rheum.* 2002; 46:3259-65.

[14] Mortensen, E. S., Rekvig, O. P. Nephritogenic potential of anti-DNA antibodies against necrotic nucleosomes. *J. Am. Soc. Nephrol.* 2009: 696-704.

[15] Culton, D. A., O'Conner, B. P., Conway, K. L. et al., Early preplasma cells define a tolerance checkpoint for autoreactive B cells. *J. Immunol.* 2006; 176: 790–802.

[16] Koarada, S., Tada, Y., Suematsu, R., Soejima, S., Inoue, H., Ohta, A., Nagasawa, K. Phenotyping of P105-negative B cell subsets in patients with systemic lupus erythematosus. *Clin. Dev. Immunol.* 2012; 2012: 198206.

[17] Grammer, A. C., Lipsky, P. E. B cell abnormalities in systemic lupus erythematosus. *Arthritis. Res. Ther.* 2003;5 Suppl. 4: S22-7.

[18] Jourdan, M., Caraux, A., De Vos, J. et al. An in vitro model of differentiation of memory B cells into plasmablasts and plasma cells including detailed phenotypic and molecular characterization. *Blood* 2009; 114: 5173-81.

[19] Hardy, Richard (2008). "Chapter 7: B Lymphocyte Development and Biology". In: Paul, William (Book). *Fundamental Immunology* (6th ed.). Philadelphia, PA: Lippincott Williams and Wilkins. pp. 237–269.

[20] Dörner, T., Goldenberg, D. M. Targeting CD22 as a strategy for treating systemic autoimmune diseases. *Ther. Clin. Risk Manag.* 2007; 3: 953-9.

[21] Ding, C., Foote, S., Jones, G. B-cell-targeted therapy for systemic lupus erythematosus: an update. *BioDrugs.* 2008; 22: 239-49.

[22] Gattei, V., Godeas, C., Degan, M., Rossi, F. M., Aldinucci, D., Pinto, A. Characterization of anti-CD138 monoclonal antibodies as tools for investigating the molecular polymorphism of syndecan-1 in human lymphoma cells. *Br. J. Haematol.* 1999 ;104: 152-62.

[23] Folzenlogen, D., Hofer, M. F., Leung, D. Y., Freed, J. H., Newell, M. K. Analysis of CD80 and CD86 expression on peripheral blood B lymphocytes reveals increased expression of CD86 in lupus patients. *Clin. Immunol. Immunopathol.* 1997; 83: 199-204.

[24] Waterhouse, P., Penninger, J. M., Timms, E., Wakeham, A., Shahinian, A., Lee, K. P., Thompson, C. B., Griesser, H., Mak, T. W. Lymphoproliferative disorders with early lethality in mice deficient in Ctla-4. *Science*. 1995; 270: 985-8.

[25] Magistrelli, G., Jeannin, P., Herbault, N., Benoit, De Coignac, A., Gauchat, J. F., Bonnefoy, J. Y., Delneste, Y. A soluble form of CTLA-4 generated by alternative splicing is expressed by nonstimulated human T cells. *Eur. J. Immunol.* 1999; 29: 3596-602.

[26] Kikuchi, Y., Koarada, S., Tada, Y., Ushiyama, O., Morito, F., Suzuki, N., Ohta, A., Horiuchi, T., Miyake, K., Nagasawa, K. Difference in B cell activation between dermatomyositis and polymyositis: analysis of the expression of RP105 on peripheral blood B cells. *Ann. Rheum. Dis*. 2001; 60: 1137-40.

[27] Koarada, S., Tada, Y., Kikuchi, Y., Ushiyama, O., Suzuki, N., Ohta, A., Nagasawa, K. CD180 (RP105) in rheumatic diseases. *Rheumatology* (Oxford). 2001; 40: 1315-6.

[28] Kikuchi, Y., Koarada, S., Nakamura, S., Yonemitsu, N., Tada, Y., Haruta, Y., Morito, F., Ohta, A., Miyake, K., Horiuchi, T., Nagasawa, K. Increase of RP105-lacking activated B cells in the peripheral blood and salivary glands in patients with Sjögren's syndrome. *Clin. Exp. Rheumatol.* 2008; 26: 5-12.

[29] MacLennan, I., Vinuesa, C. Dendritic cells, BAFF, and APRIL: innate players in adaptive antibody responses. *Immunity* 2002;17:235-8.

[30] Seyler, T. M., Park, Y. W., Takemura, S. et al. *J. Clin. Invest.* 2005;115:3083-92.

[31] Mackay, F., Schneider, P., Rennert, P., Browning, J. BAFF and APRIL: a tutorial on B cell survival. *Annu. Rev. Immunol.* 2003;21:231-64.

[32] Avery, D. T., Kalled, S. L., Ellyard, J. I. et al. BAFF selectively enhances the survival of plasmablasts generated from human memory B cells. *J. Clin. Invest.* 2003;112: 286-97.

[33] Chesnut, R. W., Grey, H. M. Studies on the capacity of B cells to serve as antigen-presenting cells. *J. Immunol.* 1981; 126:1075-9.

[34] Ron, Y., Sprent, J. T cell priming in vivo: a major role for B cells in presenting antigen to T cells in lymph nodes. *J. Immunol.* 1987; 138:2848-56.

[35] Hahne, M., Kataoka, T., Schröter, M. et al. APRIL, a new ligand of the tumor necrosis factor family, stimulates tumor cell growth. *J. Exp. Med.* 1998;188:1185-90.

[36] Thompson, J. S., Schneider, P., Kalled, S. L.,et al. BAFF binds to the tumor necrosis factor receptor-like molecule B cell maturation antigen and is important for maintaining the peripheral B cell population. *J. Exp. Med.* 2000;192:129-35.

[37] Gross, J. A., Johnston, J., Mudri, S. et al. TACI and BCMA are receptors for a TNF homologue implicated in B-cell autoimmune disease. *Nature* 2000;404:995-9.

[38] Thompson, J. S., Bixler, S. A., Qian, F. et al. BAFF-R, a newly identified TNF receptor that specifically interacts with BAFF. *Science* 2001;293:2108-11.

[39] B. Bossen, C., Schneider, P. AFF, APRIL and their receptors: structure, function and signaling. *Semin. Immunol.* 2006; 18: 263-75.

[40] Mok, M. Y. The immunological basis of B-cell therapy in systemic lupus erythematosus. *Int. J. Rheum. Dis*. 2010; 13: 3-11.

[41] Darce, J. R., Arendt, B. K., Wu, X., Jelinek, D. F. Regulated expression of BAFF-binding receptors during human B cell differentiation. *J. Immunol.* 2007;179:7276-86.

[42] Zhang, X., Park, C. S., Yoon, S. O. et al. BAFF supports human B cell differentiation in the lymphoid follicles through distinct receptors. *Int. Immunol.* 2005;17:779-88.

[43] Ng, L. G., Sutherland, A. P., Newton, R. et al. B cell-activating factor belonging to the TNF family (BAFF)-R is the principal BAFF receptor facilitating BAFF costimulation of circulating T and B cells. *J. Immunol.* 2004;173:807-17.
[44] Good, K. L., Avery, D. T., Tangye, S. G. Resting human memory B cells are intrinsically programmed for enhanced survival and responsiveness to diverse stimuli compared to naive B cells. *J. Immunol.* 2009;182:890-901.
[45] Chiu, A., Xu, W., He, B. et al. Hodgkin lymphoma cells express TACI and BCMA receptors and generate survival and proliferation signals in response to BAFF and APRIL. *Blood* 2007;109:729-39.
[46] Cucak, H., Yrlid, U., Reizis, B., Kalinke, U., Johansson-Lindbom, B. Type I interferon signaling in dendritic cells stimulates the development of lymph-node-resident T follicular helper cells. *Immunity.* 2009; 31: 491-501.
[47] Boulé, M. W., Broughton, C., Mackay, F., Akira, S., Marshak-Rothstein, A., Rifkin, I. R. Toll-like receptor 9-dependent and -independent dendritic cell activation by chromatin-immunoglobulin G complexes. *J. Exp. Med.* 2004; 199: 1631-40.
[48] Jego, G., Palucka, A. K., Blanck, J. P., Chalouni, C., Pascual, V., Banchereau, J. Plasmacytoid dendritic cells induce plasma cell differentiation through type I interferon and interleukin 6. *Immunity.* 2003; 19, 225–234.
[49] Baccala, R., Hoebe, K., Kono, D. H., Beutler, B., Theofilopoulos, A. N. TLR-dependent and TLR-independent pathways of type I interferon induction in systemic autoimmunity. *Nat. Med.* 2007;13: 543-51
[50] Andrews, B., Eisenberg, R. A., Theofilopoulos, A. N. et al. Spontaneous murine lupus-like syndromes. Clinical and immunopathological manifestations in several strains, *J. Exp. Med.* 1978; 148: 1198–1215.
[51] Casali, P., Notkins, A. L. CD5+ B lymphocytes, polyreactive antibodies and the human B-cell repertoire. *Immunol. Today.* 1989; 10: 364-8.
[52] Hayakawa, K., Hardy, R. R., Parks, D. R., Herzenberg, L. A. The "Ly-1 B" cell subpopulation in normal immunodefective, and autoimmune mice. *J. Exp. Med.* 1983; 157: 202-18.
[53] P. Wofsy, D., Chiang, N. Y. roliferation of Ly-1 B cells in autoimmune NZB and (NZB x NZW)F1 mice. *Eur. J. Immunol.* 1987; 17: 809-14.
[54] De la Hera, A., Marcos, M. A., Toribio, M. L., Marquez, C., Gaspar, M. L., Martinez, C. Development of Ly-1+ B cells in immunodeficient CBA/N mice. *J. Exp. Med.* 1987 Sep. 1;166: 804-9.
[55] Suzuki, N., Sakane, T., Engleman, E. G. Anti-DNA antibody production by CD5+ and CD5- B cells of patients with systemic lupus erythematosus. *J. Clin. Invest.* 1990; 85: 238-47.
[56] Odendahl, M., Jacobi, A., Hansen, A., Feist, E., Hiepe, F., Burmester, G. R., Lipsky, P. E., Radbruch, A., Dörner, T. Disturbed peripheral B lymphocyte homeostasis in systemic lupus erythematosus. *J. Immunol.* 2000; 165: 5970-9.
[57] Jacobi, A. M., Odendahl, M., Reiter, K., Bruns, A., Burmester, G. R., Radbruch, A., Valet, G., Lipsky, P. E., Dörner, T. Correlation between circulating CD27high plasma cells and disease activity in patients with systemic lupus erythematosus. *Arthritis. Rheum.* 2003; 48: 1332-42.

[58] Arce, E., Jackson, D. G., Gill, M. A., Bennett, L. B., Banchereau, J., Pascual, V. Increased frequency of pre-germinal center B cells and plasma cell precursors in the blood of children with systemic lupus erythematosus. *J. Immunol.* 2001; 167: 2361-9.

[59] Sims, G. P., Ettinger, R., Shirota, Y., Yarboro, C. H., Illei, G. G., Lipsky, P. E. Identification and characterization of circulating human transitional B cells. *Blood.* 2005 ; 105: 4390-8.

[60] Cappione, A. J., Pugh-Bernard, A. E., Anolik, J. H., Sanz, I. Lupus IgG VH4.34 antibodies bind to a 220-kDa glycoform of CD45/B220 on the surface of human B lymphocytes. *J. Immunol.* 2004; 172: 4298-307.

[61] Koarada, S., Ide, M., Haruta, Y. et al. Two cases of antinuclear antibody negative lupus showing increased proportion of B cells lacking RP105. *J. Rheumatol* 2005; 32:562-4.

[62] Guiducci, C., Gong, M., Xu, Z., Gill, M., Chaussabel, D., Meeker, T., Chan, J. H., Wright, T., Punaro, M., Bolland, S., Soumelis, V., Banchereau, J., Coffman, R. L., Pascual, V., Barrat, F. J. TLR recognition of self nucleic acids hampers glucocorticoid activity in lupus. *Nature.* 2010; 465: 937-41.

[63] Barrat, F. J., Coffman, R. L. Development of TLR inhibitors for the treatment of autoimmune diseases. *Immunol. Rev.* 2008; 223:271-83.

[64] Tedder, T. F. CD19: a promising B cell target for rheumatoid arthritis. *Nat. Rev. Rheumatol.* 2009; 5: 572-7.

[65] Grillo-López, A. J., White, C. A., Varns, C., Shen, D., Wei, A., McClure, A., Dallaire, B. K. Overview of the clinical development of rituximab: first monoclonal antibody approved for the treatment of lymphoma. *Semin. Oncol.* 1999; 26(5 Suppl. 14):66-73.

[66] Martin, F., Chan, A. C. B cell immunobiology in disease: evolving concepts from the clinic. *Annu. Rev. Immunol.* 2006;24:467-96.

[67] Carnahan, J., Stein, R., Qu, Z., Hess, K., Cesano, A., Hansen, H. J., Goldenberg, D. M. Epratuzumab, a CD22-targeting recombinant humanized antibody with a different mode of action from rituximab. *Mol. Immunol.* 2007; 44: 1331-41.

[68] Robak, E., Robak, T. Monoclonal antibodies in the treatment of systemic lupus erythematosus. *Curr. Drug Targets.* 2009; 10: 26-37.

[69] Leandro, M. J., Edwards, J. C., Cambridge, G., Ehrenstein, M. R., Isenberg, D. A. An open study of B lymphocyte depletion in systemic lupus erythematosus. *Arthritis Rheum.* 2002; 46: 2673-7.

[70] Anolik, J., Sanz, I., Looney, R. J. B cell depletion therapy in systemic lupus erythematosus. *Curr. Rheumatol. Rep.* 2003; 5: 350-6.

[71] Sfikakis, P. P., Boletis, J. N., Lionaki, S., Vigklis, V., Fragiadaki, K. G., Iniotaki, A., Moutsopoulos, H. M. Remission of proliferative lupus nephritis following B cell depletion therapy is preceded by down-regulation of the T cell costimulatory molecule CD40 ligand: an open-label trial. *Arthritis. Rheum.* 2005; 52: 501-13.

[72] Gottenberg, J. E., Guillevin, L., Lambotte, O., Combe, B., Allanore, Y., Cantagrel, A., Larroche, C., Soubrier, M., Bouillet, L., Dougados, M., Fain, O., Farge, D., Kyndt, X., Lortholary, O., Masson, C., Moura, B., Remy, P., Thomas, T., Wendling, D., Anaya, J. M., Sibilia, J., Mariette, X.; Club Rheumatismes et Inflammation (CRI). Tolerance and short term efficacy of rituximab in 43 patients with systemic autoimmune diseases. *Ann. Rheum. Dis.* 2005; 64: 913-20.

[73] Looney, R. J., Anolik, J. H., Campbell, D., Felgar, R. E., Young, F., Arend, L. J., Sloand, J. A., Rosenblatt, J., Sanz, I. B cell depletion as a novel treatment for systemic

lupus erythematosus: a phase I/II dose-escalation trial of rituximab. *Arthritis. Rheum.* 2004; 50: 2580-9.

[74] Van Vollenhoven, R. F., Gunnarsson, I., Welin-Henriksson, E., Sundelin, B., Osterborg, A., Jacobson, S. H., Klareskog, L. Biopsy-verified response of severe lupus nephritis to treatment with rituximab (anti-CD20 monoclonal antibody) plus cyclophosphamide after biopsy-documented failure to respond to cyclophosphamide alone. *Scand. J. Rheumatol.* 2004; 33: 423-7.

[75] Armstrong, D. J., Wright, S. A., Finch, M. B., Taggart, A. J., Bell, A. L. Active systemic lupus erythematosus successfully treated with Rituximab and oral steroid. *Clin. Exp. Rheumatol.* 2004; 22: 787-8.

[76] Merrill, J. T., Neuwelt, C. M., Wallace, D. J., Shanahan, J. C., Latinis, K. M., Oates, J. C., Utset, T. O., Gordon, C., Isenberg, D. A., Hsieh, H. J., Zhang, D., Brunetta, P. G. Efficacy and safety of rituximab in moderately-to-severely active systemic lupus erythematosus: the randomized, double-blind, phase II/III systemic lupus erythematosus evaluation of rituximab trial. *Arthrit. Rheum.* 2010; 62:222-33.

[77] Furie, R. A., Looney, J. R., Rovin, B. et al. Efficacy and safety of rituximab in patients with proliferative lupus nephritis: results from randomized, double-blind phase III LUNAR study. *Ann. Rheum. Dis.* 69 (Suppl 3):549, 2010.

[78] Hutas, G. Ocrelizumab, a humanized monoclonal antibody against CD20 for inflammatory disorders and B-cell malignancies. *Curr. Opin. Investig. Drugs.* 2008 ; 9:1206-15.

[79] Negrea, G. O., Elstrom, R., Allen, S. L., Rai, K. R., Abbasi, R. M., Farber, C. M., Teoh, N., Horne, H., Wegener, W. A., Goldenberg, D. M. Subcutaneous injections of low-dose veltuzumab (humanized anti-CD20 antibody) are safe and active in patients with indolent non-Hodgkin's lymphoma. *Haematologica.* 2011; 96: 567-73.

[80] Carnahan, J., Wang, P., Kendall, R., Chen, C., Hu, S., Boone, T., Juan, T., Talvenheimo, J., Montestruque, S., Sun, J., Elliott, G., Thomas, J., Ferbas, J., Kern, B., Briddell, R., Leonard, J. P., Cesano, A. Epratuzumab, a humanized monoclonal antibody targeting CD22: characterization of in vitro properties. *Clin. Cancer Res.* 2003; 9(10 Pt 2): 3982S-90S.

[81] Dörner, T., Kaufmann, J., Wegener, W. A., Teoh, N., Goldenberg, D. M., Burmester, G. R. Initial clinical trial of epratuzumab (humanized anti-CD22 antibody) for immunotherapy of systemic lupus erythematosus. *Arthritis. Res. Ther.* 2006; 8: R74.

[82] Jacobi, A. M., Goldenberg, D. M., Hiepe, F., Radbruch, A., Burmester, G. R., Dörner, T. Differential effects of epratuzumab on peripheral blood B cells of patients with systemic lupus erythematosus versus normal controls. *Ann. Rheum. Dis.* 2008; 67: 450-7.

[83] "FDA Sets Panel For Glaxo-Human Genome Lupus Drug." http://www.lse.co.uk/FinanceNews.asp?ArticleCode=mcjhdftaztu509yandArticleHeadline–UPDATE_2FDA_sets_panel_for_GlaxoHuman_Genome_lupus_drug.

[84] Wallace, D. J., Stohl, W., Furie, R. A., Lisse, J. R., McKay, J. D., Merrill, J. T., Petri, M. A., Ginzler, E. M., Chatham, W. W., McCune, W. J., Fernandez, V., Chevrier, M. R., Zhong, Z. J., Freimuth, W. W. A phase II, randomized, double-blind, placebo-controlled, dose-ranging study of belimumab in patients with active systemic lupus erythematosus. *Arthritis. Rheum.* 2009; 15; 61:1168-78.

[85] Navarra, S. V., Guzmán, R. M., Gallacher, A. E., Hall, S., Levy, R. A., Jimenez, R. E., Li, E. K., Thomas, M., Kim, H. Y., León, M. G., Tanasescu, C., Nasonov, E., Lan, J. L., Pineda, L., Zhong, Z. J., Freimuth, W., Petri, M. A.; BLISS-52 Study Group. Efficacy and safety of belimumab in patients with active systemic lupus erythematosus: a randomised, placebo-controlled, phase 3 trial. *Lancet*. 2011; 377: 721-31.

[86] Kayagaki, N., Yan, M., Seshasayee, D., Wang, H., Lee, W., French, D. M., Grewal, I. S., Cochran, A. G., Gordon, N. C., Yin, J., Starovasnik, M. A., Dixit, V. M. BAFF/BLyS receptor 3 binds the B cell survival factor BAFF ligand through a discrete surface loop and promotes processing of NF-kappaB2. *Immunity*. 2002.

[87] Gross, J. A., Johnston, J., Mudri, S., Enselman, R., Dillon, S. R., Madden, K., Xu, W., Parrish-Novak, J., Foster, D., Lofton-Day, C., Moore, M., Littau, A., Grossman, A., Haugen, H., Foley, K., Blumberg, H,. Harrison, K., Kindsvogel, W., Clegg, C. H. TACI and BCMA are receptors for a TNF homologue implicated in B-cell autoimmune disease. *Nature*. 2000; 404: 995-9.

[88] Dall'Era, M., Chakravarty, E., Wallace, D., Genovese, M., Weisman, M., Kavanaugh, A., Kalunian, K., Dhar, P., Vincent, E., Pena-Rossi, C., Wofsy, D. Reduced B lymphocyte and immunoglobulin levels after atacicept treatment in patients with systemic lupus erythematosus: results of a multicenter, phase Ib, double-blind, placebo-controlled, dose-escalating trial. *Arthritis. Rheum.* 2007; 56: 4142-50.

[89] Atacicept Phase II/III in Generalized Systemic Lupus Erythematosus (April SLE). http://clinicaltrials.gov/ct2/show/NCT00624338.

[90] Lee, C., Hymowitz, S., Wallweber, H. et al.: Synthetic anti-BR3 antibodies that mimic BAFF binding and target both human and murine B cells. *Blood* 2006; 108, 3103–3111.

[91] Lin, W., Gong, Q., Seshasayee, D. et al.: Anti-BR3 antibodies: a new class of B-cell immunotherapy combining cellular depletion and survival blockade. *Blood* 2007; 110, 3959–3967.

[92] Stohl, W., Merrill, J. T., Looney, R. J. et al.: Phase 1a single- and Phase 1b multiple-dose studies of AMG 623 (an anti-BAFF peptibody) in systemic lupus erythematosus (SLE). *Arthritis Rheum*. 2008; 58, S565–S566.

[93] Boumpas, D. T., Furie, R., Manzi, S., Illei, G. G., Wallace, D. J., Balow, J. E., Vaishnaw, A.; BG9588 Lupus Nephritis Trial Group. A short course of BG9588 (anti-CD40 ligand antibody) improves serologic activity and decreases hematuria in patients with proliferative lupus glomerulonephritis. *Arthritis. Rheum*. 2003; 48: 719-27.

[94] Liossis, S. N., Sfikakis, P. P. Costimulation blockade in the treatment of rheumatic diseases. *BioDrugs*. 2004; 18: 95-102.

[95] Noelle, R. J., Ledbetter, J. A., Aruffo, A. CD40 and its ligand, an essential ligand-receptor pair for thymus-dependent B-cell activation. *Immunol. Today* 1992; 13: 431–3.

[96] Nakamura, M., Tanaka, Y., Satoh, T., Kawai, M., Hirakata, M., Kaburaki, J., Kawakami, Y., Ikeda, Y., Kuwana, M. Autoantibody to CD40 ligand in systemic lupus erythematosus: association with thrombocytopenia but not thromboembolism. *Rheumatology* (Oxford). 2006; 45: 150-6.

[97] Davis, J. C. Jr, Totoritis, M. C., Rosenberg, J., Sklenar, T. A., Wofsy, D. Phase I clinical trial of a monoclonal antibody against CD40-ligand (IDEC-131) in patients with systemic lupus erythematosus. *J. Rheumatol.* 2001; 28: 95–101.

[98] IDEC Pharmaceuticals Web site. Accessed Jan. 20, 2003. URL: http://www.idecpharm.com/site/science/idec131.htm.

[99] Stebbings, R., Findlay, L., Edwards, C., Eastwood, D., Bird, C., North, D., Mistry, Y., Dilger, P., Liefooghe, E., Cludts, I., Fox, B., Tarrant, G., Robinson, J., Meager, T., Dolman, C., Thorpe, S. J., Bristow, A., Wadhwa, M., Thorpe, R., Poole, S. "Cytokine storm" in the phase I trial of monoclonal antibody TGN1412: better understanding the causes to improve preclinical testing of immunotherapeutics. *J. Immunol.* 2007; 179: 3325-31.

[100] Attarwala, H. TGN1412: From Discovery to Disaster. *J. Young Pharm.* 2010; 2: 332-6.

[101] Westhovens, R., Van Riel, P., Sibilia, J., Vratsanos, G., Nuamah, I., Becker, J. C. Abatacept (CTLA4Ig) treatment increases the remission rate in rheumatoid arthritis patients refractory to methotrexate treatment. *Arthritis. Res. Ther.* 2004; 6: 86.

[102] Finck, B. K., Linsley, P. S., Wofsy, D. Treatment of murine lupus with CTLA4Ig. *Science.* 1994; 265: 1225-7.

[103] Merrill, J. T., Burgos-Vargas, R., Westhovens, R., Chalmers, A., D'Cruz, D., Wallace, D. J., Bae, S. C., Sigal, L., Becker, J. C., Kelly, S., Raghupathi, K., Li, T., Peng, Y., Kinaszczuk, M., Nash, P. The efficacy and safety of abatacept in patients with non-life-threatening manifestations of systemic lupus erythematosus: results of a twelve-month, multicenter, exploratory, phase IIb, randomized, double-blind, placebo-controlled trial. *Arthritis. Rheum.* 2010; 62: 3077-87.

[104] Carreño, L., López-Longo, F. J., González, C. M., Monteagudo, I. Treatment options for juvenile-onset systemic lupus erythematosus. *Paediatr. Drugs.* 2002; 4: 241-56.

[105] Horowitz, D. M., Furie, R. A. Abetimus sodium: a medication for the prevention of lupus nephritis flares. *Expert Opin. Pharmacother.* 2009; 10: 1501-7.

[106] Ryan, M. C., Hering, M., Peckham, D., McDonagh, C. F., Brown, L., Kim, K. M., Meyer, D. L., Zabinski, R. F., Grewal, I. S., Carter, P. J. Antibody targeting of B-cell maturation antigen on malignant plasma cells. *Mol. Cancer Ther.* 2007; 6: 3009-18.

[107] Lee, P. Y., Reeves, W. H. Type I interferon as a target of treatment in SLE. Endocr. Metab. *Immune Disord. Drug Targets.* 2006; 6: 323-30.

[108] Yao, Y., Richman, L., Higgs, B. W., Morehouse, C. A., De los Reyes, M., Brohawn, P. et al. Neutralization of interferon-alpha/beta-inducible genes and downstream effect in a phase I trial of an anti-interferon-alpha monoclonal antibody in systemic lupus erythematosus. *Arthritis. Rheum.* 2009; 60: 1785–1796.

[109] Ikeda, H., Hideshima, T., Fulciniti, M., Lutz, R. J., Yasui, H., Okawa, Y., Kiziltepe, T., Vallet, S., Pozzi, S., Santo, L., Perrone, G., Tai, Y. T., Cirstea, D., Raje, N. S., Uherek, C., Dälken, B., Aigner, S., Osterroth, F., Munshi, N., Richardson, P., Anderson, K. C. The monoclonal antibody nBT062 conjugated to cytotoxic Maytansinoids has selective cytotoxicity against CD138-positive multiple myeloma cells in vitro and in vivo. *Clin. Cancer Res.* 2009; 15: 4028-37.

In: Lupus: Symptoms, Treatment and Potential Complications ISBN: 978-1-62081-078-1
Editors: T. D. Marquez and D. U. Neto

Chapter III

Neuropsychiatric Manifestations in Systemic Lupus Erythematosus

Aline Tamires Lapa, Mariana Postal, Fernando Augusto Peres and Simone Appenzeller*
Department of Medicine, Rheumatology Unit, Faculty of Medical Science, State University of Campinas, Cidade Universitária, Campinas SP, Brazil

Abstract

Systemic lupus erythematosus (SLE) is an autoimmune disorder that affects 0.1% of the world population. The disorder is characterized by systemic inflammation, auto-antibody production, and immune dysregulation, and it may lead to significant neurological and psychiatric morbidities. Both adults and children are diagnosed according to a set of clinical and laboratory criteria with a high sensitivity and specificity. A diagnosis of SLE in any age-group depends on excluding systemic infections or malignancies and the presence of at least 4 of 11 American College of Rheumatology (ACR) diagnostic criteria. Nephritis (leading to hypertension and renal dysfunction) and nervous system involvement are two of the more ominous manifestations in all age-groups. There are 19 case-based peripheral and central nervous syndromes that are postulated to be associated with SLE. Syndromes requiring prompt neurological evaluation include seizures, cerebrovascular accidents, demyelination, movement disorders, and peripheral neuropathies. Manifestations that may prompt psychiatric consultation include acute confusional state (delirium), affective disorders (anxiety and depression), cognitive impairment, and psychosis. Neuropsychiatric presentations may be caused by hypercoagulability in cerebral vessels (vasculopathy), proinflammatory cytokines, autoantibody effects on neuronal structures or receptors, and blood–brain barrier disruption. Alteration in the regulation of neurotransmitters such as dopamine and serotonin appear to play a role in behavioral changes seen in lupus-prone mice. We will

* Correspondence to: Simone Appenzeller-Department of Medicine, Faculty of Medical Science, State University of Campinas, Cidade Universitária, Campinas SP, Brazil, CEP 13083-970; E-mail: appenzellersimone@yahoo.com FAX: +55 19 3289-1818

review the prevalence, etiology and clinical presentation of neuropsychiatric manifestations in SLE. In addition, we will discuss treatment protocol for this serious manifestation in SLE.

Introduction

Systemic lupus erythematosus (SLE) is a chronic inflammatory, immune-mediated disease with diverse clinical manifestations, affecting 0.1% of general population. Neuropsychiatric (NP) manifestations in SLE has been more frequently recognized and reported in recent years, occurring in up to 50% of the patients during the disease course [1-4]._NP involvement may be considered primary if it results from immune-mediated injury to the central nervous system (CNS) or peripheral nervous system (PNS). NP events are secondary in nature when related to treatment, infections, metabolic abnormalities or other systemic manifestations such as hypertension [5]. The involvement is heterogeneous and may vary from subtle signs such as headache and mood disorders to severe, and life threatening conditions, such as stroke, myelopathy and acute confusional state. The diagnosis of primary NPSLE is often difficult, as both focal and diffuse manifestations may occur and a gold standard for diagnosis is still absent [5]. We will review the prevalence, etiology and clinical presentation of neuropsychiatric manifestations in SLE. In addition, we will discuss treatment protocol for this serious manifestation in SLE.

Classification Criteria

The large number of clinical studies describing NPSLE manifestations around the world has increased the awareness that there are more manifestations attributable to SLE than seizures and psychosis described in the original classification criteria by Tan et al [6].

Table 1. Central nervous system manifestation following ACR case definitions

Central nervous system Manifestations	Peripheral nervous system manifestations
Aseptic meningitis	Acute Inflammatory Demyelinating Polyradiculoneuropathy
Acute Confusional State	Autonomic Disorders
Anxiety Disorder	Cranial Neuropathy
Cerebrovascular Disease	Mononeuropathy
Cognitive Dysfunction	Myasthenia Gravis
Demyelinating Syndrome	Plexopathy
Headache	Polyneuropathy
Movement Disorder	
Mood Disorders	
Myelopathy	
Psychosis	
Seizures	

Adapted from ACR Ad hoc Committee on Neuropsychiatric Lupus Nomenclature (7).

Therefore, in 1999, the American College of Rheumatology (ACR) research committee developed case definitions that included appropriate terminology, classification criteria and complementary examinations for 19 NP syndromes [7] (Table1). These criteria were a result of a consensus meeting of experts of several subspecialties (rheumatology, neurology, immunology, and psychiatry). Furthermore, in 2001, these criteria have been validated in a cross-sectional study with a specificity of 46% [8]. However, when mild NP syndromes (mild cognitive deficit, headache, mild depression, anxiety, electroneuromyography-negative polyneuropathy) were excluded, the overall specificity increased to 91% [8].

NPSLE Epidemiology

The prevalence of NPSLE has been reported to range from 14% to over 80% in adults [2,4,5,8-14] and from 22% to 95% in children [15-17] (Table 2). This discrepancy reflects in part the lack of definitions of individual manifestations and the absence of standardization for investigation.

Table 2. Prevalence of NPSLE in studies using the 1999 ACR criteria for NP syndromes

Authors/Year	Patients (N)	Prevalence of NP (%)
Ainiala et al., 2001 [18]	46	91
Mok et al., 2001[19]	518	19
Brey et al, 2002 [12]	128	80
Sibbitt Jr et al, 2002 [15]	75*	95*
Alfreta et al., 2003 [20]	61	72
Sanna et al.,2003[21]	323	57.3
Hanly et al., 2004 [22]	111	37
Mikdashi et al.,2004 [23]	130	56,9
Appenzeller et al., 2005 [24]	72	NR
Hanly et al., 2005 [10]	53	31
Shimojima et al., 2005 [25]	25	100
Robert et al., 2006 [26]	50	78
Hanly J et al., 2009 [27]	209	NR
Borhani Haghighi A et al., 2010 [28]	407	11.3
Hawro T et al., 2010 [29]	52	NR

*Pediatric cohort.

NR: Not rated.

Most NPSLE events (40–50%) occur at onset or within the first 1– 2 years after SLE diagnosis, although cognitive dysfunction and atherosclerotic cerebrovascular disease (CVD) occur more frequently in older patients or in patients with longer disease duration [11].

The most frequent manifestations observed in adults SLE patients are headache (20–40%), cognitive dysfunction (10-20%), mood disorders (10-20%), seizures (7-10%), CVD (7-10%) and anxiety disorders (4-8%) [11]. Studies using systematic assessment of cognitive and psychiatric function found a range in the prevalence of mood disorders and cognitive dysfunction much higher comparing to studies that only evaluated symptomatic patients [8,9, 12-15].

In pediatric SLE patients, NPSLE manifestations are also commonly observed early in the course of the disease. They are not necessarily associated with disease activity in other organs (16). One prospective study demonstrated that cognitive dysfunction and headache occurred in 55% of patients followed by mood disorder in 57%, seizures in 51%, acute confusional state in 35%, peripheral nervous system impairment in 15%, psychosis in 12%, and stroke in 12% of the patients [15]. Recently, olfactory function abnormalities and sensorineural hearing loss have been described in the setting of CNS involvement in SLE [30, 31]. However, these manifestations are not included in the 1999 case definitions.

Clinical Relevance

The clinical relevance of NP manifestations in SLE has been determined by analyzing the impact of these manifestations in mortality, quality of life, overall damage scores and working disability [23, 26, 33-43]. Using mortality as indicative for poor outcome in NP manifestations, there are studies suggesting that patients with NP have increased mortality when compared to SLE patients without these manifestations [32-36]. Although some studies did not find an increased mortality among patients with CNS manifestations when compared to SLE patients without CNS manifestations and controls [36-40], the presence of CNS manifestations, independently of its etiology, seems to have a negative impact in quality of life [43], overall damage scores [44, 23, 40], higher fatigue scores [44, 45] and unemployment [40, 41,45]. The association of lower quality of life with NP events over time, independent of progression in cumulative organ damage, emphasizes the persistent negative effect of NP events in the lives of patients with SLE [43].

Fatigue is especially common in patients with NPSLE [13,23,40]. Fatigue does not only influence quality of life [10], but is also one of the main reasons for missing working hours and unemployment [41 42 46]. The ACR damage score (ACR/SLICC-DI) has been developed to determine irreversible damage in SLE patients, irrespectively if attributed to disease itself or secondary to comorbidities or medications.

In the ACR/SLICC-DI seizures, psychosis, mood disorders, CVD, neuropathy, mononeuritis multiplex, acute confusional state and myelopathy are scored in addition to several other clinical manifestations in order to determine the global damage score. Using the items of NP in order to create a NP damage score, the strongest risk factors for the development of significant NP damage was the presence of greater disease activity at the time of CNS involvement onset and the presence of antiphospholipid antibodies (aPL) [23]. Cumulative organ damage was higher in patients with NP disease because they were more likely to have received corticosteroids or immunosuppressive drugs [44].

Working disability has also been linked to the presence of NPSLE [41 42 46]. The number of cognitive spheres, and especially attention, memory, and executive functions, were important factors associated with unemployment in patients with SLE [46].

The association between memory function and employment status in patients with SLE underscores the need for judicious assessment of cognitive function and for the development of appropriate strategies that will either reverse cognitive impairment or help patients overcome obstacles they may face in daily life [41].

Risk Factors for NPSLE

Risk factors consistently associated with NPSLE events include general SLE activity or damage, previous events or other concurrent NPSLE manifestations, and the presence of persistently positive aPL antibodies [11, 23, 47-49].

Most Prevalent NP Syndromes

Psychosis due to SLE is an uncommon event that usually occurs early in the course of the disease and is associated with other clinical and biological features of SLE [49, 50]. The long-term outcome of psychosis due to SLE appears to be favorable, with 70% of the patients' archiving remission. Recurrence is rare. In addition good response to the treatment at the time of diagnosis seems to be a good prognostic marker for prolonged remission of psychotic symptoms [50]. The association between SLE and headache, including migraine, is controversial [51]. The reported prevalence of headache has varied widely between 24 and 72% but the prevalence of headache in the general population is also high, with up to 40% of individuals reporting a severe headache at least once per year. In our experience, severe migraine may be associated with disease activity, Raynaud´s phenomenon and increased organ damage [52]. Aseptic meningitis is a relatively uncommon, but well documented cause of headache in SLE and requires confirmation by analysis of cerebrospinal fluid (CSF).

Other potential causes must be considered including infection and idiosyncratic reactions to medications such as antibiotics and non-steroidal antiinflammatory drugs [51]. Thus, although headache might be a component of active SLE in individual patients, it is more likely that the majority of headaches in SLE patients are due to non-SLE causes. The most recent European consensus on treatment of NPSLE, did not consider headache a NP manifestation due to the lack of specificity [47]. Mild or moderate cognitive dysfunction is common in SLE but dementia is relatively uncommon (2–5%) and should be confirmed by neuropsychological tests in collaboration with a clinical neuropsychologist where available [11, 51]. Interestingly, the range in the prevalence of mood disorders and cognitive dysfunction is much wider, with studies using systematic assessment of cognitive and psychiatric function finding a higher prevalence [18, 41, 51, 53 54] than studies that only evaluated patients using clinical insights [53,55]. Seizures are a well recognized complication, occurring in 14–25% of SLE patients compared with 0.5–1% in the general population [56]. Although accompanying systemic and other CNS features are usually present, seizures may be one of the earliest manifestations of NP involvement, sometimes occurring several years prior to generalize SLE, understandably leading to the erroneous diagnosis of isolated epilepsy [51]. Several mechanisms may cause seizures in SLE but CSF pleocytosis in such cases raises the possibility of low grade lupus related encephalitis. Furthermore, the common finding of cerebral atrophy in SLE may also predispose to seizures [57].

SLE patients are at increased risk for CVD compared to the general population, particularly in younger and this risk cannot be fully explained by traditional cardiovascular risk factors [58]. Ischemic stroke and/or transient ischemic attack comprise >80% of cases, multifocal disease is found in 7–12%, intra-cerebral hemorrhage in 7–12%, subarachnoid hemorrhage in 3–5%, and sinus thrombosis in 2% [51]. Age, duration and activity of SLE, hypertension, and dyslipidemia are associated with increased carotid plaque and risk for stroke. aPL antibodies and valvular heart disease are strongly associated with stroke especially in patients younger than 50 years [11]. Acute confusional state has replaced what was previously called 'organic brain syndrome' and is synonymous with 'encephalopathy' and 'delirium'. It encompasses a state of impaired consciousness or level of arousal, which can progress to coma. Characteristics include the reduced ability to focus, disturbed mood and impaired cognition. It has been reported in 4–7% of SLE patients and must be distinguished from other causes, including metabolic abnormalities and hypertensive encephalopathy [51].

Ischemic stroke and/or TIA comprise over 80% of CVD cases, whereas CNS vasculitis is rare. CVD occurs commonly (50–60%) in the context of high disease activity and/or damage; other strong risk factors are persistently positive moderate-to-high titers of aPL antibodies, heart valve disease, systemic hypertension and old age [47].

SLE myelopathy presents as rapidly evolving transverse myelitis. Ischaemic/thrombotic myelopathy or inflammatory myelopathy can be observed in SLE. Patients may present with signs of grey matter (lower motor neuron) dysfunction (flaccidity and hyporeflexia) or white matter (upper motor neuron) dysfunction (spasticity and hyperreflexia) [51]. Other major NPSLE manifestations are present in one third of cases, with optic neuritis being the most common (21–48%). Acute transverse myelopathy (ATM) and chorea present acutely and are frequently associated with aPL antibodies [47, 51].

Symptoms of depression and anxiety are commonly reported in patients with SLE and are likely associated with the physical disability and stress of living with a chronic disease [59]. Psychological distress may be associated with SLE outcomes, including fatigue, physical disability, and decreased functioning. Patients with anxiety disorders often feel embarrassed to openly disclose their symptoms; other methods of assessment, such as brief self-report questionnaires may be helpful in identifying patients with these conditions, so that treatment can be delivered to alleviate psychological distress and improve overall function [60].

A sensorimotor neuropathy is the most common neuropathy and has been reported in up to 28% of SLE patients [51]. It frequently occurs independently of other disease characteristics. Other less frequent forms of neuropathy include cranial neuropathy, autonomic neuropathy, plexopathy, mononeuritis multiplexand Guillain–Barré syndrome [51]. Myasthenia gravis has been reported in SLE but is rare [51, 61].

Pathophysiology

The rationale for identifying the etiology and pathogenic mechanisms underlying NP disease in SLE is to facilitate the logical development of appropriate and effective therapies [51]. Histopathological studies of brains of SLE patients with and without CNS manifestations revealed a predominant small vessel infarction, with little signs of true vasculitis [62-65]. Multiple microinfarcts, noninflammatory thickening of small vessels with intimae proliferation, small-vessel occlusion, and intracranial embolism or hemorrhage have all been shown in SLE patients [62-65]. Microvasculopathy was formerly attributed to immune complexes deposition, but more recent studies highlight the importance of complement activation [66, 67]. Consistent with these small vessel changes, single photon emission computed tomography (SPECT) and magnetic resonance imaging (MRI) studies suggest that both cerebral atrophy and cognitive dysfunction in SLE may be related to chronic diffuse cerebral ischemia, rather than cerebral vasculitis [68, 69].

Although small vessel vasculopathy is frequently found in autopsy findings, a parallel between these and CNS symptoms were not always evident; in addition autoantibodies and inflammatory mediators may be involved in different disease expression in CNS SLE [70].

Autoantibodies directed against neurons, ribosomes and phospholipids-associated proteins have been associated with CNS manifestations and may be locally produced or cross the blood-brain barrier [62,71]. It is becoming clearer that the integrity of the blood brain-barrier (BBB) is involved in SLE related neuropathology [65]. Mechanisms leading to brain dysfunction in SLE probably involve abnormal endothelial-white blood cell interactions, allowing proteins or cells access to the CNS. BBB leakage can be stimulated by pro-inflammatory cytokines or autoantibodies that up-regulate the expression of adhesion proteins on endothelial cells, facilitating lymphocyte entry into the CNS [72]. Soluble serum levels of inter-cellular adhesion molecule 1 increases with SLE disease activity and normalizes with disease remission; strengthening the hypothesis that activated endothelial cells and a lack of integrity of the BBB might be an essential requisite for NPSLE [72-75].

Several studies have analyzed the role of inflammatory processes in NPSLE. Interleukins (IL), tumor necrosis factors (TNF) and metalloproteinase have been shown to be increased in CSF in patients with CNS manifestations and even associated with some specific clinical manifestations and MRI findings [76-80]. Among reported cytokines, IL-6 has been shown to have the strongest positive association with NPSLE and was reported to be elevated in the absence of the blood-brain barrier damage [80].CSF IL-6 might be an effective measure in diagnosing lupus psychosis, however exclusion of infectious meningoencephalitis and CVD is necessary [81].

Autoantibody production is a key feature observed in SLE. Brain-reactive antibodies have been identified in the serum of SLE patients; however the specific antigens that are recognized by these antibodies have not been identified yet, nor is their functionality known [82].

aPL antibodies are associated with both thrombosis and microvascular dysfunction [83]. Effects on platelets, coagulation proteins, and endothelial cells, including tissue factor upregulation, have been ascribed to aPL antibodies [83,84]. The majority of evidence favors a prothrombotic mechanism that amplifies thrombosis in certain settings. The incidence of aPL antibodies was reported higher in SLE patients with seizures, stroke, transverse myelitis (ATM) and cognitive dysfunction when compared to the overall incidence of aPL in SLE [48, 83-86]. aPL-induced thrombosis has been previously proposed as a pathogenetic mechanism underlying the development of ATM [86]. Such thrombosis could explain the predominance of ATM in the thoracic spine, where the longitudinal arterial trunk is considerably smaller compared with cervical and lumbar regions. However, there are no controlled trials assessing the role of aPL in patients with SLE presenting with ATM or other NP manifestations [86].

Anti-ribosomal-P (anti-P) antibodies are found in up to 25% of SLE patients. Although the association with NPSLE is still controversial, some authors have found a correlation with psychosis and depression [87-93]. In addition, more recently, an association between abnormal olfactory function and anti-P has been demonstrated [30]. This study has shown that intra-cerebra-ventricular injection of human anti-ribosomal-P induces a depression-like behavior in mice, accompanied by impaired smell capabilities [30]. However this study has not been replicated yet.

Anti-neuronal antibodies have been shown to induce memory deficits, seizures and neuropathological changes in animal models [94,95]. In SLE patients, the presence of anti-neuronal antibodies has been increased in patients with NP manifestations, although no clinical manifestations and no diagnostic specificity could be identified [51].

The N-methyl-D-aspartate receptors (NMDAR), NR2a and NR2b, have been shown to occur in patients with NP manifestations and appear to have a functional consequence leading to neuronal injury. NMDAR are receptors for the neurotransmitter glutamate, the major excitatory neurotransmitter in the brain and critically important for many brain functions [82]. The NR2A messenger RNA (mRNA) has higher concentrations in the cerebral cortex, hippocampus, and cerebellum and is widely distributed in the brain, while the NR2B transcript is selectively present in the forebrain, with higher levels of expression located in the cerebral cortex, hippocampus, septum, caudate-putamen, and olfactory bulb [82, 96]. Anti-NMDAR antibodies mediate apoptotic cell death of neurons in vitro and in vivo [97]. Many studies have attempted to correlate the presence of these antibodies in serum with aspects of NPSLE [82]. Although NMDAR antibodies have been widely studied in SLE patients there are conflicting results. Two cross-sectional studies found correlations of serum NMDAR antibodies with cognitive impairment and depression [98,99], and another study reported an association with decreased amygdala volume [100], but several other studies have found no correlations [102-103]. Studies analyzing NMDAR antibodies in CSF have reported more promising results. CSF NMDAR antibodies have been associated with diffuse NPSLE [104]. Moreover, CSF titers correlated with symptom severity [104,105]. A follow-up study analyzing serial anti-NMDAR antibodies in CSF showed a decrease, but not a total clearance of CSF anti-NMDAR antibodies [105]. Thus, antibody may be continuously present in the CSF of patients without clinically apparent CNS disease. This finding could explain why some patients present insidious manifestations of disease and others changes in cognitive function and mood, even in the absence of acute clinical CNS manifestations [82,106].

Two studies investigated the role of anti-endothelial antibodies (AECA) in CNS SLE and found a higher prevalence and concentration in patients with NP manifestations. The results of these studies suggest a relationship between AECA and a biological origin of NP manifestations [107,108].

Serum S100B protein level have also been shown to be increased in NPSLE patients. S100B levels were significantly higher in patients with defined NP syndromes than in controls and non-NPSLE patients, reflecting the presence of continuing neurological damage, and may be a useful test for the diagnosis of NPSLE, particularly in acute forms [109,110].

Gangliosides are a family of sialylated glycosphingolipids expressed in the outer leaflet of the plasma membrane and are particularly abundant in the nervous system [90]. The presence of serum anti-ganglioside M1 IgM and IgG antibodies has been associated with NP manifestations in both adult and pediatric SLE patients [90, 111].

Alteration in the regulation of neurotransmitters such as serotonin and dopamine appear to play a role in behavioral changes seen in lupus-prone MRL-*lpr* mice [112,113]. Depressive-like behavior is the most profound manifestation of autoimmunity-associated behavioral syndrome [112]. The therapeutic effectiveness of drugs specific to neurotransmitter receptors and enzymes supports the view that serotonin and dopamine play key roles in the control of affective behavior [114]. Drugs with a selective mode of action were used to probe the functional status of central serotonergic and dopaminergic systems *in vivo*. The untreated MRL-lpr and MRL +/+ mice showed increased dopamine levels in the paraventricular nucleus (PVN) and median eminence (ME), decreased concentrations of serotonin in the PVN and enhanced levels in the hippocampus [112]. Behavioral deficits correlated with the changes in PVN and median eminence. These results are consistent with the hypothesis that imbalanced neurotransmitter regulation of the hypothalamus–pituitary axis plays an important role in the etiology of behavioral dysfunction induced by systemic autoimmune disease [112].

The time of investigation is an important aspect of NPSLE studies, since most histopathology studies were performed months or years after the initial symptoms. Thus, it is not clear whether one mechanism or multiple mechanisms are responsible for these symptom complexes [115]. The strict exclusion of patients with other etiologies of CNS than SLE disease, in addition to the analysis of individual manifestations may provide a more homogenous clinical population and may favor elucidation of pathological mechanism involved in CNS manifestations in SLE.

Diagnosis

The correct diagnosis of CNS manifestations in patients with previous diagnosis of SLE, attributing individual manifestations to SLE disease activity or to a secondary cause remains a challenge in clinical practice [116, 117] (Figure 1). Because of the absence of diagnostic gold standard for most of the individual manifestations, clinical, laboratory and neuroimaging features are necessary for exclusion of alternative etiologies [116]. The approaches differ according to the presence of focal manifestations or diffuse CNS involvement (Figure 2).

The ACR nomenclature provides tools for accessing these manifestations in a systematic manner [116]. Using these guidelines, Hanly et al [21] were able to determine that 41% of the CNS manifestation in their cohort was secondary to non-SLE causes. Furthermore, several studies have shown the occurrence of subclinical NP involvement, which clinical significance has still to be determined [24,118].

Clinical and Laboratory Investigation

CNS infection should always be excluded by CSF examinations. Non-specific abnormalities may be found in the CSF of 33% of patients with NPSLE and include mild pleocytosis and elevated protein levels [119]. The clinical usefulness of measuring CSF autoantibodies, cytokines and biomarkers of neurological damage is still a subject of research [52,120].

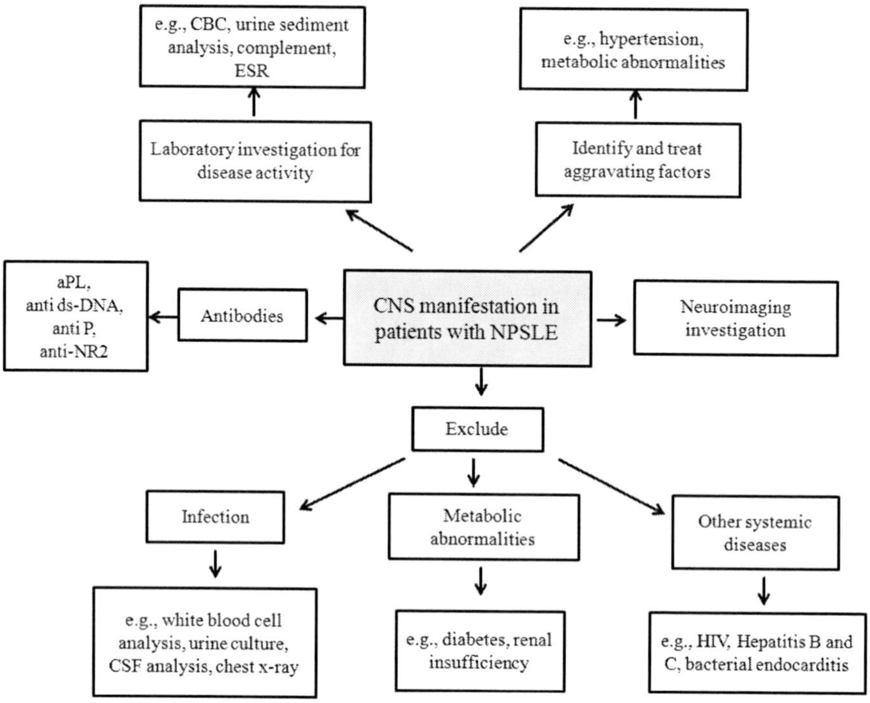

Figure 1. Investigation in patients presenting with CNS manifestations with suspected SLE and in patients with previous diagnosis of SLE.

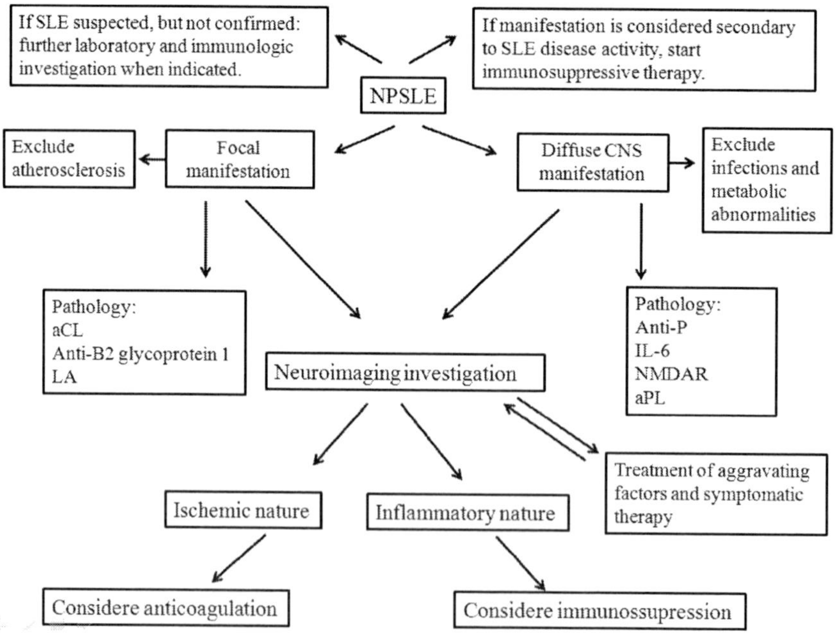

Adapted from [117].

Figure 2. Suggested investigation in a patient with CNS manifestations as initial symptom and clinical suspicion of disease and with established disease.

In considering circulating autoantibodies, those that are most likely to provide the greatest diagnostic yield are serum aPL antibodies. The value of measuring anti-P antibodies remains uncertain, given the conflicting results to date. The role of anti-NMDAR antibodies in NP-SLE is currently unknown [5].

Neuroimaging

In SLE, both structural and functional neuroimaging methods may be useful for determine CNS abnormalities. Cranial tomography (CT) may be the preferred technique in several centers for the diagnosis of gross structural abnormalities, such as infarcts, hemorrhage, tumors and abscesses. However, MRI has largely replaced CT, because of the excellent soft-tissue contrast observed with MRI and the ability to acquire multiplanar images [121]. Although MRI abnormalities may be found in 19-70% of SLE patients, its clinical significance for diagnosis of NP SLE has still to be determined, because these abnormalities may occur in both, patients with and without CNS manifestations [5].

Global and regional atrophy was described in 6-12% of SLE patients, depending upon linear or volumetric measurements have been applied (106,107). Age, disease activity, the presence of past history of CNS manifestations and the use of corticosteroid have all been associated with the occurrence of atrophy [122,123]. White matter lesions have been frequently detected SLE patients, but may occur in both symptomatic in asymptomatic patients. Although these white matter lesions are often considered nonspecific, they may be attributed to age, hypertension, disease duration, small vessel disease and the presence of NP manifestations [124].

In the presence of larger lesions, the differential diagnosis with multiple sclerosis is mandatory [121]. Therefore, in the context of SLE, these lesions are likely consequences of central nervous system damage and not mere incidental finding [124]. Patients with acute NPSLE often have normal MRI [125].

Cerebral atrophy and white matter lesions are more consistent with brain damage than active disease [93,126]. Magnetization transfer imaging (MTI) is particularly suited to the detection and quantification of diffuse brain damage [127,128], but its utility in clinical practice has still to be determined.

Diffusion weighted imaging (DWI) and perfusion MRI are highly effective in the detection of hyperacute and subacute brain injury, in particular acute ischemia following stroke [121, 129]. Magnetic resonance angiography (MRA) permits visualization of cerebral blood flow, although it is not optimum for visualization of flow in small caliber vessels that are the ones primarily involved in NPSLE [130].

Functional studies may be performed using different methods. Positron emission tomography (PET) scanning is sensitive, but practical considerations limit its applicability [5]. SPECT scanning provides semi-quantitative analysis of regional cerebral blood flow and metabolism and has shown diffuse hypoperfusion in patients with active NPSLE [68]. Magnetic resonance spectroscopy (MRS) allows the identification and quantification of brain metabolites, which reflect the quantity and integrity of neuronal cells. Several studies observed that CNS manifestations in SLE are associated with reduction in NAA/Cr ratios and NAA/Cho ratios, not only in lesions, but also in normal appearing white matter when compared to controls supporting the hypothesis of neuronal damage in SLE [69, 121].

Therapeutic Strategies in NPSLE

Due to the complexity of the disease and variability in clinical manifestations, along with its uncertain pathogenesis and lack of disease activity markers, treatment of NPSLE has remained relatively empirical [118]. In SLE patients who present with NP manifestations, the first step is to identify and treat any aggravating factors such as hypertension, infection, metabolic abnormalities, or drug adverse effects. Symptomatic therapy should be considered if appropriate, including anti-convulsants, anti-depressants, or antipsychotic medications [11] (Table 4). Patients with mild neuropsychiatric disease may be treated conservatively – even, in some cases, not treated at all – since it seems that many of these cases are spontaneously reversible [132]. Patients with mild diffuse manifestations such as anxiety and depression may benefit from symptomatic treatment only.

Table 4. Therapeutic strategies for different NPSLE syndromes

NPSLE syndrome	Therapeutic strategies
Acute confusional state	CS and/or immunosuppressants Symptomatic treatment
Cerebrovascular disease aPL antibodies Generalized SLE activity	 Anticoagulation therapy CS and/or immunosuppressant Control CV risk factors
Cognitive dysfunction	Psycho-education support Cognitive rehabilitation Control disease activity Consider ASA or anticoagulation if APS or CS if progressive
Headache	Treatment according to guidelines Consider ASA or anticoagulation if APS Consider CS if refractory and severe
Myelopathy	CS and/or immunosuppressive therapy Consider anticoagulation if APS
Movement disorders	Symptomatic treatment ASA or anticoagulation if APS CS
Psychosis	Symptomatic treatment CS or immunossupressants Exclude secondary causes
Seizures Abnormal MRI/EEG/aPL Lupus activity aPL	Antiepileptic therapy High risk for recurrence: consider long-term antiepileptic therapy CS and/or immunosuppressive therapy ASA or long-term anticoagulation therapy if recurrence

ASA: aspirin; APS: antiphospholipid syndrome; CS: Corticosteroids; CV: cardiovascular.

It is often difficult to decide whether anxiety/depression are due to SLE or simply related to having a chronic debilitating disease [132]. Long-term anti-epileptic therapy may be considered for recurrent seizures. The presence of positive aPL, abnormal electroencephalography and/or MRI are markers for recurrent seizures [56]. If new onset seizures are thought to reflect an acute inflammatory event or if a concomitant lupus flare exists, corticosteroids alone or in combination with immunosuppressive therapy may be considered [11]. There is no evidence to suggest that established SLE is aggravated by the use of anticonvulsant medication, even though these agents may occasionally cause drug-induced lupus. However, patients need to be close monitored for possible hematologic side effects, bone marrow suppression, drug-induced rashes and hepatotoxicity [132].

Although most headaches are clearly not attributed to SLE, in some cases they can suggest brain pathology. In absence of high-risk features from the history (explosive onset, severe headache, age>50 years, fever or concomitant infection, immunosuppression, aPL antibodies/APS, use of anticoagulants) and the physical examination (focal neurological signs, decreased level of consciousness, meningismus, overt lupus activity), headache alone in a patient with SLE does not require additional investigation beyond the evaluation needed for an individual without SLE [11,47].

The treatment for NPSLE is mostly empirical and corticosteroids alone, or in combination with other immunomodulators (including cyclophospamide, azathioprine, mycophenolate mofetil, and methotrexate), demonstrating variable improvement to complete remission [131, 133, 134]. Up to date there is one single randomized controlled clinical trial for NPSLE (133). In this study, long-term use of cyclophosphamide and methylprednisolone showed a better overall therapeutic control of SLE-related neurological manifestations (refractory seizures, peripheral and cranial neuropathy, ATM, and optic neuritis) than intravenous methylprednisolone alone [133].

Although the approach to corticosteroid therapy for CNS lupus remains largely empirical, they continue to represent the first line of treatment for NPSLE [134]. High dose oral prednisolone (1–2mg/kg/day) or intravenous methylprednisolone (0.5–1g/day for 3 days), followed by oral prednisone, are indicated for acute severe CNS manifestations [132,135,136]. Corticosteroid have also shown efficacy in mild NP symptoms and inactive SLE, showing that improvement in cognition and mood can be observed relatively low doses of corticosteroids (0.5mg/kg/day) [128]. Corticosteroids have also been used for the treatment of aseptic meningitis and psychosis not responsive to antipsychotic treatment [132,137]. Furthermore intrathecal corticosteroids may also be an option in patients with severe diffuse involvement and without response to systemic corticosteroid administration [138].

The use of intravenous cyclophosphamide is currently recommended for acute severe CNS disease, in those refractory to corticosteroids or when a steroid-sparing effect is desired [132,133,136,138-140]. There is one controlled trial [140] and one randomized controlled clinical trial [133] to support the therapeutic regimen with cyclophosphamide [133]. In addition, animal studies have shown that immunosuppression with cyclophosphamide prevents neuronal atrophy, reduces levels of autoantibodies and attenuates leukocytes in the brain while improving behavioral abnormalities [141]. More recently, an MRI study has shown that cyclophosphamide prevents cerebral atrophy in SLE patients [142].

Plasmapheresis is useful to remove free antibodies, complement components and circulating immune complexes [132]. Better response is observed in patients with severe disease activity, refractory to corticosteroids and cyclophosphamide therapy, and with the highest levels of circulating immune complexes [132]. The efficacy of plasmapheresis is anecdotal and there are no controlled studies to confirm its efficacy. Combination therapy with synchronized plasmapheresis and subsequent cyclophosphamide in severe SLE has been proposed by some authors, however higher rates of fatal infections were observed [143].

Intravenous immunoglobulin (IVIg) has proved useful in the treatment of peripheral neuropathy, myasthenia gravis, MS and Guillain–Barré syndrome, associated or not with SLE. In addition there are reports of successful treatment with IVIg in acute severe diffuse CNS disease and psychosis, although no randomized control trial is available. [143-147].

Intrathecal administration of methotrexate can be a treatment option in NPSLE in patients not responsive to conventional steroid therapy [134,135]. Side effects including itching sensation of lower limbs, headache and incontinence were mild and transient, however further studies are necessary [132].

Reports using azathioprine in NPSLE have shown beneficial effects, especially in patients unable to tolerate cyclophosphamide [148,149]. Mycophenolate mofetil (MMF) has also been used in the treatment of NPSLE. Clinical and imaging improvement was reported in more than two thirds of the patients with MMF (1g/day) [150]. Rituximab (anti-CD20 mAb) has been reported to improve NPSLE, especially acute confusional state, cognitive dysfunction, psychosis and seizure and reduced the SLEDAI score [150,151]. Rituximab is a chimeric mouse/human monoclonal antibody that binds to the CD20 antigen that is expressed on the surface of B cells from the pre-B cell through memory B cell stages. Importantly, CD20 is not expressed on B cell precursors or plasma cells. Because of the putative role of B cells in the pathogenesis of SLE, Rituximab was viewed as an appealing treatment option for SLE. Treatment with rituximab results in rapid depletion of B cells. Several uncontrolled studies suggested that Rituximab might be beneficial across a broad range of manifestations of SLE, including lupus nephritis [150]. However to control trials failed to demonstrate this benefits [152]. There is good safety data, as rituximab has been used since the 1990's in patients with lymphoma and since 2002 in SLE [153]. Adverse event rates in SLE are comparable to placebo – the only differences being leucopenia (12.3%vs4.2%), neutropenia (5.5%vs1.4%) and hypotension (11%vs4.2%) [154]. However, rare but serious side effects include serum-sickness-like reactions, tumor lysis syndrome, and progressive multifocal leukoencephalopathy. The latter became a concern in 2006 when rituximab-treated patients developed this progressive CNS demyelinating disease caused by JC virus reactivation [155]. The acute management of SLE stroke or TIA is similar to that in the general population. A stroke specialist consultation is necessary to identify patients who are candidates for thrombolytic or surgical therapy; unless contraindicated, aspirin should be initiated. Secondary prevention includes tight control of cardiovascular risk factors, antiplatelet therapy and carotid endarterectomy when indicated. Generalized lupus activity may be controlled with glucocorticoids and/or immunosuppressive therapy [47]. Anti-coagulation therapy is recommended for NPSLE related to aPL antibodies, especially for thrombotic CVD. Anti-coagulation may be superior to anti-platelet therapy for secondary prevention of arterial events (including stroke) in aPL antibody syndrome (APS) [132, 151,152]. This therapy has also been used in aPL–associated ischemic optic neuropathy and chorea, as well as in AMT refractory to immunosuppressive therapy with good results (response rates 50–60%) [156]. The titers and persistence of aPL and the Ž findings on brain MRI scanning are of major importance when deciding anticoagulant treatment. Minimum treatment requires antiaggregant therapy as a prophylactic measure, but long-term anticoagulation with warfarin may be indicated in previous thrombotic events. Although efficacy has been shown to be similar, there is no consensus among aPL specialists [157]. Intensive warfarin therapy with an international normalized ratio (INR) 3 seems to be the most effective antithrombotic treatment in APS [154].

Conclusion

NP manifestations are a frequent finding in SLE. Its etiology is multifactorial, including vasculopathy, proinflammatory cytokines, autoantibody effects on neuronal structures or receptors, and blood–brain barrier disruption. Alteration in functional status of central serotonergic and dopaminergic systems appear to play a role in behavioral changes seen in lupus-prone mice. The advancement in technology employing MRI may be capable in distinguishing a subgroup of patients with worse prognosis, based on hippocampal atrophy. Treatment is still controversial, in part because of the lack of controlled studies and draws upon the experience in the management of other serious organ involvement such as lupus nephritis.

Acknowledgments

Grants: Fundação de Amparo à Pesquisa do Estado de São Paulo (FAPESP 08/020917-0 and 2010/13639-1 and 09/11076-2) and Conselho Nacional Pesquisa Desenvolvimento-Brasil CNPq (300447/2009-4).

References

[1] Kozora E, Arciniegas DB, Filley CM, et al. Cognition, MRS neurometabolites, and MRI volumetrics in nonneuropsychiatric systemic lupus erythematosus: preliminary data. *Cogn. Behav. Neurol.* 2005; 18: 159-62.

[2] West SG. Neuropsychiatric lupus. *Rheum. Dis. Clin. North Am.* 1994; 20: 129-58.

[3] Hanly JG, Walsh NM, Sangalang V. Brain pathology in systemic lupus erythematosus. *J. Rheumatol.* 1992; 19: 732-41.

[4] Johnson RT, Richardson EP. The neurological manifestations of systemic lupus erythematosus. Medicine Baltimore. 1968; 47: 337-69.

[5] Hanly JG. Neuropsychiatric lupus. *Rheum. Dis. Clin. North Am.* 2005; 31: 273-98, vi.

[6] Tan EM, Cohen AS, Fries JF, et al. The 1982 revised criteria for the classification of systemic lupus erythematosus. *Arthritis. Rheum.* 1982; 25: 1271-7.

[7] The American College of Rheumatology nomenclature and case definitions for neuropsychiatric lupus syndromes. *Arthritis. Rheum.* 1999; 42: 599-608.

[8] Ainiala H, Loukkola J, Peltola J, et al. The prevalence of neuropsychiatric syndromes in systemic lupus erythematosus. *Neurology* 2001; 57: 496-500.

[9] Brey RL. Neuropsychiatric lupus: clinical and imaging aspects. *Bull NYU Hosp. Jt. Dis.* 2007; 5: 194-9.

[10] Hanly JG, Fisk JD, McCurdy G, et al. Neuropsychiatric syndromes in patients with systemic lupus erythematosus and rheumatoid arthritis. *J. Rheumatol.* 2005; 32: 1459-6.

[11] Bertsias GK, Boumpas DT. Pathogenesis, diagnosis and management of neuropsychiatric SLE manifestations. *Nat. Rev. Rheumatol.* 2010; 6: 358-67.

[12] Brey RL, Holliday SL, Saklad AR, et al. Neuropsychiatric syndromes in lupus: prevalence using standardized definitions. *Neurology* 2002; 58: 1214-20.

[13] Hanly JG, McCurdy G, Fougere L, et al. Neuropsychiatric events in systemic lupus erythematosus: attribution and clinical significance. *J. Rheumatol.* 2004; 31: 2156-62.

[14] Hanly JG, Urowitz MB, Sanchez-Guerrero J, et al. Neuropsychiatric events at the time of diagnosis of systemic lupus erythematosus: an international inception cohort study. *Arthritis. Rheum.* 2007; 56: 265-73.

[15] Sibbitt Jr WL, Brandt JR, Johnson CR, et al. The incidence and prevalence of neuropsychiatric syndromes in pediatric onset systemic lupus erythematosus. *J. Rheumatol.* 2002; 29: 1536-42.

[16] Harel L, Sandborg C, Lee T, et al. Neuropsychiatric manifestations in pediatric systemic lupus erythematosus and association with antiphospholipid antibodies. *J. Rheumatol.* 2006; 33: 1873-7.

[17] Yu HH, Lee JH, Wang LC, et al. Neuropsychiatric manifestations in pediatric systemic lupus erythematosus: a 20-year study. *Lupus* 2006; 15: 651-7.

[18] Ainiala H, Hietaharju A, Loukkola J, et al. Validity of the new American College of Rheumatology criteria for neuropsychiatric lupus syndromes: a population-based evaluation. *Arthritis. Rheum.* 2001: 45; 419-423.

[19] Mok CC, Lau CS, Wong RW. Neuropsychiatric manifestations and their clinical associations in southern Chinese patients with systemic lupus erythematosus. *J. Rheumatol.* 2001:28; 766-71.

[20] Afeltra A, Garzia P, Mitterhofer AP, et al. Neuropsychiatric lupus syndromes, relationship with antiphospholipid antibodies. *Neurology.* 2003: 61; 108-10.

[21] Sanna G, Bertolaccini ML, Cuadrado MJ, et al. Neuropsychiatric manifestations in systemic lupus erythematosus: prevalence and association with antiphospholipid antibodies. *J. Rheumatol.* 2003: 30; 985-92.

[22] Hanly JG, McCurdy G, Fougere L, et al. Neuropsychiatric events in systemic lupus erythematosus: attribution and clinical significance. *J. Rheumatol.* 2004;31:2156–62.

[23] Mikdashi J, Handwerger B. Predictors of neuropsychiatric damage in systemic lupus erythematosus: data from the Maryland lupus cohort. *Rheumatology Oxford.* 2004;43:1555–60.

[24] Appenzeller S, Carnevalle AD, Li LM, Costallat LT, Cendes F. Hippocampal atrophy in systemic lupus erythematosus. *Ann. Rheum. Dis.* 2006;65:1585-9.

[25] Shimojima Y, Matsuda M, Gono T, et al. Relationship between clinical factors and neuropsychiatric manifestations in systemic lupus erythematosus. *Clin. Rheumatol.* 2005: 24; 469-75.

[26] Robert M, Sunitha R, Thulaseedharan NK. Neuropsychiatric manifestations systemic lupus erythematosus: a study from South India. *Neurol. India.* 2006:54;75-7.

[27] Hanly J, Su L, Farewell V, et al. Prospective study of neuropsychiatric events in systemic lupus erythematosus. *J. Rheumatol.* 2009: 36; 1449-59.

[28] Borhani Haghighi A, Haza SG. Neuropsychiatric manifestations of systemic lupus erythematosus: Iranian experience. *Ann. Indian Acad. Neurol.* 2010;13:108-11.

[29] Hawro T, Krupińska-Kun M, Rabe-Jabłońska J, et al. Psychiatric disorders in patients with systemic lupus erythematosus: association of anxiety disorder with shorter disease duration. *Rheumatol. Int.* 2010 Dec 7. (Epub ahead of print).

[30] Kivity S, Tsarfaty G, Agmon-Levin N, et al. Abnormal olfactory function demonstrated by manganese-enhanced MRI in mice with experimental neuropsychiatric lupus. *Ann. N. Y. Acad. Sci.* 2010; 1193: 70-7.

[31] Maciaszczyk K, Durko T, Waszczykowska E, et al. Auditory function in patients with systemic lupus erythematosus. *Auris Nasus Larynx* 2011; 38: 26-32.

[32] Feng PH; Cheah PS; Lee YK. Mortality in systemic lupus erythematosus: a 10-year review. *Br. Med. J.,* 1973, 4, 772-4.

[33] Cheatum DE; Hurd ER; Strunk SW; Ziff M. Renal histology and clinical course of systemic lupus erythematosus. A prospective study. *Arthritis. Rheum.,* 1973, 16, 670-6.

[34] Lee P; Urowitz MB; Bookman AA; et al. Systemic lupus erythematosus. A review of 110 cases with reference to nephritis, the nervous system, infections, aseptic necrosis and prognosis. *Q. J. Med.* 1977, 46, 1-32.

[35] Ginzler EM; Diamond HS; Weiner M; et al. A multicenter study of outcome in systemic lupus erythematosus. I. Entry variables as predictors of prognosis. *Arthritis. Rheum.* 1982, 25, 601-611.

[36] Sibley JT; Olszynski, WP; Decotea, WE; Sundaram MB. The incidence and prognosis of central nervous system disease in systemic lupus erythematosus. *J. Rheumatol.* 1992, 19, 47-52.

[37] Sergent JS; Lockshin MD; Klempner MS; Lipsky BA. Central nervous system disease in systemic lupus erythematosus. Therapy and prognosis. *Am. J. Med.* 1975, 58, 644-54.

[38] Feinglass EJ; Arnett FC; Dorsch CA; Zizic TM; Stevens MB. Neuropsychiatric manifestations of systemic lupus erythematosus: diagnosis, clinical spectrum, and relationship to other features of the disease. *Medicine*, Baltimore.. 1976, 55, 323-39.

[39] Kovacs JA; Urowitz MB; Gladman DD. Dilemmas in neuropsychiatric lupus. *Rheum. Dis. Clin. North Am.*, 1993, 19, 795-814.

[40] Jonsen A; Bengston AA; Nived O; Rayberg, B; Sturfelt, G. Outcome of neuropsychiatric systemic lupus erythematosus within a defined Swedish population: increased morbidity but low mortality. *Rheumatology*, 2002, 41, 1308-12.

[41] Panopalis P; Julian L; Yazdany J; et al. Impact of memory impairment on employment status in persons with systemic lupus erythematosus. *Arthritis. Rheum.*, 2007, 57, 1453-60.

[42] Baker K; Pope J. Employment and work disability in systemic lupus erythematosus: a systematic review. *Rheumatology Oxford* 2009, 48, 281-4.

[43] Hanly JG; Su L; Farewell V; et al. Prospective study of neuropsychiatric events in systemic lupus erythematosus. *J. Rheumatol.*, 2009, 36, 1449-59.

[44] Hanly JG; McCurdy G; Fougere L; et al. Neuropsychiatric events in systemic lupus erythematosus: attribution and clinical significance, *J. Rheumatol.,* 2004, 31, 2156-62.

[45] Appenzeller S; Cendes F; Costallat LT. Cognitive impairment and employment status in systemic lupus erythematosus: a prospective longitudinal study. *Arthritis. Rheum.*, 2009, 61, 680-7.

[46] Appenzeller S, Cendes F, Costallat LT. Cognitive impairment and employment status in systemic lupus erythematosus: a prospective longitudinal study. *Arthritis. Rheum.* 2009; 61: 680-7.

[47] Bertsias GK, Ioannidis JP, Aringer M, et al. EULAR recommendations for the management of systemic lupus erythematosus with neuropsychiatric manifestations: report of a task force of the EULAR standing committee for clinical affairs. *Ann. Rheum. Dis.* 2010; 69: 2074-82.

[48] Appenzeller S, Cendes F, Costallat LT. Epileptic seizures in systemic lupus erythematosus. *Neurology* 2004; 63: 1808-12.

[49] Appenzeller S, Cendes F, Costallat LT. Acute psychosis in systemic lupus erythematosus. *Rheumatol. Int.* 2008; 28: 237-43.

[50] Pego-Reigosa JM, Isenberg DA. Psychosis due to systemic lupus erythematosus: characteristics and long-term outcome of this rare manifestation of the disease. *Rheumatology Oxford.* 2008; 47: 1498-502.

[51] Hanly JG, Harrison MJ. Management of neuropsychiatric lupus. *Best Pract. Res. Clin. Rheumatol.* 2005; 5: 799-821.

[52] Appenzeller S, Costallat LT. Clinical implications of migraine in systemic lupus erythematosus: relation to cumulative organ damage. Cephalalgia 2004; 24: 1024-30.

[53] Davey R, Bamford J, Emery P. The ACR classification criteria for headache disorders in SLE fail to classify certain prevalent headache types. *Cephalalgia* 2008; 28: 296-9.

[54] Zhou HQ, Zhang FC, Tian XP, et al. Clinical features and outcome of neuropsychiatric lupus in Chinese: analysis of 240 hospitalized patients. *Lupus* 2008; 17: 93-9.

[55] Muscal E, Brey RL. Neurologic manifestations of systemic lupus erythematosus in children and adults. *Neurol. Clin.* 2010; 28: 61-73.

[56] Joseph FG, Scolding NJ. *Neurolupus. Pract. Neurol.* 2010; 10: 4-15.

[57] Bessant R, Hingorani A, Patel L, et al. Risk of coronary heart disease and stroke in a large British cohort of patients with systemic lupus erythematosus. *Rheumatology Oxford.* 2004; 43: 924-9.

[58] Seawell AH, Danoff-Burg S. Psychosocial research on systemic lupus erythematosus: a literature review. *Lupus* 2004; 13: 891-9.

[59] Bachen EA, Chesney MA, Criswell LA. Prevalence of mood and anxiety disorders in women with systemic lupus erythematosus. *Arthritis. Rheum.* 2009; 61: 822-9.

[60] Appenzeller S, Veilleux M, Clarke A. Third cranial nerve palsy or pseudo 3rd nerve palsy of myasthenia gravis? A challenging diagnosis in systemic lupus erythematosus. *Lupus* 2009; 18: 836-40.

[61] Carlomagno S, Migliaresi S, Ambrosone L, et al. Cognitive impairment in systemic lupus erythematosus: a follow-up study. *J. Neurol.* 2000; 247: 273-9.

[62] Ellis SG, Verity MA. Central nervous system involvement in systemic lupus erythematosus: a review of neuropathologic findings in 57 cases, 1955-1977. *Sem. Arthritis. Rheum.* 1979; 8: 212-21.

[63] Zvaifler NJ, Bluestein HG. The pathogenesis of central nervous system manifestations of systemic lupus erythematosus. *Arthritis. Rheum.* 1982; 25: 862-6.

[64] Abbott NJ, Mendonca LL, Dolman DE. The blood-brain barrier in systemic lupus erythematosus. *Lupus* 2003; 12: 908-15.

[65] Brooks WM, Sibbitt Jr WL, Kornfeld M, et al. The histopathologic associates of neurometabolite abnormalities in fatal neuropsychiatric systemic lupus erythematosus. *Arthritis. Rheum.* 2010; 62: 2055-63.

[66] Belmont HM, Abramson SB, Lie JT. Pathology and pathogenesis of vascular injury in systemic lupus erythematosus: interactions of inflammatory cells and activated endothelium. *Arthritis. Rheum.* 1996; 39: 9-22.

[67] Appenzeller S, Amorim BJ, Ramos CD, et al. Voxel-based morphometry of brain SPECT can detect the presence of active central nervous system involvement in systemic lupus erythematosus. *Rheumatology Oxford.* 2007; 46: 467-72.

[68] Appenzeller S, Li LM, Costallat LT, et al. Evidence of reversible axonal dysfunction in systemic lupus erythematosus: a proton MRS study. Brain 2005; 128: 2933-40.

[69] Postal M, Appenzeller S. Central nervous system manifestations in systemic lupus erythematosus: diagnosis to treatment. In: Columbus F, editor. Autoimmune diseases: *symptoms, diagnosis and treatment.* New York NY.: Nova Science Publishers, Inc., 2001: 209-31.

[70] Karpiak SE, Graf L, Rapport MM. Antiserum to brain gangliosides produces recurrent epileptiform activity. *Science* 1976; 194: 735-7.

[71] Zaccagni H, Fried J, Cornell J, et al. Soluble adhesion molecule levels, neuropsychiatric lupus and lupus-related damage. *Front Biosci.* 2004; 9: 1654-9.

[72] Matsuda J, Gohchi K, Gotoh M, et al. Circulating intercellular adhesion molecule-1 and soluble interleukin 2- receptor in patients with systemic lupus erythematosus. *Eur. J. Haematol.* 1994; 52: 302-3.

[73] Sfikakis PP, Charalambopoulos D, Vayiopoulos G, et al. Increased levels of intercellular adhesion molecule-1 in the serum of patients with systemic lupus erythematosus. *Clin. Exp. Rheumatol.* 1994; 12: 5-9.

[74] Spronk PE, Bootsma H, Huitema MG, et al. Levels of soluble VCAM-1, soluble ICAM-1, and soluble E-selectin during disease exacerbations in patients with systemic lupus erythematosus SLE.; a long term prospective study. *Clin. Exp. Rheumatol.* 1994; 97: 439-44.

[75] Trysberg E, Carlsten H, Tarkowski A. Intrathecal cytokines in systemic lupus erythematosus with central nervous system involvement. *Lupus* 2000; 9: 498-503.

[76] Shiozawa S, Kuroki Y, Kim M, et al. Interferon-alpha in lupus psychosis. *Arthritis. Rheum.* 1992; 35: 417-22.

[77] Faber-Elmann A, Sthoeger Z, Tcherniack A, et al. Activity of matrix metalloproteinase-9 is elevated in sera of patients with systemic lupus erythematosus. *Clin. Exp. Immunol.* 2002; 127: 393-8.

[78] Ainiala H, Hietaharju A, Dastidar P, et al. Increased serum matrix metalloproteinase 9 levels in systemic lupus erythematosus patients with neuropsychiatric manifestations and brain magnetic resonance imaging abnormalities. *Arthritis. Rheum.* 2004; 50: 858-65.

[79] Hirohata S, Kanai Y, Mitsuo A, et al. NPSLE Research Subcommittee. Accuracy of cerebrospinal fluid IL-6 testing for diagnosis of lupus psychosis: a multicenter retrospective study. *Clin. Rheumatol.* 2009; 28: 1319-23.

[80] Okamoto H, Kobayashi A, Yamanaka H. Cytokines and chemokines in neuropsychiatric syndromes of systemic lupus erythematosus. *J. Biomed. Biotechnol. Epub.* 2010 Jun 29.

[81] Aranow C, Diamond B, Mackay M. Glutamate receptor biology and its clinical significance in neuropsychiatric systemic lupus erythematosus. *Rheum. Dis. Clin. North Am.* 2010; 36: 187-201.

[82] Sabet A, Sibbitt Jr WL, Stidley CA, et al. Neurometabolite markers of cerebral injury in the antiphospholipid antibody syndrome of systemic lupus erythematosus. *Stroke* 1998; 29: 2254-60.

[83] Afeltra A, Garzia P, Mitterhofer AP, et al. Neuropsychiatric lupus syndromes: relationship with antiphospholipid antibodies. *Neurology* 2003; 61: 108-10.

[84] Pierangeli SS, Harris EN. Antiphospholipid antibodies in an in vivo thrombosis model in mice. *Lupus* 1994; 3: 247-51.

[85] Katsiari CG, Giavri I, Mitsikostas DD, et al. Acute transverse myelitis and antiphospholipid antibodies in lupus: no evidence for anticoagulation. *Eur. J. Neurol.* 2011; 18: 556-63.

[86] Karassa FB, Afeltra A, Ambrozic A, et al. Accuracy of anti-ribosomal P protein antibody testing for the diagnosis of neuropsychiatric systemic lupus erythematosus: an international meta-analysis. *Arthritis. Rheum.* 2006; 54: 312-24.

[87] Gerli R, Caponi L, Tincani A, et al. Clinical and serological associations of ribosomal P autoantibodies in systemic lupus erythematosus: prospective evaluation in a large cohort of Italian patients. *Rheumatology Oxford* 2002; 41: 1357-66.

[88] Ghirardello A, Briani C, Lucchetta M, et al. Antiribosomal P protein antibodies and neuropsychiatric systemic lupus erythematosus: cross-sectional vs. prospective studies. *Lupus* 2010; 19: 771-3.

[89] Mostafa GA, Ibrahim DH, Shehab AA, et al. The role of measurement of serum autoantibodies in prediction of pediatric neuropsychiatric systemic lupus erythematosus. *J. Neuroimmunol.* 2010; 227: 195-201.

[90] Nery FG, Borba EF, Viana VS, et al. Prevalence of depressive and anxiety disorders in systemic lupus erythematosus and their association with anti-ribosomal P antibodies. *Prog. Neuropsychopharmacol. Biol. Psychiatry* 2008; 32: 695-700.

[91] Bonfa E, Golombek SJ, Kaufman LD, et al. Association between lupus psychosis and anti-ribosomal P protein antibodies. *N. Engl. J. Med.* 1987; 317: 265-71.

[92] Hanly JG, Urowitz MB, Siannis F, *et al.* Autoantibodies and neuropsychiatric events at the time of systemic lupus erythematosus diagnosis: results from an international inception cohort study. *Arthritis. Rheum.* 2008; 58: 843-53.

[93] Kobiler D, Allweis C. The effect of antisynaptosomal plasma membrane antibodies on memory. *Brain Res.* 1976; 115: 129-38.

[94] Morris RG, Anderson E, Lynch GS, *et al.* Selective impairment of learning and blockade of long-term potentiation by an N-methyl-D-aspartate receptor antagonist, AP5. *Nature* 1986; 319: 774-6.

[95] Skerry TM, Genever PG. Glutamate signalling in nonneuronal tissues. Trends *Pharmacol. Sci.* 2001; 22: 174-81.

[96] DeGiorgio LA, Konstantinov KN, Lee SC, *et al.* A subset of lupus anti-DNA antibodies cross-reacts with the NR2 glutamate receptor in systemic lupus erythematosus. *Nat. Med.* 2001; 7: 1189-93.

[97] Lapteva L, Nowak M, Yarboro CH, *et al.* Anti-N-methyl- D-aspartate receptor antibodies, cognitive dysfunction, and depression in systemic lupus erythematosus. *Arthritis. Rheum.* 2006; 54: 2505-14.

[98] Omdal R, Brokstad K, Waterloo K, *et al.* Neuropsychiatric disturbances in SLE are associated with antibodies against NMDA receptors. *Eur. J. Neurol.* 2005; 12: 392-8.

[99] Emmer BJ, van der Grond J, Steup-Beekman GM, et al. Selective involvement of the amygdala in systemic lupus erythematosus. *PLoS Med* 2006; 3: e499.

[100] Hanly JG, Robichaud J, Fisk JD. Anti-NR2 glutamate receptor antibodies and cognitive function in systemic lupus erythematosus. *J. Rheumatol.* 2006; 33: 1553-8.

[101] Harrison MJ, Ravdin LD, Lockshin MD. Relationship between serum NR2a antibodies and cognitive dysfunction in systemic lupus erythematosus. *Arthritis. Rheum.* 2006; 54: 2515-22.

[102] Steup-Beekman G, Steens S, van Buchem M, *et al.* Anti- NMDA receptor autoantibodies in patients with systemic lupus erythematosus and their first degree relatives. *Lupus* 2007; 16: 329-34.

[103] Arinuma Y, Yanagida T, Hirohata S. Association of cerebrospinal fluid anti-NR2 glutamate receptor antibodies with diffuse neuropsychiatric systemic lupus erythematosus. *Arthritis. Rheum.* 2008; 58: 1130-5.

[104] Yoshio T, Onda K, Nara H, *et al.* Association of IgG anti- NR2 glutamate receptor antibodies in cerebrospinal fluid with neuropsychiatric systemic lupus erythematosus. *Arthritis. Rheum.* 2006; 54: 675-8.

[105] Fragoso-Loyo H, Cabiedes J, Orozco-Narvaez A, *et al.* Serum and cerebrospinal fluid autoantibodies in patients with neuropsychiatric lupus erythematosus: implications for diagnosis and pathogenesis. *PLoS One* 2008; 3: e3347.

[106] Conti F, Alessandri C, Bompane D, *et al.* Autoantibody profile in systemic lupus erythematosus with psychiatric manifestations: a role for antiendothelial-cell Abs. *Arthritis. Res. Ther.* 2004; 6: 366-72.

[107] Song J, Park YB, Lee WK, *et al.* Clinical associations of anti-endothelial cell Abs in patients with systemic lupus erythematosus. *Rheumatol. Int.* 2000; 20: 1-7.

[108] Schenatto CB, Xavier RM, Bredemeier M, *et al.* Raised serum S100B protein levels in neuropsychiatric lupus. *Ann. Rheum. Dis.* 2006; 65: 829-31.

[109] Yang XY, Lin J, Lu XY, *et al.* Expression of S100B protein levels in serum and cerebrospinal fluid with different forms of neuropsychiatric systemic lupus erythematosus. *Clin. Rheumatol.* 2008; 27: 353-7.

[110] Costallat LT, de Oliveira RM, Santiago MB, *et al.* Neuropsychiatric manifestations of systemic lupus erythematosus: the value of anticardiolipin, antigangliosides and antigalactocerebrosides antibodies. *Clin. Rheumatol.* 1990; 9: 489-97.

[111] Jonsen A, Bengtsson AA, Nived O, *et al.* The heterogeneity of neuropsychiatric systemic lupus erythematosus is reflected in lack of association with cerebrospinal fluid cytokine profiles. *Lupus* 2003; 12: 846-50.

[112] Sakic B, Lacosta S, Denburg JA, *et al.* Altered neurotransmission in brains of autoimmune mice: pharmacological and neurochemical evidence. *J. Neuroimmunol.* 2002 Aug;1291-2.:84-96.

[113] Ballok DA, Earls AM, Krasnik C, *et al.* Autoimmune-induced damage of the midbrain dopaminergic system in lupus-prone mice. *J. Neuroimmunol.* 2004 Jul;1521-2.:83-97.

[114] Kandel, ER., 1991. Disorders of mood: depression, mania, and anxiety disorders. In: Kandel, E.R., Schwartz, J.H., Jessell, T.M. Eds.., *Principles of Neural Science.* Appleton and Lange, Norwalk, CT, pp. 869– 883.

[115] Small P, Mass MF, Kohler PF, *et al.* Central nervous system involvement in SLE: diagnostic profile and clinical features. *Arthritis Rheum* 1977; 20: 869-78.

[116] Hanly, JG. Neuropsychiatric lupus. *Rheum. Dis. Clin. North Am.* 2005, 31, 273-98.

[117] Postal M, Costallat LT, Appenzeller S. Neuropsychiatric manifestations in systemic lupus erythematosus: epidemiology, pathophysiology and management. *CNS Drugs*. 2011 Sep 1;259.:721-36.

[118] Hanly, JG; Harrison, MJ. Management of neuropsychiatric lupus. *Best Pract. Res. Clin. Rheumatol.* 2005, 19, 799-821.

[119] Trysberg E, Nylen K, Rosengren LE, *et al.* Neuronal and astrocytic damage in systemic lupus erythematosus patients with central nervous system involvement. *Arthritis. Rheum.* 2003; 48: 2881-7.

[120] Appenzeller S, Pike GB, Clarke AE. Magnetic resonance imaging in the evaluation of central nervous system manifestations in systemic lupus erythematosus. *Clin. Rev. Allergy Immunol.* 2008; 34: 361-6.

[121] Appenzeller S, Rondina JM, Li LM, *et al.* Cerebral and corpus callosum atrophy in systemic lupus erythematosus. *Arthritis. Rheum.* 2005; 52: 2783-9.

[122] Appenzeller S, Bonilha L, Rio PA, *et al.* Longitudinal analysis of gray and white matter loss in patients with systemic lupus erythematosus. *Neuroimage* 2007; 34: 694-701.

[123] Appenzeller S, Vasconcelos Faria A, Li LM, *et al.* Quantitative magnetic resonance imaging analyses and clinical significance of hyperintense white matter lesions in systemic lupus erythematosus patients. *Ann. Neurol.* 2008; 64: 635-43.

[124] Luyendijk J, Steens SC, Ouwendijk WJ, *et al.* Neuropsychiatric SLE: lessons learned from MRI. *Arthritis. Rheum.* 2011; 63: 722-32.

[125] Rovaris M, Viti B, Ciboddo G, et al. Brain involvement in systemic immune mediated diseases: magnetic resonance and magnetisation transfer imaging study. *J. Neurol. Neurosurg. Psychiatry.* 2000; 68: 170-7.

[126] Bosma GP, Rood MJ, Zwinderman AH, *et al.* Evidence of central nervous system damage in patients with neuropsychiatric systemic lupus erythematosus, demonstrated by magnetization transfer imaging. *Arthritis. Rheum.* 2000; 43: 48-54.

[127] Moritani T, Shrier DA, Numaguchi Y, *et al.* Diffusionweighted echo-planar MR imaging of CNS involvement in systemic lupus erythematosus. *Acad. Radio.* 2001; 8: 741-53.

[128] Demaerel P, De Ruyter N, Maes F, *et al.* Magnetic resonance angiography in suspected cerebral vasculitis. *Eur. Radiol.* 2004; 14: 1005-12.

[129] Efthimiou P, Blanco M. Pathogenesis of neuropsychiatric systemic lupus erythematosus and potential biomarkers. *Mod. Rheumatol.* 2009; 19: 457-68.

[130] Sanna G, Bertolaccini ML, Mathieu A. Central nervous system lupus: a clinical approach to therapy. *Lupus* 2003; 12: 935-42.

[131] Barile-Fabris L, Ariza-Andraca R, Olguin-Ortega L, *et al.* Controlled clinical trial of IV cyclophosphamide versus IV methylprednisolone in severe neurological manifestations in systemic lupus erythematosus. *Ann. Rheum. Dis.* 2005; 64: 620-5.

[132] Mok CC, Lau CS, Wong RW. Treatment of lupus psychosis with oral cyclophosphamide followed by azathioprine maintenance: an open-label study. *Am. J. Med.* 2003; 115: 59-62.

[133] Cuadrado MJ, Khamashta MA, Ballesteros A, *et al.* Can neurologic manifestations of Hughes antiphospholipid. syndrome be distinguished from multiple sclerosis? Analysis of 27 patients and review of the literature. *Medicine Baltimore* 2000; 79: 57-68.

[134] Baca V, Lavalle C, Garcia R, *et al.* Favorable response to intravenous methylprednisolone and cyclophosphamide in children with severe neuropsychiatric lupus. *J. Rheumatol.* 1999; 26: 432-9.

[135] Chatham WW, Kimberly RP. Treatment of lupus with corticosteroids. *Lupus* 2001; 10: 140-7.

[136] Boumpas DT, Yamada H, Patronas NJ, *et al.* Pulse cyclophosphamide for severe neuropsychiatric lupus. *Q. J. Med.* 1991; 81: 975-84.

[137] Takada K, Illei GG, Boumpas DT. Cyclophosphamide for the treatment of systemic lupus erythematosus. *Lupus* 2001; 10: 154-61.

[138] Ramos PC, Mendez MJ, Ames PR, *et al.* Pulse cyclophosphamide in the treatment of neuropsychiatric systemic lupus erythematosus. *Clin. Exp. Rheumatol.* 1996; 14: 295-9.

[139] Sakic B, Kolb B, Whishaw IQ, *et al.* Immunosuppression prevents neuronal atrophy in lupus-prone mice: evidence for brain damage induced by autoimmune disease? *J. Neuroimmunol.* 2000; 111: 93-101.

[140] Xu J, Cheng Y, Chai P, *et al.* White-matter volume reduction and the protective effect of immunosuppressive therapy in systemic lupus erythematosus patients with normal appearance by conventional magnetic resonance imaging. *Rheumatol.* 2010; 37: 974-86.

[141] Schroeder JO, Euler HH. Treatment combining plasmapheresis and pulse cyclophosphamide in severe systemic lupus erythematosus. *Adv. Exp. Med. Biol.* 1989; 260: 203-13.

[142] Kazatchkine MD, Kaveri SV. Immunomodulation of autoimmune and inflammatory diseases with intravenous immune globulin. *N. Engl. J. Med.* 2001; 345: 747-55.

[143] Hughes RA, Raphael JC, Swan AV, et al. Intravenous immunoglobulin for Guillain-Barre syndrome. *Cochrane. Database. Syst. Rev.* 2001; 2.: CD002063.

[144] Sherer Y, Levy Y, Langevitz P, *et al.* Successful treatment of systemic lupus erythematosus cerebritis with intravenous immunoglobulin. *Clin. Rheumatol.* 1999; 18: 170-3.

[145] Tomer Y, Shoenfeld Y. Successful treatment of psychosis secondary to SLE with high dose intravenous immunoglobulin. *Clin. Exp. Rheumatol* 1992; 10: 391-3.

[146] Valesini G, Priori R, Francia A, *et al.* Central nervous system involvement in systemic lupus erythematosus: a new therapeutic approach with intrathecal dexamethasone and methotrexate. *Springer Semin. Immunopathol.* 1994; 16: 313-21.

[147] Dong Y, Zhang X, Tang F, *et al.* Intrathecal injection with methotrexate plus dexamethasone in the treatment of central nervous system involvement in systemic lupus erythematosus. *Chin. Med. J. Engl.* 2001; 114: 764-6.

[148] Grisanti M, Nader A, Cacciuttolo R. Central nervous system involvement due to systemic lupus erythematosus/ antiphospholipid syndrome: successful treatment with mycophenolate mofetil. *Lupus* 2001; 10: S31.

[149] Dall'Era M, Wofsy D. Biologic therapy for systemic lupus erythematosus. *Discov. Med.* 2010; 9: 20-3.

[150] Tokunaga M, Saito K, Kawabata D, *et al.* Efficacy of rituximab anti-CD20. for refractory systemic lupuserythematosus involving the central nervous system. *Ann. Rheum. Dis.* 2007; 66: 470-5.

[151] Merrill JT, Neuwelt CM, Wallace DJ, *et al.* Efficacy and safety of rituximab in moderately-to-severely active systemic lupus erythematosus: the randomized, double-blind, phase II/III systemic lupus erythematosus evaluation of rituximab trial. *Arthritis. Rheum.* 2010; 62: 222-33.

[152] Murray E, Perry M. Off-label use of rituximab in systemic lupus erythematosus: a systematic review. *Clin. Rheumatol.* 2010; 29: 707-16.

[153] Turner-Stokes T, Lu TY, Ehrenstein MR, et al. The efficacy of repeated treatment with B-cell depletion therapy in systemic lupus erythematosus: an evaluation. *Rheumatology Oxford* 2011; 50: 1401-8.

[154] Genentech, Inc. and Biogen Idec. Study of Rituxan rituximab. in lupus nephritis misses primary endpoint (online). Available from URL: http://www.newsmedical.net/news/2009/03/11/46787.aspx (Accessed 2011 Jul 4).

[155] Heinlein AC, Gertner E. Marked inflammation in catastrophic longitudinal myelitis associated with systemic lupus erythematosus. *Lupus* 2007; 16: 823-6.

[156] Crowther MA, Ginsberg JS, Julian J, et al. A comparison of two intensities of warfarin for the prevention of recurrent thrombosis in patients with the antiphospholipid antibody syndrome. *N. Engl. J. Med.* 2003; 349: 1133-8.

[157] Ruiz-Irastorza G, Hunt BJ, Khamashta MA. A systematic review of secondary thromboprophylaxis in patients with antiphospholipid antibodies. *Arthritis. Rheum.* 2007; 57: 1487-95.

In: Lupus: Symptoms, Treatment and Potential Complications ISBN: 978-1-62081-078-1
Editors: T. D. Marquez and D. U. Neto

Chapter IV

Treatment in Systemic Lupus Erythematosus

Mariana Postal* and Simone Appenzeller
Department of Medicine, Rheumatology Unit, Faculty of Medical Science, State University of Campinas, Cidade Universitária, Campinas SP, Brazil

Abstract

Systemic lupus erythematosus (SLE) is a prototypic inflammatory autoimmune disorder characterized by multisystem involvement and fluctuating disease activity. Symptoms range from rather mild manifestations such as rash or arthritis to life-threatening end-organ manifestations such as nephritis. Despite new and improved therapy having positively impacted the prognosis of SLE, a subgroup of patients do not response to therapy. Moreover, the risk of fatal outcomes and the damaging side effects of immunosuppressive therapies in SLE call for an improvement in the current therapeutic management of SLE. New therapeutic approaches are focused on B-cell targets, T-cell downregulation and co-stimulatory blockade, cytokine inhibition, or the modulation of complement. Several biological agents have been used in recent and ongoing studies, but this encouraging news follows several disappointments in trials of other biologic therapies. We will review potential therapeutics in SLE and reflect on where we stand, what we have learned, and what may lie ahead.

Introduction

Systemic lupus erythematosus (SLE) is an autoimmune, multisystemic, relapsing and remitting disease that is characterized by the production of antibodies against nuclear antigens

* Correspondence to: Simone Appenzeller-Department of Medicine, Faculty of Medical Science, State University of Campinas, Cidade Universitária, Campinas SP, Brazil, CEP 13083-970; Email: appenzellersimone@yahoo.com, FAX: +55 19 3289-1818

[1]. The pathogenesis includes genetic, environmental, and hormonal factors, but the cause of SLE remains unclear. It is a highly heterogeneous disorder and patients differ significantly in terms of both organ involvement and disease severity. Disease manifestations range from fatigue, skin rash and arthralgias to central nervous system involvement, nephritis, pneumonitis and cardiac disease [2]

The current treatment options include the use of corticosteroids, hydroxychloroquine and other immunosuppressive medications (e.g. azathioprine, mycophenolate and cyclophosphamide) [3,4].

Due to earlier diagnosis and better treatment options of both disease and complications, the prognosis has markedly improved in the last decades. The 5-year survival of patients with SLE has exceeded 90% in most centers [5,6]. However, morbidity, especially renal failure, and mortality from cardiovascular events after long-term follow-up are still an important issue [6].

In the last decade new treatment strategies have been developed. Advanced knowledge of the pathogenesis of SLE has led to new therapeutic approaches targeting specific molecules [5]. Beside autoantibody production, B-cells are the key for the activation of the immune system, particularly through cytokines and as antigen-presenting cells. An important part of B-cells are activated in a T-cell dependant manner. This article will review potential therapeutics in SLE, including biologic therapies.

Conventional Therapies

Our limited understanding of the precise pathogenesis of SLE, the lack of reliable outcome measures, the propensity of lupus patients to have bad outcomes and to react to medicines in unusual ways and the heterogeneity of the patient population means that the majority of treatments is still broadly immunosuppressive in action, and hence carries a significant risk of adverse effects [7].

It is necessary first to identify and treat potential aggravating factors such as hypertension, infection and metabolic abnormalities and second, symptomatic therapy should be considered, such as anticonvulsants, antidepressants and antipsychotic medications, when necessary [8].

Salicylate and Nonsteroidal Therapy

Nonsteroidal anti-inflammatory drugs (NSAIDs) are among the most commonly prescribed drugs in the world. NSAIDs are able to produce analgesia, inhibit platelet aggregation, and reduce fever and inflammation.

Despite the fact of that the Food and Drug Administration (FDA) has not approved the commercial promotion of NSAIDs in the management of SLE, these agents have been used for the treatment of fever, arthritis, pleuritis and pericarditis. NSAIDs can interact with other medications; NSAIDs blunt the antihypertensive effects of loop and thiazide diuretics [9].

Antimalarial Therapies

Unlike other disease-modifying therapeutic agents that are used to treat SLE, antimalarials do not suppress the bone marrow or increase the risk for opportunistic infections [10]. Chloroquine is 90% absorbed by the gastrointestinal tract. Renal excretion (50%) is increased by acidification and decreased by alkalinization. The drug is bound by plasma proteins and largely deposited into tissues. It is used to cutaneous lesions, arthritis-arthralgias, fatigue, and serositis. The only serious complication of the chloroquine is retinotoxicity, which is observed in 10% of patients in chloroquine and in 3% of those on hydroxychloroquine [11].

Hydroxychloroquine has a hydroxyl group at the end of a side chain, therefore differs from chloroquine, but it has similar pharmacokinectics. Hydroxychloroquine has been shown to decrease the probability of flares, the accrual of damage, to possibly protect patients with SLE from the occurrence of vascular and thrombotic events and to facilitate the response to other agents in patients with renal involvement [12-18]. Therefore, chloroquine and hydroxychloroquine have been shown to exert a protective effect on survival in a cohort of 232 patients with SLE.

In this study, patients treated with either of these compounds experienced a better survival rate than those not treated with either agent, even after adjusting for patient characteristics, as patients treated with hydroxychloroquine or chloroquine generally tend to have milder disease than untreated patients [19]. In addition, use of hydroxychloroquine and antihypertensive medication reduced

Retrospective analyses have suggested that in adults with SLE, hydroxychloroquine is associated with lower total cholesterol, LDL-c, VLDL-c and triglycerides [20,21]. This effect is most notable when corticosteroids are co-administered.Given its beneficial impact on lipids and SLE disease activity, hydroxychloroquine is recommended for all children and adolescents with SLE. It is dosed for children at 6–7 mg/kg/day given as single daily dose and can be made into a suspension [22].

Glucocorticoid Therapy

The biologic effects of glucocorticois (GC) are multiple, affect all tissues and are essential for body homeostasis during normal or stress conditions. Although in clinical medicine GCs are used to suppress inflammation and pathologic immune responses [23, 24]. It seems that endogenous GCs have an important overall regulatory role in modulating immune responses that develop to such stressors as infections [23].

The most common anti-inflammatory effects of GCs are mediated via their receptors and correlate with dose and duration of treatment. At the level of blood vessels, GCs inhibit vasodilatation and vascular permeability, limiting therefore erythema, plasma exudation, and swelling. Neutrophils are affected primarily in their ability to migrate to inflammatory area. Consequently, GCs inhibit chemokine synthesis and adhesion molecule expression. There is inhibition of synthesis of inflammatory mediators such as eicosanoids by downregulating phospholipase A2 and COX-2. An alteration between cytokines anti-inflammatory cytokines [Interleukin (IL) 10, Transforming growth factor β] and proinflammatory cytokines [tumor necrosis factor alpha (TNF-α), IL-1β] happens during the treatment with GCs [25].

Immunosuppressive effects also happen. They include lymphopenia, inhibition of signal transduction events critical for T-cell activation, downregulation of cell surface molecules (important for full T-cell activation and function), inducting of T-cell apoptosis and inhibition of antigen-presenting cell function [26].

Immunosuppressive Drug Therapy

Immunosuppressive agents are widely used to treat SLE despite the relative paucity of controlled trials showing their efficacy, especially with regard to prolongation of survival.

Methotrexate

Methotrexate (MTX) appears to have multiple anti-inflammatory effects including increased adenosine levels at the local of inflammation, inhibition of leukotriene B2 formation, IL-1 effects, fibroblast proliferation, and preferential cyclooxygenase-2 inhibition. Side effects of MTX are hepatotoxicity and cytopenias [27].

Azathioprine

Azathioprine (AZA), a purine analogue has a major role in the treatment SLE patients, especially as a corticosteroid-sparing agent [28]. AZA is inactive until it is metabolized to mercaptopurine by the liver and erythrocytes, at which point it inhibits DNA synthesis and therefore prevents cell proliferation in the immune system. Adverse effects include toxicity to the gastrointestinal tract, oral ulcers, nausea, vomiting, diarrhea, and epigastric pain [28]. Dose-related toxicity to the bone marrow results in leukopenia and, less commonly, thrombocytopenia and anemia. Although it has superior efficacy to corticosteroids in the treatment of diffuse proliferative lupus nephritis, it is less effective than cyclophosphamide [28, 29].

Mycophenolate Mofetil

Mycophenolate Mofetil (MMF) has established itself as a successful immunosuppressive drug in multiple applications and has a unique mode of action that may be particularly applicable to control of SLE. MMF is the 2-morpholinoethyl ester derivative of mycophenolic acid (MPA), a weak organic acid produced by several Penicillium species [30]. MMF has excellent oral bioavailability of 94.1% in healthy volunteers [31]. After absorption, MMF is rapidly converted to its active metabolite, MPA by various plasma, liver and renal esterases. Several factors including renal dysfunction, hypoalbuminemia, accumulation of glucuronide and hemoglobin levels have been shown to affect MPA pharmacokinetics and pharmacodynamics [31]. MMF has several effects on the immune system. The best described of these is its selective inhibition of inosine monophosphate dehydrogenase (IMPDH), an enzyme involved in purine biosynthesis. IMPDH exists in two isoforms – type I, which is seen in most cell types and type II, which has greatly increased expression in activated lymphocytes [31]. MMF inhibits the type II isoform nearly 5 times as much compared with the type I isoform, hence conferring its specificity for activated lymphocytes [32].

The principal adverse effects include gastrointestinal symptoms particularly diarrhea, nausea and vomiting and abdominal cramps. There is a suggestion that the gastrointestinal side effects may occur more frequently in the transplant setting compared with its use in inflammatory disease [33].

Cyclosporine

Cyclosporine has complex immunologic effects, mainly inhibition of T-cell gene activation, transcription of cytokine genes and lymphokine release. Besides, it inhibits the recruitment of antigen-presenting cells [34]. A major adverse effect is nephrotoxicity.

Reduction of glomerular filtration may be underestimated because of compensatory hyperfiltration and the increasing contribution of tubular secretion of creatinine to the measured creatinine clearance as renal function declines [35]. In small controlled trials of intermediate duration low dose cyclosporine has also been found effective as a maintenance therapy after cyclophosphamide and even as an induction therapy [36, 37].

Cyclophosphamide

Cyclophosphamide is inactive when administrated. It is metabolized by mitochondrial cytochrome P-450 enzymes in the liver to a variety of active metabolites, an increasing number of which have been shown to have both therapeutic and toxic effects.

This medication can cause hematologic alterations as lymphopenia (dose-related). It is toxic to the granulose cell and, as consequence, reduces serum estradiol levels and progesterone production, inhibits the maturation of oocytes and reduces the number of ovarian follicles, resulting in ovarian failure [38]. Patients who are receiving cyclophosphamide may develop transient amenorrhea. The risk of osteoporosis is increased by amenorrhea regardless of its cause. It is also a potent teratogen, which can cause severe birth defects after administration of as little as 200 mg during early pregnancy (39,40).

B-Cell Targeting

Despite the fact that the pathogenesis of the disease has not yet been fully defined there is no doubt on the central role of B-cells at multiple levels as shown by research in mice and humans. Autoantibody production leads to the formation of immune complexes resulting in an inflammatory reaction, stimulates toll-like receptors and influences cytokine production like IL-1, IL-2, TNF and interferon-α (IFN-α) via innate immune cells. Antibody-independent B-cell functions include T-cell activation, antigen presentation and effects on dendritic cells. [41-43]. B-cell targeted therapies, including anti-CD20 monoclonal antibody (Rituximab) and anti-B lymphocyte stimulator (BLyS), are at forefront of new SLE therapies [43, 44].

Anti-CD20 Antibody

Rituximab was first B-cell depleting biological used in SLE. It is a chimeric murine/human monoclonal antibody against CD20 (Figure 1). Rituximab administration results in rapid depletion of CD20-positive B-lymphocytes [42,45, 46]. After rituximab treatment some patients reconstitute with naive B cells and enter remission. Others, however, do not deplete B cells completely and they reconstitute with memory B cells and might therefore benefit from rituximab retreatment [47]. Two recent open-label studies confirmed that repeated cycles of rituximab are effective in treating refractory SLE, may produce a sustained clinical response and have a favorable safety profile [47,48].

Abbreviations: TNF-α: tumor necrosis factor alpha, IFN-α/γ: interferon alpha and interferon gamma, IL: interleukin, mAb: monocloral antibodies, BLyS: B lymphocyte stimulator, APRIL: proliferation inducing ligand, CTLA-4: Cytotoxic T lymphocyte–associated antigen 4. Rituximab has been used in open trials and improvements in disease activity has been observed [49,50]. In addition it has been shown to be safe and well-tolerated [49, 51, 52]. Two large multicenter randomized placebo-controlled trials with rituximab in moderately to severely active SLE (EXPLORER) [53] and in proliferative lupus nephritis patients (LUNAR) [54] could not demonstrate a significant benefit of rituximab when compared to placebo.

The inclusion of milder forms of SLE, the ethnic background of patients, the concomitant use of steroids and other immunosuppressive drugs and the short follow-up (52 weeks) could explain in part why no benefit could be demonstrated for rituximab in these studies [52-54] Despite the lack of evidence in randomized trials, rituximab has been used in refractory patients and improvement in up to 89% of the patients has been observed [55-69]. Adverse events associated with the use of rituximab are most often mild, but infusion reactions (30–35%), neutropenia (8%) and human anti-chimeric antibodies (9%) production have been observed [47].

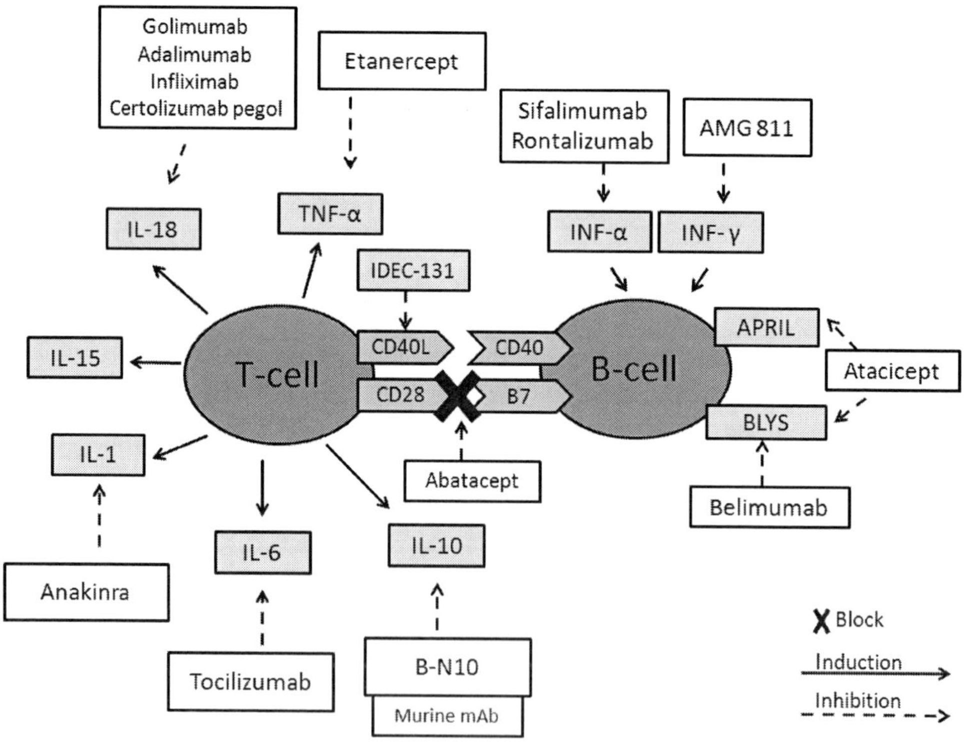

Figure 1. Potential targets and relevant drugs in connection with B and T-cells in the management of SLE.

In addition, two cases of fatal progressive multifocal leukoencephalopathy (lethal encephalitis caused by the polyomavirus JC) in SLE patients after rituximab treatment have been reported [48]. Ocrelizumab is a new monoclonal anti-CD20 antibody. It is a recombinant humanized monoclonal anti-CD20 antibody has been studied in Phase III trials in extrarenal SLE (BEGIN study) [60] and lupus nephritis (BELONG study) (38). However, treatment with ocrelizumab has been suspended in SLE trials, following the negative outcome of a similar study design with the anti-CD20 antibody and also due to an increase in serious in the treatment group [60-62].

Anti-CD22 Antibodies

Epratuzumab is a fully humanized antibody against CD22. CD 22 is 128a 135-kD B-lymphocyte restricted type I transmembrane sialoglycoprotein of the Ig superfamily and modulates B-cell function without B-cell depletion [44,63]. Epratuzumab was evaluated in randomized controlled trials in patients with moderate-to-severe SLE flares [64].

An improvement in BILAG scores and reduction in corticosteroid doses with a good safety profile was observed, however the trial was interrupted due to problems in the biologic supply [39]. Two studies are currently evaluating the efficacy of epratuzumab in a subset of serologically active SLE, and results have yet not been presented [65, 66].

B-Lymphocyte Tolerogens

Abetimus (LJP-394) is a B-cell tolerogen. It consists of four double-stranded DNA (dsDNA) epitopes on a polyethylene glycol platform [28]. It cross-links anti-dsDNA surface immunoglobulin receptors on B-cells, leading to anergy or apoptosis. It also reduces titers of anti-dsDNA antibodies [67]. Abetimus was the first B-cell tolerogen developed for SLE and was studied in human trials for the treatment of non-renal lupus and lupus nephritis [67]. Initial trials suggested a reduction in renal flares in patients who have high-affinity antibodies to the DNA epitope contained within the abetimus molecule [5,67]. After an analysis of a phase III Abetimus Sodium in patients with a history of lupus nephritis (ASPEN) trial, the trial was terminated when interim efficacy analysis indicated no benefit to continue [68].

Another tolerogen, TV-4710 (Edratide) a peptide composed of 19 aminoacids based on the complementarily determining regions (CDR1) of a human anti-dsDNA antibody, was tested in a phase II trial [69]. This study has been concluded but there are yet no results released [69].

BLyS Blockers

The B cell survival molecule B lymphocyte stimulator (BLyS) also known as B cell activation factor of the TNF family (BAFF) plays a key role in the activation and differentiation of B-cells [5]. BLyS represents, therefore, an excellent target for interventions in SLE. High serum levels of soluble BLyS, and its homolog APRIL (a proliferation inducing ligand), are found in SLE patients and in murine lupus. Selective blockade of BLyS reduces transitional type 2 follicular and marginal-zone B-cells, and significantly attenuates immune activation [5,44].

Belimumab is a fully human monoclonal antibody that binds to BLyS and inhibits its biological activity (Figure 1). Efficacy, tolerability and safety of three different doses of belimumab in SLE were evaluated in a multicenter phase II study [70]. After 52 weeks of analysis, belimumab was associated with a reduction in activity and new flares. Two Phase III trials (BLISS-52 and BLISS-76) showed that belimumab plus standard care achieved a significant improvement in patient response rate, and increased time to-first-flare compared with placebo plus standard care [70,71]. Based on these results, FDA recently approved Belimumab for the treatment of SLE [72].

An alternative blocker to BlyS is atacicept (also known as TACI-Ig). It is a soluble transmembrane activator and calcium-modulator and cyclophilin ligand interactor (TACI) receptor, which binds both BAFF and APRIL (Figure 1). In a phase I trial in SLE patients, atacicept was well tolerated [73].

Atacicept is of interest in SLE because of its profound effects on plasma cells, but its use leads to significant decrease in IgM and IgG immunoglobulin levels [74,75]. A phase II study of atacicept plus mycophenolate in SLE nephritis was terminated because of an increased number of infections [74]. The increased number of infection could be explained by the fact that plasma cells require APRIL and so serum Ig was reduced. A phase II/III trial of atacicept for generalized SLE (April SLE) is still ongoing [76].

T-Cell Targeting and Co-Stimulatory Blockade

Co-stimulatory molecules provide the necessary second signal for T-cell activation by antigen-presenting cells. The inhibition of this mechanism has been demonstrated to be effective in murine lupus models [77, 78]. The most important antigen-independent signal for T-cell activation is the CD28:B7 co-stimulatory interaction [5]. CD28 is expressed on T-cells, whereas the ligands B7-1 and B7-2 (CD80 and CD86) are found on antigen presenting cells [5]. CTLA4 inhibits T-cell activation by binding to B7-1 and B7-2 (CD80 and CD86) expressed on antigen-presenting cells. Therefore CTLA4 interacts with B7 but inhibits T-cell activation, by preventing the co-stimulatory signal CD28–B7 interaction necessary for T-cell activation [5] (Figure 1).

Abatacept is a soluble receptor or fusion protein encoded by fusion of CTLA-4 with the Fc portion of IgG1. Abatacept blocks CD28–B7 interaction and subsequent T-cell-dependent B cell function [79,80] (Figure 1). In murine model, abatacept prevents initiation but not evolution of anti-phospholipid syndrome in NZW/BXSB mice [81]. In SLE patients, abatacept has been tested in phase I to III trials [81, 82].

CD40-CD40 ligand (CD40L) is another important co-stimulatory pair that induces T-cell dependent B-cell proliferation and antibody production. CD40 is expressed on B- cells, endothelial cells and antigen-presenting cells and binds to CD40L (or CD154) on CD4+ T helper cells [5] (Figure 1). In lupus-prone mice with nephritis treated with anti-CD40L antibodies reduction in anti-dsDNA antibody, milder renal disease and increased survival was observed [83]. Unfortunately, anti- CD40L monoclonal antibody (mAb) (IDEC-131) did not prove to be clinically effective in human SLE compared with placebo [84]. Another study (BG9588) was terminated prematurely after a few patients demonstrated life-threatening prothrombotic events despite improvement in serologic activity [85].

Efalizumab is a monoclonal antibody directed against CD11a, the alpha-subunit of the leukocyte-functioning antigen-1. It plays an important role in T-cell activation, re-activation, extravasation and trafficking from the circulation into the skin, through its binding to intercellular adhesion molecules (Figure 1). Efalizumab seems to reduce cutaneous manifestations in SLE patients [86]. The majority of patients with difficult lupus discoid had an important response to treatment with the mean time to response being 5.5 week [86]. However, this study evaluated only a small number of patients. There is a need for more prospective studies with long-term follow up to better define the efficacy and safety of efalizumab in SLE.

The inducible costimulator (ICOS) is a T cell–specific molecule structurally and functionally related to CD28. ICOS regulates T cell activation and T-helper cell differentiation and is mainly involved in humoral immune responses and, thus, autoantibody production. A fully humanized anti-B7RP1 antibody (AMG557) is currently being investigated and may represent a further target for SLE therapy [87].

Mammalian target of rapamycin (mTOR) has multiple regulatory functions in T and B-cell intracellular signaling [88]. It controls the expression of T-cell receptor-associated signaling proteins through increased expression of the endosome recycling regulator genes and enhances intracellular calcium flux [89].

Rapamycin (Sirolimus) interacts with mTOR by influencing gene transcription and multiple cellular metabolic pathways. This interaction has been proven to be beneficial in murine lupus [90]. Rapamycin appeared to be a safe and effective therapy for refractory SLE in a small pilot study [91].

Anticytokines Therapy

As cytokine dysregulation can be demonstrated in murine and in SLE patients, an anticytokine approach seems promising in this autoimmune disease [92]. Cytokines such as TNF-α, IFN-α/-γ and IL 1, 6, 10,15, 18 are upregulated in SLE and play important roles in the inflammatory processes that leads to tissue and organ damage [92]. These cytokines have been considered potential targets for the reduction of chronic inflammation in SLE (Figure 1).

Anti-TNF-α

TNF-α is a pleiotropic cytokine that exerts several functions in the immune system and can either promote or reduce autoimmunity. In SLE, its role is controversial. TNF-α promotes apoptosis and significantly affects the activity of B and T-cells and dendritic cells (DCs). In different strains of lupus mice, the expression of TNF-α is often variable, and beneficial effects on the disease can be observed either after administration of TNF-α or upon TNF-α blockade [93, 94-96]. TNF-α blockers are associated with the development of autoantibodies, such as antinuclear, anti-dsDNA and anticardiolipine, as well as with rare cases of drug-induced lupus-like syndromes, all of which disappear after therapy is discontinued [92].

There are several TNF-α inhibitors available for clinical use such as infliximab, adalimumab, golimumab and certolizumab pegol and a fusion protein that acts as a "decoy receptor" for TNF-α (etanercept) [93,97] (Figure 1).

TNF-α inhibitors are usually well tolerated, however their use may increase the overall risk of opportunistic infections, in particular the re-activation of latent tuberculosis [98, 99]. The appearance of neutralizing antibodies has been described in patients treated with infliximab, which is a chimeric human/mouse mAb, as well as in those treated with adalimumab, in spite of its fully human sequence [99]. The concomitant use of an immunosuppressive drug like methotrexate has been shown to prevent the development of neutralizing antibodies [100].

Anti-IFN-α/-γ

IFN-α plays a significant role in the pathogenesis of SLE. IFN-γ is elevated in (New Zealand Black [NZB] × New Zealand White [NZW]) F1 (NZB/W) lupus mice, and a correlation with disease activity has been observed [101, 102]. In addition, administration of IFN-γ accelerates murine lupus, while anti-IFN-γ antibody (or soluble IFN-γ receptor or IFN-γ receptor-immunoglobin) delays the disease [103-105]. Finally, it has been demonstrated that late treatment with IFN-γ in MRL/lpr mice accelerates SLE, while early treatment protects disease progression [106]. IFN-α levels are increased in SLE patients and correlate with disease activity and kidney involvement [107].

In addition an increased expression of interferon-regulated inflammatory genes in the peripheral blood mononuclear cells of the SLE patients (known as 'interferon signature') has been observed [108,109].

Sifalimumab (MEDI-545) is a monoclonal human antibody that blocks multiple IFN-α subtypes. It is currently being tested in Phase I /II clinical trials to evaluate safety and tolerability of multiple intravenous and subcutaneous doses in SLE [110] (Figure 1). Rontalizumab, a humanized mAb against IFN-α (rhuMAb IFN-α) is in a phase II, randomized, double-blind, placebo-controlled trial that evaluates the efficacy and safety in patients with moderately to severely active SLE [111] (Figure 1).

AMG 811, a human mAb to IFN-γ is under investigation in a phase Ib, randomized, multicenter study in SLE patients with and without glomerulonephritis [112].

Anti-IL-1

IL-1 levels are increased by serum TNF levels and by anti-dsDNA antibody. The increase in serum IL-1 level is associated with lupus disease activity and a low level of IL-1 receptor antagonist is seen in patients with lupus nephritis [113,114]. Anakinra, a nonglycolated version of the human IL-1Ra (IL-1 receptor antagonist), neutralizes the biological activity of IL-1 (Figure 1).

It has been used as an alternative in individual patients with lupus arthritis not responding to conventional treatments [115]. Anakinra has shown both safety and efficacy in improving arthritis in an open trial on four SLE patients, however short-lasting therapeutic effects were observed in two patients (115).

Anti–IL-6

IL-6 induces B-cell differentiation to plasma cells, hyperactivity and secretion of antibodies, and also promotes T-cell proliferation, cytotoxic T-cell differentiation and local inflammation [92]. IL-6 is highly expressed in patients with lupus nephritis. IL-6 is induced in DCs by nucleic acid containing immune complexes, as well as by multiple cytokines, including TNF, IL-1, and IFN-γ. In NZB/W mice IL-6 promotes disease, and anti–IL-6 therapy delays lupus nephritis, suggesting that IL-6 blockade might also be beneficial in SLE patients [116].

Tocilizumab is a humanized IgG1 antibody directed to human IL-6 receptor that inhibits IL-6 signaling [117] (Figure 1). An open-label, dose escalating phase I study of tocilizumab in SLE patients has recently been published [118]. Although neutropenia may limit the maximum dosage of tocilizumab in SLE patients, the observed clinical and serologic responses are promising and warrant further studies to establish the optimal dosing regimen and efficacy [118].

Anti-IL-10

IL-10 is produced by Th2 cells and considered an inhibitory cytokine for T-cells and contrasts the activity of other proinflammatory cytokines such as TNF-α and IFN-γ. In SLE patients, IL-10 levels are increased in sera and are associated with disease activity [28]. NZB/W mice treated with anti-IL-10 mAb have reduced anti-dsDNA antibody titers and a delay in the onset of proteinuria and glomerulonephritis [119].

In the absence of a humanized mAb to IL-10, the murine anti-IL-10 mAb (B-N10) was used to inhibit the activity of IL-10 in a small uncontrolled, open-label study in SLE patients with relatively mild disease [120] (Figure 1). Disease activity improved and inactivity was observed in SLE patients up to 6 months after treatment. However, all patients developed antibodies against the murine mAb [120].

Anti–IL-15

IL-15 is mainly produced by the macrophage/monocyte cell line [121]. High serum levels of IL-15 are found in 40% of SLE patients; however it´s levels are not directly associated with disease activity [122]. IL-15 might be responsible for some immune abnormalities of the disease, such as stimulating lymphocytic expression of B-cell lymphoma 2 (Bcl-2) and CD25 (in both B and T-cells) [122]. Therapeutic agents against IL-15 are currently being tested in other autoimmune diseases.

Anti-IL-18

IL-18 is a proinflammatory cytokine closely related to IL-1. Several groups have observed increased serum levels of IL-18 in SLE patients, which appear to be associated with TNF levels [123-125]. IL-18 is overexpressed in the nephritic kidneys of MRL/lpr mice. Moreover, MRL/lpr mice benefit from targeting IL-18 [126]. Until now, IL-18 blockade has not been used in human SLE (Figure 1).

Complement Inhibition

The complement system consists of 3 pathways and more than 30 proteins, including those with biological activity that directly or indirectly mediate complement effects, plus a set of regulatory proteins necessary to prevent inadvisable complement activation [33]. The complement system appears to have a protective effect in SLE, since homozygous deficiencies of classic pathway components are associated with an increased risk for SLE. The deposition of immune complexes, however, observed in human and animal models, leads to an activation of the complement system, amplifying the inflammatory response. Pathologic evidence of immune complex-mediated activation of complement in affected tissues is clearly evident in both experimental and human SLE [127].

Two complement inhibitors, soluble complement receptor 1 (TP10) and a monoclonal anti-C5 antibody (Eculizumab) have been shown to inhibit complement safely and now are being investigated in a variety of clinical conditions [44]. Eculizumab has shown to reduce hemolysis and has been approved by the FDA in paroxysmal nocturnal hemoglobinuria [116].Although still no clinical trial has been performed in SLE, they hold promise to be used therapeutically in SLE [128].

Conclusion

In recent years advances in our understanding of the mechanisms of SLE has offered better drug targets for treatment. Over the next years, we will test the efficacy of many new therapeutic agents. The knowledge on how to divide patients into subsets according to genetic susceptibility, pathogenetic mechanisms, and phases of the disease will maximize the therapeutic effect of each agent and minimize its toxicity.

Acknowledgments

Grants: Fundação de Amparo À Pesquisa Estado São Paulo-Brasil (FAPESP 2008/02917-0 and 2009/06049-6 and 2009/11076-2), Conselho Nacional Pesquisa Desenvolvimento-Brasil CNPq (300447/2009-4).

References

[1] Rahman A, Isenberg DA. Systemic lupus erythematosus. *N. Engl. J. Med.* 2008;358:929-39.

[2] Ermann J, Bermas BL. The biology behind the new therapies for SLE. *Int. J. Clin. Pract.* 2007;61:2113-9.

[3] Hahn BH. Targeted therapies in systemic lupus erythematosus: successes, failures and future. *Ann. Rheum. Dis.* 2011;70(Suppl 1):i64–i66.

[4] Wong M, La Cava A. Lupus, the current therapeutic approaches. *Drugs Today.* 2011;47:289-302.

[5] Haubitz M. New and emerging treatment approaches to lupus. *Biologics*. 2010;4: 263-71.

[6] Trager J, Ward MM. Mortality and causes of death in systemic lupus erythematosus. *Curr. Opin. Rheumatol.* 2001;13:345–351.

[7] Manson JJ, Rahman A. Systemic lupus erythematosus. *Orphanet J. Rare Dis.* 2006;1:6.

[8] Hanly, JG. Neuropsychiatric lupus. *Rheum. Dis. Clin. North. Am.* 2005;31: 273-9.

[9] Nishihara KK, Furst DE. Aspirin and other nonsteroidal anti-inflammatory drugs. In: Koopman WJ, ed. Arthritis and allied conditions: *a textbook of rheumatology.* Baltimore: Williams and Wilkins, 1997:611-654.

[10] Wallace DJ. Antimalarials- the `real' advance in lupus. *Lupus* 2001;10:385-387.

[11] Portnoy JZ, Callen JP. Ophthalmologic aspects of chloroquine and hydroxychloroquine therapy. *Int. Dermatol.* 1983;22:273-278.

[12] Canadian Hydroxychloroquine Study Group. A randomized study of the effect of withdrawing hydroxychloroquine sulfate in systemic lupus erythematosus. *N. Engl. J. Med.* 1991;324:150–4.

[13] Petri M. Hydroxychloroquine use in the Baltimore lupus cohort: effects on lipids, glucose and thrombosis. Lupus 1996;1:S16–22.

[14] Wallace DJ. Antimalarials—the ‘real’ advance in lupus. *Lupus* 2001;10:385–7.

[15] Tsakonas E, Joseph L, Esdaile JM, Choquette D, Senecal JL, Cividino A, et al. A long-term study of hydroxychloroquine withdrawal on exacerbations in systemic lupus erythematosus. Canadian Hydroxychloroquine Study Group. *Lupus* 1998;7:80–5.

[16] Wang C, Fortin PR, Li Y, Panaritis T, Gans M, Esdaile JM. Discontinuation of antimalarial drugs in systemic lupus erythematosus. *J. Rheumatol.* 1999;26:808–15.

[17] Fessler BJ, Alarcon GS, McGwin G Jr, Roseman J, Bastian HM, Friedman AW, et al. Systemic lupus erythematosus in three ethnic groups. XVI: Association of hydroxychloroquine use with reduced risk of damage accrual, *Arthritis Rheum.* 2005;52:1473–80.

[18] Kasitanon N, Fine DM, Haas M, Magder LS, Petri M. Hydroxychloroquine use predicts complete renal remission within 12 months among patients treated with mycophenolate mofetil therapy for membranous lupus nephritis. *Lupus*.

[19] Ruiz-Irastorza G, Egurbide MV, Pijoan JI, Garmendia M, Villar I, MartinezBerriotxoa A, et al. Effect of antimalarials on thrombosis and survival in patients with systemic lupus erythematosus. *Lupus* 2006;15:577–83.

[20] Brindley DN. Role of glucocorticoids and fatty acids in the impairment of lipid metabolism observed in the metabolic syndrome. *Int. J. Obes. Relat. Metab. Disord.* 1995; 19: 69S–75S.

[21] Boots JM, Christiaans MH, van Hooff JP. Effect of immunosuppressive agents on long-term survival of renal transplant recipients: focus on the cardiovascular risk. *Drugs* 2004; 64: 2047–2073.

[22] Ardoin SP, Sandborg C, Schanberg LE. Management of dyslipidemia in children and adolescents with systemic lupus erythematosus. *Lupus*. 2007;16:618-26.

[23] Chrousos GP. The hypothalamic-pituitary-adrenal axis and immune-mediated inflammation. *N. Engl. J. Med.* 1995; 332:1351-62.

[24] Sapolsky RM, Romero LM, Munk AU. How do glucocorticoids influence stress responses? Integrating permissive, suppressive, stimulatory, and preparative actions. *Endocr. Rev.* 2000;21:55-89.

[25] O'Banion Mk, Winn VD, Young DA. cDNA cloning and functional activity of a glucocorticoid-regulated inflammatory cyclooxygenase. *Proc. Natl. Acad. Sci. USA* 1992;89:4888-92.

[26] Paliogianni F, Ahuja SS, Yamada H, et al. Glucocorticoid inhibit T cell proliferation by downregulating proliferative signals mediated through both T cell antigen and interleukin-2 receptors. *Arthritis Rheum.* 1992;35:S127.

[27] Mello S, Barros D, Silva A, et al. Methotrexate as a preferential cyclooxygenase-2 inhibition in whole blood of patients with rheumatoid arthritis. *Rheumatology* (Oxf) 2000;39:533-536.

[28] Yildirim-Toruner C, Diamond B. Current and novel therapeutics in the treatment of systemic lupus erythematosus. *J. Allergy. Clin. Immunol.* 2011;127:303-12.

[29] Sztenjnbok M, Stewart A, Diamond H. Azathioprine in the treatment of systemic lupus erythematosus: a controlled study. *Arthritis Rheum.* 1971;14:639-645.

[30] Allison AC, Eugui EM. Mycophenolate mofetil and its mechanisms of action. *Immunopharmacology* 2000; 47:85–118.

[31] Bullingham RE, Nicholls AJ, Kamm BR. Clinical pharmacokinetics of mycophenolate mofetil. *Clin. Pharmacokinet.* 1998;34: 429–55.

[32] Carr SF, Papp E, Wu JC, et al. Characterization of human type I and type II IMP dehydrogenases. *J. Biol. Chem.* 1993; 268:27286–90.

[33] Goldblum R. Therapy of rheumatoid arthritis with mycophenolate mofetil. *Clin. Exp. Rheumatol.* 1993; 11(Suppl 8):S117–S19.

[34] McCune WJ, Friedman AW. Immunosuppressive drug therapy for rheumatic disease. *Curr. Opin. Rheumatol.* 1993;5:282-292.

[35] DeMattos A, Olvaei A, Bennett W. Nephrotoxicity of immunosuppressive: long-term consequences and challenges for the future. *Am. J. Kidney Dis.* 2000;35:333-346.

[36] Moroni G, Doria A, Mosca M, et al. A randomized pilot trial comparing cyclosporine and azathioprine for maintenance therapy in diffuse lupus nephritis over four years. *Clin. J. Am. Soc. Nephrol.* 2006; 1: 925–932.

[37] Zavada J, Pesickova S, Rysava R, et al. Cyclosporine A or intravenous cyclophosphamide for lupus nephritis: the Cyclofa-Lune study. *Lupus* 2010; 19: 1281–1289.

[38] Lynch J, McCune W. Immunosuppressive and cytotoxic pharmacotherapy for pulmonary disorders: state of the art. *Am. J. Respir. Crit. Care. Med.* 1997;155: 395-420.

[39] Gilchrist DM, Friedman JM. Teratogenesis and IV cyclophosphamide (letter). *J. Rheumatol.* 1989;16:1008-1009.

[40] Kirshon B, Wasserstrum N, Willis R. Teratogenic effects of first trimester cyclophophamide therapy. *Obstet. Gynecol.* 1988;72:462.

[41] Anolik J, Sanz I. B cells in human and murine systemic lupus erythematosus. *Curr. Opin. Rheumatol.* 2004; 16: 505–512.

[42] Sabahi R, Anolik JH. B-cell-targeted therapy for systemic lupus erythematosus. *Drugs*. 2006;66:1933-48.

[43] Ding C, Foote S, Jones G. B-cell-targeted therapy for systemic lupus erythematosus: an update. *BioDrugs*. 2008;22:239-49.

[44] Murdaca G, Colombo BM, Puppo F. Emerging biological drugs: A new therapeutic approach for Systemic Lupus Erythematosus. An update upon efficacy and adverse events. *Autoimmun. Rev.*. 2011;11:56-60.

[45] Perosa F, Favoino E, Caragnano MA, et al. CD20: a target antigen for immunotherapy of autoimmune diseases. *Autoimmun. Rev.* 2005;4:526–31.

[46] Grillo-López AJ, White CA, Dallaire BK, et al. Rituximab: the first monoclonal antibody approved for the treatment of lymphoma. *Curr. Pharm. Biotechnol.* 2000;1: 1-9.

[47] Roccatello D, Sciascia S, Rossi D, et al. Intensive short-term treatment with rituximab, cyclophosphamide and methylprednisolone pulses induces remission in severe cases of SLE with nephritis and avoids further immunosuppressive maintenance therapy. *Nephrol. Dial Transplant.* 2011 Mar 8. [Epub ahead of print].

[48] Rituxan warning. FDA *Consum* 2007;41:3.

[49] Abud-Mendoza C, Moreno-Valdés R, Cuevas-Orta E, et al. Treating severe systemic lupus erythematosus with rituximab. An open study. *Reumatol. Clin.* 2009;5:147-52.

[50] Leandro MJ, Edwards JC, Cambridge G, et al. An open study of B lymphocyte depletion in systemic lupus erythematosus. *Arthritis Rheum*. 2002 ;46:2673-7.

[51] García-Carrasco M, Jiménez-Hernández M, Escárcega RO, et al. Use of rituximab in patients with systemic lupus erythematosus: an update. *Autoimmun Rev.* 2009;8: 343–8. 434.

[52] Lu TYT, Ng KP, Combrodge G, et al. A retrospective seven-year analysis of the use of B cell depletion therapy in systemic lupus erythematosus at university college London hospital: the first fifty patients. *Arthritis Rheum*. 2009;61:482–487.

[53] Merrill JT, Neuwelt CM, Wallace DJ, et al. Efficacy and safety of rituximab in moderately-to-severely active systemic lupus erythematosus. *Arthritis Rheum.* 2010;62:222–233.

[54] Clinicaltrials.gov. A Study to Evaluate the Efficacy and Safety of Rituximab in Subjects With ISN/RPS Class III or IV *Lupus Nephritis* (LUNAR) (NCT00282347).

[55] Pinto LF, Velásquez CJ, Prieto C, et al. Rituximab induces a rapid and sustained remission in colombian patients with severe and refractory systemic lupus erythematosus. *Lupus*. 2011 Jul 22. [Epub ahead of print].

[56] Terrier B, Amoura Z, Ravaud P, et al. Safety and efficacy of rituximab in systemic lupus erythematosus: results from 136 patients from the French AutoImmunity and Rituximab registry. *Arthritis Rheum*. 2010;62:2458-66.

[57] Reynolds JA, Toescu V, Yee CS, et al. Effects of rituximab on resistant SLE disease including lung involvement. *Lupus*. 2009;18:67-73.

[58] Turner-Stokes T, Lu TY, EhrensteinMR, et al. The efficacy of repeated treatment with B-cell depletion therapy in systemic lupus erythematosus: an evaluation. *Rheumatology* (Oxford). 2011;50:1401-8.

[59] Anolik JH, Aringer M. New treatments for SLE: cell-depleting and anti-cytokine therapies. *Best Pract. Res. Clin. Rheumatol* 2005;19:859–78.

[60] ClinicalTrials.gov. *Study to Evaluate Two Doses of Ocrelizumab in Patients With Active Systemic Lupus Erythematosus* (BEGIN) (NCT00539838). http://www.clinicaltrials.gov/ct2/show/NCT00539838? term=Ocrelizumabandrank=10. Accessed August 15, 2011.

[61] ClinicalTrials.gov. *A Study to Evaluate Ocrelizumab in Patients With Nephritis Due to Systemic Lupus Erythematosus* (BELONG) (NCT00626197). http://www.clinicaltrials.gov/ct2/show/NCT00626197?term=Ocrelizumabandrank=12. Accessed August 15,2011.

[62] Lateef A, Petri M. Biologics in the treatment of systemic lupus erythematosus. *Curr. Opin. Rheumatol*. 2010;22:504-9.

[63] Wallace DJ, Hobbs K, Houssiau F, et al. Randomized controlled trials of epratuzumab (anti-CD-22MAB targeting B cells) reveal clinically meaningful reductions in corticosteroid use with favorable safety profile in moderate and severe flaring SLE patients. *Ann. Rheum. Dis*. 2008; 67 (Suppl II):212.

[64] Petri MA, Hobbs K, Gordon C, et al. Randomized controlled trials of epratuzumab (anti-CD-22MAB targeting B cells) reveal clinically meaningful improvements in patients with moderate and severe SLE flares. *Ann. Rheum. Dis*. 2008; 67 (Suppl II):53.

[65] ClinicalTrials.gov. *Study of epratuzumab in serologically-positive systemic lupus erythematosus patients with active disease* (NCT00624351). http://www.clinicaltrials.gov/ct2/show/NCT00624351? term=NCT00624351andrank=1. Accessed August 15, 2011.

[66] ClinicalTrials.gov. *Open-label study of epratuzumab in serologically-positive systemic lupus erythematosus patients with active disease* (NCT00660881). http://www.clinicaltrials.gov/ct2/show/NCT00660881? term=NCT00660881andrank=1. Accessed August 15, 2011.

[67] Cardiel MH, Tumlin JA, Furie RA, et al. Abetimus sodium for renal flare in systemic lupus erythematosus: results of a randomized, controlled phase III trial. *Arthritis Rheum* 2008;58:2470-80.

[68] ClinicalTrials.gov. *Study of LJP 394 in Lupus Patients with History of Renal Disease* (ASPEN) (NCT00089804). http://www.clinicaltrials.gov/ct2/show/NCT00089804? term=Study+of+LJP+394+in+lupus+patients+with+history+of+renal+disease+%28AS PEN%29.andrank=1. Accessed August 15, 2011.

[69] ClinicalTrials.gov. *A Study to Evaluate the Tolerability, Safety and Effectiveness of Edratide in the Treatment of Lupus* (PRELUDE) (NCT00203151). http://www.clinicaltrials.gov/ct2/show/NCT00203151?term=Edratideandrank=1.Access ed August 15, 2011.

[70] Wallace DJ, Stohl W, Furie RA, et al. A phase II, randomized, double-blind, placebo-controlled, dose-ranging study of belimumab in patients with active systemic lupus erythematosus. *Arthritis Rheum* 2009; 61:1168–1178.

[71] ClinicalTrials.gov. *A Study of Belimumab in Subjects With Systemic Lupus Erythematosus* (SLE) (BLISS-76) (NCT00410384). http://www.clinicaltrials.gov/ct2/show/study/NCT00410384?term=BLISS-76andrank=1. Accessed August 15, 2011.

[72] Human Genome Sciences. *Human Genome Sciences and GlaxoSmithKline announce FDA priority review designation for Benlysta (belimumab) as a potential treatment for systemic lupus erythematosus.* http://www.hgsi.com/belimumab.html. Accessed October 1, 2011.

[73] Dall'Era M, Chakravarty E,Wallace D, et al. Reduced B lymphocyte and immunoglobulin levels after atacicept treatment in patients with systemic lupus erythematosus: results of a multicenter, phase Ib, double-blind, placebo-controlled, dose-escalating trial. *Arthritis Rheum* 2007;56:4142-50.

[74] ClinicalTrials.gov. *The Efficacy and Safety of Atacicept in Combination With Mycophenolate Mofetil Used to Treat Lupus Nephritis.* (NCT00573157). http://www.clinicaltrials.gov/ct2/show/NCT00573157?term=The+efficacy+and+safety+of+atacicept+in+combination+with+mycophenolate+mofetilandrank=1. Accessed in August 19, 2011.

[75] Gayed M, Gordon C. Novel treatments for systemic lupus erythematosus. Curr Opin Investig Drugs. 2010;11:1256-64.

[76] ClinicalTrials.gov. *Atacicept Phase II/III in Generalized Systemic Lupus Erythematosus* (April SLE) (NCT00624338). http://www.clinicaltrials.gov/ct2/show/NCT00624338?term=April+SLEandrank=1. Accessed in August 19, 2011.

[77] Schiffer L, Sinha J, Wang X, et al. Short term administration of costimulatory blockade and cyclophosphamide induces remission of systemic lupus erythematosus nephritis in NZB/W F1 mice by a mechanism downstream of renal immune complex deposition. *J. Immunol.* 2003;171:489–497.

[78] Navarra SV. Immune therapy of lupus: what is on the horizon? *Nephrol. Dial. Transplant.* 2006;21:579-81.

[79] Merrill JT, Burgos-Vargas R, Westhovens R, et al. The efficacy and safety of abatacept in patients with non-life-threatening manifestations of systemic lupus erythematosus: results of a twelve-month, multicenter, exploratory, phase IIb, randomized, double-blind, placebo-controlled trial. *Arthritis Rheum*. 2010;62:3077-87.

[80] Akkerman A, Huang W, Wang X, et al. CTLA4Ig prevents initiation but not evolution of anti-phospholipid syndrome in NZW/BXSB mice. *Autoimmunity*. 2004;37:445-51.

[81] ClinicalTrials.gov. *Abatacept and Cyclophosphamide Combination Therapy for Lupus Nephritis* (ACCESS) (NCT00774852). http://www.clinicaltrials.gov/ct2/show/NCT00774852?term=abatacept+sleandrank=4a Accessed in August 23,2011

[82] ClinicalTrials.gov. *Efficacy and Safety Study of Abatacept to Treat Lupus Nephritis* (NCT00430677).http://www.clinicaltrials.gov/ct2/show/NCT00430677?term=abatacept+sleandrank=2. Accessed in August 23,2011.

[83] Wang X, Huang W, Schiffer LE et al. Effects of anti-CD154 treatment on B cells in murine systemic lupus erythematosus. *Arthritis Rheum* 2003; 48: 495–506.

[84] Kalunian KC, Davis Jr. JC, Merrill JT et al. Treatment of systemic lupus erythematosus by inhibition of T cell costimulation with anti-CD154: a randomized, double-blind, placebo-controlled trial. *Arthritis Rheum* 2002; 46:3251–3258.

[85] Boumpas DT, Furie R, Manzi S et al. A short course of BG9588 (anti-CD40 ligand antibody) improves serologic activity and decreases hematuria in patients with proliferative lupus glomerulonephritis. *Arthritis Rheum* 2003; 48: 719–727.

[86] Usmani N, Goodfield M. Efalizumab in the treatment of discoid lupus erythematosus. *Arch. Dermatol.* 2007;143:873–7.

[87] ClinicalTrials. *A Study of AMG 557 in Adults With Systemic Lupus Erythematosus.* (NCT00774943). http://www.clinicaltrials.gov/ct2/show/NCT00774943?term=AMG557andrank=2. Accessed in October 1, 2011.

[88] Fernandez DR, Telarico T, Bonilla E, et al. Activation of mammalian target of rapamycin controls the loss of TCRzeta in lupus T cells through HRES-1/Rab4-regulated lysosomal degradation. *J. Immunol* 2009; 182:2063–2073.

[89] Perl A. Systems biology of lupus: mapping the impact of genomic and environmental factors on gene expression signatures, cellular signaling, metabolic pathways, hormonal and cytokine imbalance, and selecting targets for treatment. *Autoimmunity* 2010;43: 32–47.

[90] Warner LM, Adams LM, Sehgal SN. Rapamycin prolongs survival and arrests pathophysiologic changes in murine systemic lupus erythematosus. *Arthritis Rheum* 1994; 37:289–297.

[91] Fernandez D, Bonilla E, Mirza N, et al. Rapamycin reduces disease activity and normalizes T cell activation-induced calcium fluxing in patients with systemic lupus erythematosus. *Arthritis Rheum* 2006; 54:2983–2988.

[92] La Cava A. Anticytokine therapies in systemic lupus erythematosus. *Immunotherapy.* 2010;2:575-82.

[93] Aringer M, Houssiau F, Gordon C, et al. Adverse events and efficacy of TNF-alpha blockade with infliximab in patients with systemic lupus erythematosus: long-term follow-up of 13 patients. *Rheumatology* (Oxford). 2009;48:1451-4.

[94] Jacob C, McDevitt H. Tumour necrosis factor-α in murine autoimmune 'lupus' nephritis. *Nature* 1988;331:356–358.

[95] Brennan D, Yui M, Wuthrich R, Kelley V. Tumor necrosis factor and IL-1 in New Zealand Black/White mice. Enhanced gene expression and acceleration of renal injury. *J. Immunol.* 1989;143:3470–3475.

[96] Edwards C, Zhou T, Zhang J, et al. Inhibition of superantigen-induced proinflammatory cytokine production and inflammatory arthritis in MRL-lpr/lpr mice by a transcriptional inhibitor of TNF-α. *J. Immunol.* 1996;157:1758–1772.

[97] Tracey D, Klareskog L, Sasso EH, et al. Tumor necrosis factor antagonist mechanisms of action: a comprehensive review. *Pharmacol. Ther.* 2008;117:244–79.

[98] HochbergMC, LebwohlMG, Plevy SE, et al. The benefit/risk profile of TNF-blocking agents: findings of a consensus panel. *Semin. Arthritis. Rheum.* 2005;34:819–36. 564.

[99] Rosenblum H, Amital H. Anti-TNF therapy: safety aspects of taking the risk. *Autoimmun Rev.* 2011;10:563–8.

[100] Bender NK, Heilig CE, Dröll B, et al. Immunogenicity, efficacy and adverse events of adalimumab in RA patients. *Rheumatol. Int.* 2007;27:269–74.

[101] Braun D, Geraldes P, Demengeot J. Type I Interferon controls the onset and severity of autoimmune manifestations in lpr mice. *J. Autoimmun.* 2003;20:15-25.

[102] Santiago-Raber ML, Baccala R, Haraldsson KM, et al. Type-I interferon receptor deficiency reduces lupus-like disease in NZB mice. *J. Exp. Med.* 2003;197:777–88.

[103] Balomenos D, Rumold R, Theofilopoulos A. Interferon-γ is required for lupus-like disease and lymphoaccumulation in MRL-lpr mice. *J. Clin. Invest.* 1998;101:364–371.

[104] Jacob C, van der Meide P, McDevitt H. In vivo treatment of (NZB × NZW)F1 lupus-like nephritis with monoclonal antibody to γ interferon. *J. Exp. Med.* 1987;166: 798–803.

[105] Lawson B, Prud'homme G, Chang Y, et al. Treatment of murine lupus with cDNA encoding IFN-γR/Fc. *J. Clin. Invest.* 2000;106:207–215.

[106] Nicoletti F, Di Marco R, Zaccone P, et al. Dichotomic effects of IFN-γ on the development of systemic lupus erythematosus-like syndrome in MRL-lpr/lpr mice. *Eur. J. Immunol.* 2000;30:438–447.

[107] Koutouzov S, Mathian A, Dalloul A. Type-I interferons and systemic lupus erythematosus. *Autoimmun Rev.* 2006;5:554-62.

[108] Rönnblam l, Eloranta ML, Alm GV. The type I interferon system in systemic lupus erythematosus. *Arthritis Rheum.* 2006;54:408–420.

[109] Baechler EC, Batliwalla FM, Karypis G, et al. Interferon-inducible gene expression signature in peripheral blood cells of patients with severe lupus. *Proc. Natl. Acad. Sci. USA* 2003;100:2610–2615.

[110] Wallace DJ, Petri MA, Olsen M et al. MEDI-545, an anti-interferon alpha monoclonal antibody, shows evidence of clinical activity in systemic lupus erythematosus. *Arthritis Rheum.* 2007;56:526–527.

[111] ClinicalTrials.gov. *A Study to Evaluate the Efficacy and Safety of Rontalizumab in Patients With Moderately to Severely Active Systemic Lupus Erythematosus* (ROSE)(NCT00962832). http://www.clinicaltrials.gov/ct2/show/NCT00962832?term=Rontalizumabandrank=1. Accessed in August 19, 2011.

[112] ClinicalTrials.gov. *Safety Study of AMG 811 in Subjects with Systemic Lupus Erythematosus With and Without Glomerulonephritis* (NCT00818948). http://www.clinicaltrials.gov/ct2/show/NCT00818948?term=AMG+811andrank=2. Accessed in August 19, 2011.

[113] Suzuki H, Takemura H, Kashiwagi H. Interleukin-1 receptor antagonist in patients with active systemic lupus erythematosus. Enhanced production by monocytes and correlation with disease activity. *Arthritis Rheum.* 1995;38:1055-9.

[114] Sturfelt G, Roux-Lombard P, Wollheim FA, et al. Low levels of interleukin-1 receptor antagonist coincide with kidney involvement in systemic lupus erythematosus. *Br. J. Rheumatol.* 1997;36:1283-9.

[115] Ostendorf B, Iking-Konert C, Kurz K, et al. Preliminary results of safety and efficacy of the interleukin 1 receptor antagonist anakinra in patients with severe lupus arthritis. *Ann. Rheum. Dis.* 2005;64:630–633.

[116] Finck BK, Chan B, Wofsy D. Interleukin 6 promotes murine lupus in NZB/NZW F1 mice. *J. Clin. Invest.* 1994;94:585-91.

[117] Tak PP, Kalden JR. Advances in rheumatology: new targeted therapeutics. *Arthritis Res. Ther.* 2011;13 Suppl 1:S5.

[118] Illei GG, Shirota Y, Yarboro CH, et al. Tocilizumab in systemic lupus erythematosus: data on safety, preliminary efficacy, and impact on circulating plasma cells from an open-label phase I dosage-escalation study. *Arthritis Rheum* 2010;62:542-52.

[119] Ishida H, Muchamuel T, Sakaguchi S, et al. Continuous administration of anti-interleukin 10 antibodies delays onset of autoimmunity in NZB/W F1 mice. *J. Exp. Med.* 1994;179:305–310.

[120] Llorente L, Richaud-Patin Y, García-Padilla C, et al. Clinical and biologic effects of antiinterleukin-10 monoclonal antibody administration in systemic lupus erythematosus. *Arthritis Rheum* 2000;43:1790–1800.

[121] Aringer M, Stummvoll GH, Steiner G, et al. Serum interleukin-15 is elevated in systemic lupus erythematosus. *Rheumatology* (Oxford) 2001;40:876-81.

[122] Aringer M, Stummvoll GH, Steiner G, et al. Serum interleukin-15 is elevated in systemic lupus erythematosus. *Rheumatology* (Oxford). 2001;40:876-81.

[123] Park MC, Park YB, Lee SK. Elevated interleukin-18 levels correlated with disease activity in systemic lupus erythematosus. *Clin. Rheumatol.* 2004;23:225-9.

[124] Ogata A, Kitano M, Fukamizu M, et al. Increased serum interleukin-18 in a patient with systemic lupus erythematosus and T-cell large granular lymphocytic leukemia. *Mod. Rheumatol.* 2004;14:267-70.

[125] Favilli F, Anzilotti C, Martinelli L, et al. IL-18 activity in systemic lupus erythematosus. *Ann. N.Y. Acad. Sci.* 2009;1173:301-9.

[126] Bossu P, Neumann D, Del Giudice E, et al. IL-18 cDNA vaccination protects mice from spontaneous lupus-like autoimmune disease. *Proc. Natl. Acad. Sci. USA* 2003;100:14181-6.

[127] Bao L, Quigg RJ. Complement in lupus nephritis: the good, the bad, and the unknown. *Semin Nephrol.* 2007;27:69–80.

[128] Dmytrijuk A, Robie-Suh K, Cohen MH, et al. FDA report: eculizumab (Soliris) for the treatment of patients with paroxysmal nocturnal hemoglobinuria. *Oncologist.* 2008;13:993-1000.

In: Lupus: Symptoms, Treatment and Potential Complications ISBN: 978-1-62081-078-1
Editors: T. D. Marquez and D. U. Neto

Chapter V

Hematologic Manifestations of Systemic Lupus Erythematosus

***Kam Newman*[1], *Ihab El-Hemaidi*[2] *and Mojtaba Akhtari*[3,*]**

[1]Department of Internal Medicine, Jamaica Hospital Medical Center, Van Wyck Expressway, Jamaica, NY, US
[2]Hematology Department, Queen Elizabeth Hospital, Stadium Road, London, UK
[3]Division of Hematology and Oncology, Department of Internal Medicine, University of Nebraska Medical Center, Nebraska Medical Center Omaha, NE, US

A chronic disorder with unknown etiology, systemic lupus erythematosus (SLE) is the most diverse autoimmune disorder with a relapsing and remitting course that may affect any organ in the body. SLE has a broad spectrum of clinical presentations with higher mortality than general population. These diverse clinical manifestations are mainly due to SLE complex immunopathology in which B cells produce autoantibodies against mainly intracellular auto antigen targets, and form complement fixing immune complex deposits resulting in irreversible organ damage. More than one hundred autoantibodies have been found in SLE, but only few of them are associated with the SLE manifestations.

There are almost always autoantibodies against one or more cell components in the blood of SLE patients. Hematologic complications of SLE are among the most common manifestations of this disorder, and almost all patients have hematologic abnormality at some stage of the disease.

In 1971, American college of rheumatology established the SLE criteria in which hemolytic anemia, leukopenia, and thrombocytopenia were the individual criterion. In revised version in 1982, these criteria classified as a group in hematologic system:

* Corresponding author: Tel: 402-559-3834. Fax: 402-559-6520. Email: mojtaba.akhtari@unmc.edu.

- Hemolytic anemia with reticulocytosis
- Leukopenia with leukocyte count less than 4 x 10^9/l on two or more occasions
- Lymphopenia with lymphocyte count less than 1.5 x 10^9/l on two or more occasions
- Thrombocytopenia with platelet count lees than 100 x 10^9/l in the absence of offending drugs

Presence of one or more of these abnormalities consider as a single hematologic criterion [1-3]. In this chapter, we review most clinical and laboratory manifestations of lupus, and discuss their diagnostic and prognostic significance.

Anemia

Anemia is common in about 50% of SLE patients, and may have immune or non-immune etiology. Anemia in SLE can be secondary to anemia of chronic disorder, iron deficiency anemia, and autoimmune hemolytic anemia or less commonly may be seen secondary to chronic kidney disease or myelosuppressor drugs. Anemia of chronic disorder (ACD) is essentially a non-immune hypoproliferative process, and the most common type of anemia that clinicians are faced in SLE. ACD is often a mild to moderate normocytic normochromic anemia that commonly seen in chronic inflammatory disorders, and has multifactorial pathogenesis. Transferrin saturation, serum iron, and transferrin level are low, ferritin is normal or high, reticulocyte count is normal or low, and bone marrow iron store is normal or increased while bone marrow myeloid erythroid ratio (M/E) is normal. The prevalence of ACD in SLE is about 46%, ranging from 37% to 73% in different studies. ACD may coexist with other types of anemia in SLE but does not have any correlation with disease activity [4-6]. There is a large body of evidences that suggests there is resistance to erythropoietin (EPO) proliferative action secondary to increased inflammatory cytokines which plays an important part in ACD pathogenesis. Interleukins, tumor necrosis factor α, interferon α, interferon β, interferon γ, and transforming growth factor β are only some of the cytokines involved in blunt response of EPO in SLE, in addition to suppression of EPO production. It has been shown that the major contributor of ACD in SLE patients is an inadequate response of EPO to anemia. Anti-EPO antibody which is detected in 21% of SLE patients with anemia is another possible mechanism that explains resistance to EPO and prevents sufficient supply to erythroid progenitor cells [7, 8]. Interestingly, low level of EPO in patients with anti-EPO antibody is not associated with lower levels of hemoglobin and may not interfere with EPO function. Most anti-EPO antibodies are not functional, and do not have any relation with the degree of anemia. It has been reported that the presence of anti-EPO antibody is correlated with younger age, and SLE disease activity markers [9].

Interleukin 6 (IL6), a product of inflammatory cells, is a potent stimulator of lymphoid and myeloid cells. It has been shown that IL6 levels are increased in SLE patients, and has a direct relation with overall disease activity. It has been postulated that by suppression of EPO, IL6 can inhibit erythroid progenitor cell proliferation [10].

The production of hepcidin, a dominant regulator of iron absorption in duodenum is increased in the liver of SLE patients. Hepcidin inhibits iron absorption in duodenum, and blocks iron release from macrophage. The current evidence point to the presence of an iron deficiency anemia due to hepcidin overproduction in ACD [11, 12].

Iron deficiency anemia (IDA) is the second most common anemia in SLE patients, and may be secondary to NSAID use, gastrointestinal hemorrhage, and menometrorrhagia. Serum iron is low in SLE patients with ACD, but ferritin above 20 μg/dl almost never happens in IDA.

Autoimmune hemolytic anemia (AIHA) is the third most common type of anemia in SLE patients, and in two-third of patients the first hemolytic crisis occurs at the presentation. The prevalence of AIHA is about 8-28% in patients with SLE, and recurrence rate is as low as 3-5% per year in treated patients. Isolated AIHA may be the only presenting sign of SLE, or even can present before subsequent development of the SLE. In 25% of patients, AIHA is a sign of an underlying disease and therefore, it is warranted to search for SLE related antibodies in unexplained AIHA. AIHA is considered a complication of SLE and amongst the 11criteria for SLE by American College of Rheumatology. AIHA is more common in younger SLE patients' population, African-American ethnicity, azathioprine usage, more frequent in men than women, and is a sign of disease activity. It has been shown that renal involvement, seizures, pericarditis, and pleuritis are more prevalent with AIHA, and SLE patients with AIHA should follow closely for other organ involvements. Death rate increases two-fold in AIHA and SLE regardless of presence at presentation or the course of disease [13]. The possibility of positive anti-dsDNA antibody in the absence of thrombocytopenia is two times more common in SLE patients with AIHA. Anti-dsDNA antibodies are more common in moderate to severe AIHA [14-17]. Venous thrombosis is more common in SLE patients with AIHA, and has high mortality. AIHA associated with frequent arterial/venous thrombosis, thrombocytopenia, IgG anticardiolipin antibodies (aCL) and recurrent fetal loss is a common phenomenon as part of antiphospholipid syndrome (APS) in 74% of Coombs positive SLE patients. The pathogenesis of AIHA related to SLE patients with APS is unclear, but it has been suggested that aCL has an anti RBC activity in some SLE patients with APS [18]. IgG aCL is positive in about 74% of SLE patients with Coombs positive AIHA, and titer of anti-dsDNA and aCL antibody are higher in this subset of patients [19].

The direct antiglobulin test (Coombs' test) is positive in 18-65% of patients without any evidence of hemolysis, which is typically due to epitope-specific warm type autoantibodies (IgG isotypes).

AIHA due to cold type autoantibodies is rare in SLE. Pathogenic IgG isotypes in SLE mainly belong to IgG1, and IgG3 subclasses that fix first component of complement. Positive direct antiglobulin test (DAGT) is usually due to deposition of complement (mostly C3 or C4) and IgG on the RBC surface and deposition of IgG or complement alone is rare. AIHA is the final result of RBCs opsonization by either autoantibodies or deposition of complement on RBCs and adherence to the Fcγ receptors (FCGR) on the macrophages of the reticuloendothelial system.

Rh determinants specific IgG autoantibodies have the capability to activate complement cascade. Spleen is the main place for opsonized RBCs destruction, and spherocyte formation is the end result of RBC phagocytosis in moderate to severe hemolysis. However, interestingly macrophages of SLE patients with AIHA have less phagocytic activity. Hemoglobinuria due to direct complement hemolysis is rare in the presence of warm antibodies. There are suggestive evidences that expression of complement regulatory proteins

CD55, CD59, or both are decreased on the RBCs of some SLE patients with AIHA, and enhance susceptibility to complement mediated lysis. These glycoprotein I anchor proteins regulate complement activity, and prevents damage to self; their congenital deficiency leads to paroxysmal nocturnal hemoglobinuria (PNH). CD55, also called decay accelerating factor (DAF), dissociates complement component C3 and C5 convertases and prevents activation of complement cascade. CD59 blocks C8 and C9 binding, and subsequent formation of membrane attack complex (MAC).

This deficiency is probably due to increased cleavage or decrease production of these anchor proteins [20, 21]. CD55 and CD59 expression on RBCs are quite constant, and their regulatory mechanisms are not fully understood.

AIHA is usually associated with mild to moderate anemia, seldom is life threatening and rarely can be fatal. Patients may present with signs and symptoms of anemia such as pallor, dizziness, shortness of breath, easy fatigability, tachycardia, chest pain and heart failure. Mild to moderate splenomegaly and jaundice are common, but sometimes in severe cases patients present with hepatosplenomegaly, severe jaundice, and heart failure exacerbations. Reticulocyte counts increase in mild cases, and reticulocytosis is an early sign of AIHA. Unconjugated hyperbilirubinemia, low haptoglobin levels, and high serum LDH are commonly seen in AIHA [22]. AIHA is a major clinical sign of SLE activity and is significantly associated with decreased survival [23].

Other types of anemia secondary to hematopoietic failure such as aplastic anemia, pure red cell aplasia, hemophagocytic syndrome, myelofibrosis, and pernicious anemia are seldom reported, but are serious complications of SLE. Aplastic anemia is rare in SLE, and only sporadic cases have been reported. Aplastic anemia is characterized by presence of pancytopenia, reticulocytopenia, with a decreased bone marrow progenitor cells. Pancytopenia secondary to peripheral destruction of cells are common in SLE, and may obscure aplastic anemia diagnosis.

Aplastic anemia may antedate SLE diagnosis, and therefore possibility of SLE should be ruled out in aplastic anemia patients. The exact nature of aplastic anemia in SLE patients has not been well understood, and dramatic response to immunosuppressive therapy suggests an immune mechanism.

Aplastic anemia in SLE patients can be fatal and usually needs immunosuppression [24, 25]. Pure red cell aplasia (PRCA) is a normochromic, normocytic anemia, and reticulocytopenia associated with decreased number of erythroid progenitor cells in an otherwise normal bone marrow. PRCA may be associated with other hematologic and non-hematologic conditions, and even may precede other SLE manifestations. Most cases respond to corticosteroids and immunosuppressive therapy [26-28].

Reactive hemophagocytosis syndrome (HPS) is a rare condition characterized by peripheral pancytopenia, high grade fever, hepatosplenomegaly, lymphadenopathy, elevated liver enzymes and bone marrow infiltration by benign looking histiocytes in the setting of serious infections or lymphoma. HPS is very rare in systemic diseases, and can be life threatening. High triglyceride and ferritin levels associated with pancytopenias are uncommon in SLE and highly suggestive of HPS [29].

Secondary myelofibrosis is a rare cause of anemia in SLE and can be potentially fatal. Clinical signs and symptoms of SLE may not present at the time of diagnosis and bone marrow phenotype is not helpful, but lack of splenomegaly and other features of myeloproliferative disorders is a clue to differentiate from autoimmune myelofibrosis [30].

Leukopenia

It is a very well-known fact that leukopenia is common in SLE and persistent leukopenia has been observed in as many as half of SLE patients that may be a sign of disease activity. At least part of the leukopenia is due to circulating anti-lymphocyte and anti-granulocyte antibodies produced by patient's own immune system against antigens on the surface of these cells. Leukopenia can be due to glucocorticoid and immunosuppressive therapy or SLE activity. In one recent study WBC abnormalities were seen in 36.3% of patients but sever leukopenia was uncommon [31].

Leukopenia is more common in pediatric than adult SLE population, and more seen in SLE patients with skin and mucosal involvement [5]. Infection is 5-10 times more prevalent in SLE patients comparing to similar patients with nephrotic syndrome and rheumatoid arthritis, and in a cohort of 1000 SLE patients it was the second most common cause of death (28.9%) [32]. Increased risk of infection is mainly related to SLE treatment with corticosteroids or immunosuppressants, however, leukopenia per se does not increase the risk and even may be protective [33].

Lymphopenia

Lymphopenia – lymphocyte count less than $1500/mm^3$ - is the most common hematologic finding at the time of diagnosis, and almost all SLE patients have lymphopenia at presentation or at some point in the course of disease. Lymphopenia can occur independently from leukopenia, and is less common in other autoimmune disorders. It is more frequent in older SLE population, more common in men than in women, and African-Latino American than European ancestry. Unlike leukopenia, lymphopenia seems to be a risk factor for infection in SLE patients. Active SLE is a known risk factor for infection which may be due to lymphopenia of active disorder. In one cohort study, the most common involved organs were lungs and urinary tract, and E. coli and S. aureus were leading causative pathogens [34]. Absolute lymphocyte count may return to normal levels after SLE inactivation.

Different studies showed that besides having diagnostic implication, moderate to severe lymphopenia is a sign of disease activity, organ damage, and poor prognosis. Along with anemia and ANA level, lymphopenia is one of the best predictors of SLE flare up, and monitoring its activity in the next year of follow up [35]. Certain manifestations of SLE such as lupus nephritis, neurologic involvement, high anti ds-DNA antibodies, and anti-Ro antibodies have strong association with lymphopenia [36, 37]. Anti-SSa, anti-Ro, anti-La, anti-dsDNA, anti-RNP, and anti-ribosomal P protein (anti-P) are autoantibodies that recognize intracellular antigens, and present in high titers in lymphopenic SLE patients, but their direct role in lymphopenia has not well known yet. However, there is a subset of SLE that may not develop lymphopenia throughout the course of disease, and has better prognosis [38]. Increased lymphocyte apoptosis and/or anti lymphocyte antibodies are possible explanation for SLE lymphopenia, and both of them related to active disease. However, antibodies against lymphocyte surface antigens are the most likely pathogenic mechanism.

Marked B lymphocytopenia and reduced number of $CD27^-$ is characteristic of both SLE and immunosuppressive therapy. It is a very well-known fact that regardless of significant B lymphocytopenia in SLE, peripheral and bone marrow B lymphocytes are the source of polyclonal autoantibodies against self-antigens [39].

Lymphopenia-induced proliferation (LIP) is homeostatic proliferation of T cells in response to T cell depletion. T cell expansion occurs in response to both foreign and self-antigens, and can be homeostatic which is slow and dependent on interleukin 7 or spontaneous which is rapid and independent of interleukin 7. In lymphopenic state, regulatory T cells (T_{reg}) proliferation depends on effector cells, which are increased in lymphopenic patients. This might be due to increased conversion of T_{reg} cells to effector cells. In SLE patients with lymphopenia, decreased number of $CD4^{+}T_{reg}$ correlates with disease activity and maintenance of systemic autoimmunity. Decreased number of $CD4^{+}T_{reg}$ increases resistance of effector T cells which is related to lymphopenia in lymphopenic SLE patients [40]. It has been shown that there is a high titer of anti CD4 antibody in 17.2% of SLE patients that has direct clinical significance which correlates with lymphopenia and active neuropsychiatric disease. These antibodies are both IgG and IgM isotypes, but their exact pathogenic potential is not clearly understood [41]. Anti-ribosomal P protein antibodies are cytotoxic to lymphocytes, and are associated with SLE neuropsychosis.

As mentioned earlier, CD-55 and CD-59 are glycosylated anchor proteins that regulate complement system properties. It has been found that the expression of CD55 and CD59 on both T and B cells in lymphopenic SLE patients are less than control group, and most likely increases lymphocytes susceptibility to complement cytolysis activity [42, 43].

Galectins are immune response regulator proteins that modulate cell adhesion, migration, and growth, and may induce apoptosis of different type of cells. Anti-galactin-8 (Gal-8) has been reported in 30% of SLE patients (vs. 7% in healthy population), and this association is even higher in SLE patients with lymphopenia and malar rash. There is a possibility that anti Gal-8 antibodies might provoke apoptosis of T cells, and induce lymphopenia [44].

Higher rate of lymphocyte apoptosis has been reported in SLE patients as a possible cause of lymphocytopenia, and is associated with active disease and neuropsychiatry manifestations. Little is known how autologous serum of neuropsychiatry SLE patients increases the neglect-apoptosis induced lymphocyte death. However, findings suggest that exposure to phospholipids and released nucleosomes during the apoptosis increases antiphospholipid antibody production that may contribute in enhancement of lymphocyte neglect-apoptosis rate [45].

Neutropenia

Neutropenia is a common hematologic finding in SLE, and has been found in 47% of patients, but severe neutropenia is not common. Neutropenia is a marker of SLE activity, and about two third of patients have anti neutrophil antibodies. This antibody usually is IgG, and more common in anti-Ro antibody positive patients. It has been shown that anti-SSB/La is an anti-neutrophil antibody that can bind to SSB/La on the surface of neutrophil. However, part of the neutropenia is due to bone marrow failure secondary to drug toxicity, and study shows that drug toxicity and not disease activity is the most common reason of neutropenia in SLE. There is an association between neutropenia, aCL, and CNS involvement in SLE patients [46, 47].

Thrombocytopenia

Thrombocytopenia is a frequent SLE manifestation and its incidence is about 10-40%. Sever thrombocytopenia causing bleeding is not a common finding in SLE, but it is associated with a subset of patients with serious organ involvements including CNS, AIHA, renal disease, and a poor prognosis. Thrombocytopenia is associated with less skin rash in SLE [48, 49]. Thrombocytopenia can be due to antiplatelet antibodies, anti-thrombopoietin antibodies (anti-TPO), antiphospholipid antibody, thrombotic microangiopathy, hemophagocytic syndrome, and defective megakaryopoiesis among others.

About 62% of SLE patients are positive for antiplatelet antibodies, and its presence per se is not correlated to disease activity. Specific antiplatelet antibodies targeting platelet membrane glycoprotein complex IIb/IIIa is the most common pathologic mechanism in SLE patients, and can lead to platelet destruction by complement system. C3 or CH50 levels are lower in SLE patients with thrombocytopenia. However, there is no direct correlation between platelet autoantibodies and platelet count, and not all platelet autoantibody positive patients develop thrombocytopenia. Antiplatelet antibody levels are undetectable in patients with normal platelet count after response to therapy, and reappear in relapse [50]. Anti-TPO antibodies are detected in 39% of patients in a cohort study, but it is not associated directly with thrombocytopenia and its exact pathologic role is not clear [51]. CD40 ligand (CD40L), also called CD154, is expressed on $CD4^+$ cells and platelets, and presence of IgG anti CD40L is strongly associated with thrombocytopenia in a subset of SLE patients with antiphospholipid syndrome (APS) and ITP. CD40L is expressed only on activated platelets, and it is possible that anti CD40L autoantibody production happens after destruction of platelets by pathogenic antiplatelet antibodies. In one study, all anti CD40L antibody positive patients were positive for the pathogenic antiplatelet antibodies, anti GPIIb/IIIa [52].

APS initially described in SLE, and there are different antiphospholipid antibodies, mainly IgG isotype, that their pathogenic role in thrombocytopenia is not clear. aCL is positive in about 39% of SLE patients and levels higher than 5 standard deviation (SD) above the mean increases risk of thrombosis two folds. Lupus anticoagulant antibody (LAC) presents in about 22% of SLE patients and its presence increases the risk of clot formation by six fold increases. In a prospective study of 100 consecutive patients with SLE, 42% of patients with high D dimer levels were at increased risk of thrombosis and combination of high D dimer levels and positive aCL/LAC were 100% sensitive for clot formation in all patients. Studies show that 70% of APS patients with thrombocytopenia have circulating autoantibodies against platelet surface glycoproteins. It has been suggested that anti GPIIb/IIIa autoantibody plays a major role in SLE patients with APS and thrombocytopenia [53-55]. On the other hand, only 10% of APS patients without thrombocytopenia have circulating autoantibodies against platelet membrane glycoproteins. 75% of patients with idiopathic thrombocytopenic purpura (ITP) are positive for antiphospholipid antibodies (aPL) but its presence does not have any relation with clinical features [56]. In ITP, patients develop IgG isotype autoantibodies against platelet surface proteins. ITP can be primary (idiopathic) or secondary to autoimmune disorders (SLE, APS), chronic infections (HIV, HCV, H pylori), lymphoproliferative disorders, thyroid disease, or certain drugs. Although ITP patients are commonly ANA positive, only 15-20% develops SLE.

First described by Moschowitz in 1924, thrombotic thrombocytopenic purpura (TTP) is a rare but serious multisystem disorder which affects various systems. The complete syndrome is characterized by pentad of severe thrombocytopenia, hemolytic anemia, renal impairment, fever, and neurological features. Respiratory failure is uncommon in TTP. Waiting for the full pentad to evolve could prove fatal. The female to male ratio is 3:2 with median age of 35 years.

The prevalence of idiopathic TTP is 1 per million but TTP may coexist in 2-3% of SLE patients. In one study, TTP presented 3 months to 12 years after diagnosis of SLE with a median of one year. Presence of TTP in SLE may be a sign of disease activity, and TTP subsides with remission of SLE. However, TTP occurs in both active and inactive SLE. Some elements of TTP are the same as SLE, and diagnosis of TTP as a separate syndrome from SLE may be easily missed due to overlapping features of two disorders [57-59]. Characteristic features of active SLE are the same as TTP pentad; however, presence of microangiopathic hemolytic anemia (presence of schistocytes in the peripheral blood smear) is more in favor of TTP.

Management of SLE patients with thrombocytopenia is different from TTP, and it is crucial to recognize TTP in SLE patients. Platelet aggregation in TTP leads to occlusive microangiopathy. In patients with TTP and SLE direct Coombs test is positive, but this is not the case in idiopathic TTP. In one study, SLE was diagnosed in 73% of patients before the TTP onset, and 15% had synchronous presentation of SLE and TTP. Concomitant presentation of SLE and TTP appears to be more common in children than in adults. In 12% of patients TTP preceded the diagnosis of SLE. Idiopathic TTP has many histological changes of SLE, and a positive Coombs test does not rule out TTP in SLE patients. It has been shown that active stage of SLE or renal impairment is risk factors for TTP in SLE. Infection is an independent risk factor for SLE patients with TTP, and has higher mortality rate [60-63].

As mentioned above, differentiation of thrombocytopenia, renal involvement, and neurologic manifestations in a patient with SLE from APS, TTP, SLE exacerbation and malignant hypertension as possible explanations is challenging. The pathogenesis of thrombocytopenia in SLE and APS are immune mediated while in malignant hypertension and TTP are consumptive.

Both SLE and TTP primarily involve arterioles but the pathology in SLE is inflammation with vasculitis while in TTP consists of platelet-rich thrombi without overt inflammation with a propensity for the brain blood vessels.

The mortality rate in coexistence of SLE and TTP is about 33% which is higher than each disease alone. The histopathology in APS is small vessel occlusion [64-66]. Microangiopathic hemolytic anemia (MAHA) without TTP is very rare in SLE, and it has been proposed that presence of MAHA in SLE is secondary to lupus nephritis.

In a case series of 3, all patients had significant proteinuria with normal level of Von Willebrand Factor cleaving protease (VWF-CP), and responded well to immunosuppressive therapy instead of plasma exchange [67].

Endothelial cells are activated by inflammatory cytokines during acute inflammation, and release von Willebrand factor (vWF) into the plasma. As a consequence of endothelial cell activation, high level of plasma vWF is associated with increased mortality in systemic inflammatory disorders. von Willebrand factor protease inhibitor, a disintegrin-like and metalloproteinase with thrombospondin type I motif 13 (ADAMTS13), specifically cleaves newly released plasma vWF, and vWF is the only known substrate of ADAMS13. Newly released vWF is a large molecule known as ultralarge vWF multimers (UL-VWFMs) that can accumulate in the body and form microvascular thrombi. It has been shown that neutrophils can oxidize and inactivate the vWF processing enzyme ADAMTS13, and induce acquired ADAMTS13 deficiency. ADAMTS13 and vWF have reciprocal relationship. Increased level of plasma vWF is in part due to reduced activity of ADAMTS13 in acute pancreatitis, sepsis induced DIC, acute systemic inflammation caused by endotoxin, sepsis induced organ dysfunction, and other systemic inflammatory disorders.

In acute systemic inflammation such as TTP impaired processing of UL-VWFMs because of decreased ADAMTS13 activity and increased secretion of UL-VWFMs due to endothelial cell activation increases plasma UL-VWFMs and the risk of platelet aggregation by hyperadhesive UL-VWFMs [68]. Upshaw-Schulman is congenital deficiency of ADAMTS13 (<5%) which is mostly asymptomatic during childhood but due to disequilibrium between ADAMTS13 and its substrate -UL-VWFMs- presents with TTP episodes in adulthood.

Although some SLE patients with TTP have IgG autoantibodies against ADAMTS13, its level is almost normal or slightly decreased in most SLE patients with TTP. Different studies show that low level of ADAMTS13 activity has a better prognosis in SLE patients with TTP. It has been suggested that higher shear stress due to vasculitis in SLE generates extensive platelet aggregation and thrombi formation which are characteristic of TTP [69, 70].

The prognosis of idiopathic TTP is much better than TTP associated with SLE, and symptoms are more diverse. Cases of recurrent TTP in patients with SLE have been reported, and owing to a shortage of reports, the role of ADAMTS13 is still unclear in SLE with TTP [71].

APS consists of different subset of manifestations. APS and TTP are both prothrombotic, and vascular endothelial cell activation and platelet aggregation are central pathology of both conditions. In one study serum activity of ADAMTS13 in 33% of patients was lower and IgG anti ADAMTS13 was present in more than half of patients. ADAMTS13 activity was mild to moderately low in 1/3 of patients. However, the presence of these findings and their relationship with pathogenesis and clinical symptoms of TTP is not clear [72, 73].

Bone Marrow as a Target Organ in SLE

Like any other organ, bone marrow is an important target organ in SLE. Inflammatory cytokines and autoantibodies not only involve destruction of peripheral blood cells but also act on bone marrow progenitor cells and its microenvironment.

Bone marrow findings may be part of SLE manifestation or associated with cytotoxic therapy and various infections. Bone marrow hypocellularity and granulocytic hypoplasia are characteristic manifestations of bone marrow biopsy in SLE, but bone marrow necrosis and stromal changes are other common findings.

Hematopoietic and medullary stromal necrosis- known as necrosis of bone marrow- is due to vascular obstruction and dilated sinuses, and has been seen in 19% of patients. Aplastic anemia, myelofibrosis, and increased fibrillar reticulin are other bone marrow alterations in SLE [74, 75].

Hematological Manifestations, SLE Subsets and Prognosis

SLE is a heterogeneous disease with the most diverse clinical manifestations among autoimmune disorders, which makes it difficult to relate initial clinical presentation to prognosis. Assessing the disease activity, response to treatment, and outcome in short term is challenging. The objective outcome measures are better understood in SLE patients with renal involvement and hematologic abnormalities.

There are many SLE subphenotypes with several risk alleles with strong association with anti-dsDNA production and immunologic disorder activity. It has been shown that there are three different SLE subphenotypes with strong association with known susceptibility loci: 1) subphenotypes most associated with the number of risk alleles and cumulative genetic risk score (GRS). Age at diagnosis, hematologic disorder, immunologic disorder, oral ulcers (protective), and anti-dsDNA antibodies are part of this subset, 2) subphenotypes influenced by single known genes.

This subset includes renal disorder and arthritis (protective). Renal disorder is strongly associated with HLA-DR3, but there is a protective effect of integrin alpha M (ITGAM) locus for arthritis, and 3) subphenotypes which potentially are non-genetic including malar rash, discoid rash, photosensitivity, serositis, and neurologic disorder [76, 77].

SLE can be divided into different clinical clusters with specific organ involvement. The relationship between these clinical clusters and organ damage index, survival, remission, and relapse rate has been widely evaluated. In a cohort study of 600 patients with SLE, renal involvement was more associated with hemolytic anemia and anti-dsDNA antibodies, CNS involvement was related to thrombocytopenia, IgG aCL, and LAC antibodies, and myositis was accompanied by anemia and anti RNP antibodies [78].

In a retrospective study of 542 patients, the long term prognosis of SLE was evaluated according to the clinical manifestation at the time of presentation. The remission rate was lower in patients with nephropathy or leucopenia, and patients with nephropathy and thrombocytopenia had a poor prognosis. Bleeding was cause of death in most patients with thrombocytopenia [79].

References

[1] Budman DR, Steinberg AD. Hematologic aspects of systemic lupus erythematosus. Current concepts. Ann Intern Med. 1977; 86: 220-229.

[2] Keeling DM, Isenberg DA. Haematological manifestations of systemic lupus erythematosus. *Blood Rev*. 1993; 7: 199-207.

[3] Kao AH, Manzi S, Ramsey-Goldman R. Review of ACR hematologic criteria in systemic lupus erythematosus. *Lupus*. 2004; 13: 865-868.

[4] Voulgaris M, Kokori SIG, Ioannidis JPA, Tzioufas AG, Kyriaki D, Moutsopoulos HM. Anaemia in systemic lupus erythematosus: aetiological profile and the role of erythropoietin. *Ann. Rheum. Dis*. 2000; 59: 217-222.

[5] Beyan E, Beyan C, Turan M. Hematological presentation in systemic lupus erythematosus and its relationship with disease activity. *Hematology*. 2007; 12(3): 257-261.

[6] Fietta P, Delsanta G, Quaini F. Hematologic manifestation of connective autoimmune diseases. *Clin. Exp. Rheumatol*. 2009; 27: 140-154.

[7] Giannouli S, Voulgarelis M, Ziakas PD, Tziofas AG. Anaemia in systemic lupus erythematosus: from pathophysiology to clinical assessment. *Ann. Rheum. Dis*. 2006; 65: 144-148.

[8] Tzioufas AG, Kokori SI, Petrovas CI, Moutsopoulos HM. Autoantibodies to human recombinant erythropoietin in patients with systemic lupus erythematosus: correlation with anemia. *Arthritis Rheum*. 1997; 40 (12): 2212-6.

[9] Schett G, Firbas U, Furder W, Hiesberger H, Winkler S, Wachauer D, Koller M, Kapiotis S, Smolen J. decreased serum erythropoietin and its relation to anti-erythropoietin antibodies in anaemia of systemic lupus erythematosus. *Rheumatology*. 2001; 40: 424-431.

[10] Ripley BJM, Goncalves B, Isenberg DA, Latchman DS, Rahman A. Raised levels of interleukin 6 in systemic lupus erythematosus correlate with anaemia. *Ann. Rheum. Dis*. 2005; 64: 849-853.

[11] Ganz T. Hepcidin, a key regulator of iron metabolism and mediator of anemia of inflammation. *Blood*. 102: 783-788.

[12] Levine AB, Erkan D. Clinical assessment and management of cytopenia in lupus patients. *Curr. Rheumatol. Rep*. 2011. 13: 291-299.

[13] Kasitanon N, Magder LS, Petri M. predictors of survival in systemic lupus erythematosus. *Medicine* (Baltimore). 2006; 85: 147-156.

[14] Jeffries M, Hamadeh F, Aberle T, Glenn S, Kamen DL, Kelly JA, Reichlin M, Harley JB, Sawalha AH. Haemolytic anaemia in a multi-ethnic cohort of lupus patients: a clinical and serological perspective. *Lupus*. 2008; 17: 739-743.

[15] Kokori SIG, Ioannidis PA, Voulgarelis M, Tzioufas AG, Moutsopoulos HM. Autoimmune hemolytic anemia in patients with systemic lupus erythematosus. *Am. J. Med*. 2000; 108: 198-204.

[16] Sultan SM, Begum S, Isenberg DA. Prevalence, patterns of disease and outcome in patients with systemic lupus erythematosus who develop sever haematological problems. *Rheumatology* (Oxford). 2003; 42: 230-234.

[17] Duran S, Apte M, Alarcon GS, Marion MC, Edberg JC, Kimberly RP, Zhang J, Langefeld CD, Vila LM, Reveille JD. Features associated with, and the impact of, hemolytic anemia in patients with systemic lupus erythematosus: LX, results from a multiethnic cohort. *Arthritis and Rheumatism*. 2008; 59 (9): 1332-1340.

[18] Rottem M, Krause I, Fraser A, Stojanovich L, Rovensky J, Shoenfeld Y. autoimmune hemolytic anemia in the Antiphospholipid syndrome. *Lupus*. 2006; 15: 473-477.

[19] Domiciano DS, Shinjo SK. Autoimmune hemolytic anemia in systemic lupus erythematosus: association with thrombocytopenia. *Clin. Rheumatol*. 2010; 29: 1427-1431.

[20] Richaud-Patin Y, Perez-Romano B, Carrillo-Maravilla E, Rodriguez AB, Simon AJ, Cabiedes J, Jakez-Ocampo J, Llorente L, Ruiz-Arguelles A. Deficiency of red cell bound CD55 and CD59 in patients with systemic lupus erythematosus. *Immunology Letters*. 2003; 88: 95-99.

[21] Ruiz-Delgado GJ, Vazquez-Garza E, Mendez-Ramirez N, Gomez-Almaguer D. Abnormalities in the expression of CD55 and CD59 surface molecules on peripheral blood cells are not specific to paroxysmal nocturnal hemoglobinuria. *Hematology*. 2009; 14(1): 33-37.

[22] Packman CH. Hemolytic anemia due to warm autoantibodies: new and traditional approaches to treatment. *Clin. Adv. Hematol. Oncol.* 2008; 6 (10): 739-741.

[23] Jacobsen S, Petersen J, Ullman S, Junker P, Voss A, Rasmussen JM, Tarp U, Poulsen LH, van Overeem Hansen G, Skaarup B, Hansen TM, Podenphant J, Halberg P. a multicentre study of 513 Danish patients with systemic lupus erythematosus. II. Disease mortality and clinical factors of prognostic value. *Clin. Rheumatol.* 1998; 17: 478-484.

[24] Tagoe C, Shah A, Yee H, Belmont HM. Aplastic anemia in systemic lupus erythematosus: a distinct presentation of acquired aplastic anemia? *J. Clin. Rheumatol.* 2001; 7: 377-383.

[25] Singh NP, Prakash A, Garg D, Makhija A, Pathania A, Prakash N, Kubba S, Agarwal SK. aplastic anemia complicating systemic lupus erythematosus: successful management with cyclosporine. *Rheumatol. Int.* 2004; 24(1): 40-2.

[26] Hara A, Wada T, Kitajima S, Toyama T, Okumura T, Kitagawa K, Iwata Y, Sakai N, Furuichi K, Higuchi M, Kaneko S. cpmbined pure red cell aplasia and autoimmune hemolytic anemia in systemic lupus erythematosus with anti-erythropoietin autoantibodies. *Am. J. Hematol.* 2008; 83: 750-752.

[27] Habib GS, Saliba WR, Froom P. Pure red cell aplasia and lupus. *Semin. Arthritis. Rheum.* 2002; 31: 279-283.

[28] Jimeno Sainz A, Blazquez Encinar JC, Conesa V. Pure red cell aplasia as the first manifestation of systemic lupus erythematosus. *Am. J. Med.* 2001; 111 (1): 78-9.

[29] Lambotte O, Khellaf M, Harmouche H, Bader-Meunier B, Manceron V, Goujard C, Amoura Z, Godeau B, Piette JC, Delfraissy JF. Characteristic and long-term outcome of 15 episodes of systemic lupus erythematosus-associated hemophagocytic syndrome. *Medicine* (Baltimore). 2006; 85 (3): 169-182.

[30] Paquette RL, Meshkinpour A, Rosen PJ. A steroid-responsive cause of bone marrow fibrosis associated with systemic lupus erythematosus. *Medicine* (Baltimore). 1994; 73 (3): 145-152.

[31] Dias AM, do Couto MC, Duarte CC, Ines LP, Malcata AB. White blood cell abnormalities and infections in one-year follow-up of 124 patients with SLE. *Ann. N. Y. Acad. Sci.* 2009; 1173: 103-107.

[32] Cervera R, Khamashta MA, Font J, Sebastiani GD, Gil A, Lavilla P, Aydintug AO, Jedryka-Goral A, De Ramon E, Fernandez-Nebro A, Geleazzi M, Haga HJ, Mathieu A, Houssiau F, Ruiz-Irastorza G, Ingelmo M, Hughes GR. Morbidity and mortality in systemic lupus erythematosus during a 5-year period. *Medicine* (Baltimore). 1999; 78: 167-75.

[33] Ward MM, Pyun E, Studenski S. mortality risks associated with specific clinical manifestations of systemic lupus erythematosus. *Arch. Intern. Med.* 1996; 156(12): 1337-44.

[34] NG WL, Chu CM, Wu AKL, Cheng VCC, Yuen KY. Lymphopenia at presentation is associated with increased risk of infections in patients with systemic lupus erythematosus. *Q. J. Med.* 2006; 99: 37-47.

[35] Mirzayan MJ, Schmidt RE, Witte T. prognostic parameters for flare in systemic lupus erythematosus. *Rheumatology* (Oxford). 39 (12): 1316-9.
[36] Vila LM, Alarcon GS, McGwin G, Bastian HM, Fessler BJ, Reveille JD. Systemic lupus erythematosus in a multiethnic US cohort, XXXVII: association of lymphopenia with clinical manifestations, serologic abnormalities, disease activity, and damage accrual. *Arthritis. Rheum.* 2006; 55 (5): 799-806.
[37] Yu HH, Wang LC, Lee JH, Lee CC, Yang YH, Chiang BL. Lymphopenia is associated with neuropsychiatric manifestations and disease activity in paediatric systemic lupus erythematosus patients. *Rheumatology*. 2007; 46: 1492-1494.
[38] Rivero SJ, Diaz-Jouanen E, Alarcon-Segovia D. lymphopenia in systemic lupus erythematosus. Clinical, diagnostic, and prognostic significance. *Arthritis. Rheumat.* 1978; 21 (3): 295-305.
[39] Odendahl M, Jacobi A, Hansen A, Feist E, Hiepe F, Burmester GR, Lipsky PE, Radbruch A, Dorner T. Disturbed peripheral B lymphocyte homeostasis in systemic lupus erythematosus. *The journal of immunology*. 2000; 165: 5970-5979.
[40] Gomez-Martin D, Diaz-Zamudio M, Vanoye G, Crispin JC, Alcocer-Varela J. quantitative and functional profiles of CD4+ lymphocytes subsets in systemic lupus erythematosus patients with lymphopenia. *Clin. Exp. Immunol.* 2011; 164 (1): 17-25.
[41] Lenert P, Lenert G, Senecal J. CD-$ reactive antibodies in systemic lupus erythematosus. *Human Immunology*. 1996; 49: 38-48.
[42] Alegretti AP, Mucenic T, Merzoni J, Faulhaber GA, Silla LM, Xavier RM. Expression of CD55 and CD59 on peripheral blood cells from systemic lupus erythematosus (SLE) patients. *Cellular Immunology*. 2010; 265: 127-132.
[43] Garcia-Valladares I, Atisha-Fregoso, Richaud-Patin Y, Jakez-Ocampo J, Soto-Vega E, Elias-Lopez D, Carrillo-Maravilla E, Cabiedes J, Ruiz-Arguelles A, Llorente L. *Lupus*. 2006; 15: 600-605.
[44] Massardo L, Metz C, Pardo E, Mezzano V, Babul M, Jarpa E, Guzman AM, Andre S, Kaltner H, Gabius HJ, Jacobelli S, Gonzalez A, Soza A. Autoantibodies against galectin-8: their specificity, association with lymphopenia in system lupus erythematosus and detection in rheumatoid arthritis and acute inflammation. *Lupus*. 18: 539-546.
[45] Silva LM, Garcia AB, Bonadi EA. Increased lymphocyte death by neglect-apoptosis is associated with lymphopenia and autoantibodies in lupus patients presenting with neuropsychiatric manifestations. *J. Neurol.* 2002; 249: 1048-1054.
[46] Martinez-Banos D, Crispin JC, Lazo-Langner A, Sanchez-Guerrero J. Moderate and sever neutropenia in patients with systemic lupus erythematosus. *Rheumatology*. 2006; 45: 994-998.
[47] Newman KA, Akhtari M. Management of autoimmune neutropenia in Felty's syndrome and systemic lupus erythematosus. *Autoimmune Rev.* 2011; 10: 432-437.
[48] Zhao H, Li S, Yang R. Thrombocytopenia in patients with systemic lupus erythematosus: significant in the clinical implication and prognosis. *Platelets*. 2010; 21 (5): 380-385.
[49] Ziakas PD, Giannouli S, Zintzaras E, Tziofas AG, Voulgarelis M. Lupus thrombocytopenia: clinical implications and prognostic significance. *Ann. Rheum. Dis.* 2005; 64: 1366-1369.

[50] Pujol M, Ribera A, Vilardell M, Ordi J, Feliu E. High prevalence of platelet autoantibodies in patients with systemic lupus erythematosus. *Br. J. Haematol.* 1995; 89: 137-141.

[51] Ziakas PD, Giannouli S, Tasidou A, Tziofas AG, Voulgarelis M. Suspects in the tale of lupus-associated thrombocytopenia. *Clin. Exp. Immunol.* 2006; 145 (1): 71-80.

[52] Nakamura M, Tanaka Y, Satoh T, Kawai M, Hirakata M, Kaburaki J, Kawakami Y, Ikeda Y, Kuwana M. Autoantibody to CD40 ligand in systemic lupus erythematosus: association with thrombocytopenia but not thromboembolism. *Rheumatology* (Oxford). 2006; 45: 150-156.

[53] Macchi L, Rispal P, Clofent-Sanchez G, Pellegrin J, Nurden P, Leng B, Nurden AT. Anti-platelet antibodies in patients with systemic lupus erythematosus and the primary antiphospholipid antibody syndrome: their relationship with the observed thrombocytopenia. *B. J. Haematology.* 1997; 98: 336-341.

[54] Clines DB, Liebman H, Stasi R. Pathophysiology of secondary immune thrombocytopenia. *Semin. Hematol.* 46 (1 suppl 2): S2-14.

[55] Wu H, Birmingham DJ, Rovin B, Hackshaw KV, Haddad N, Haden D, Yu CY, Hebert LA. D-dimer level and the risk for thrombosis in systemic lupus erythematosus. *Clin. J. Am. Soc. Nephrol.* 2008; 3: 1628-1636.

[56] Uthman I, Godeau B, Taher A, Khamashta M. The hematologic manifestations of the antiphospholipid syndrome. *Blood Rev.* 2008; 22: 187-194.

[57] Vaidya S, Abul-ezz S, Lipsmeyer E. Thrombotic thrombocytopenic purpura and systemic lupus erythematosus. *Scand. J. Rheumatol.* 2001; 30: 308-10.

[58] Vasoo S, Thumboo J, Fong K-Y. Thrombotic thrombocytopenic purpura in systemic lupus erythematosus: disease activity and the use of cytotoxic drugs. *Lupus.* 2002; 11: 443-450.

[59] Musio F, Bohen EM, Yuan CM, Welch PG. Review of thrombotic thrombocytopenic purpura in the setting of systemic lupus erythematosus. *Semin. Arthrit. Rheumat.* 1998; 28 (1): 1-19.

[60] Kwok SK, Ju JH, Cho CS, Kim HY, Park SH. Thrombotic thrombocytopenic purpura in systemic lupus erythematosus: risk factors and clinical outcome: a single centre study. *Lupus.* 2009; 18: 16-21.

[61] Aleem A, Al-Sugair S. Thrombotic thrombocytopenic purpura associated with systemic lupus erythematosus. *Acta Haematol.* 2006; 115: 68-73.

[62] Nesher G, Hanna VE, Moore TL, Hersh M, Osborn TG. Thrombotic microangiopathic hemolytic anemia in systemic lupus erythematosus. *Semin. Arthrit. Rheumat.* 1994; 24 (3): 165-172.

[63] Dold S, Singh R, Sarwar H, Menon Y, Candia L, Espinoza LR. Frequency of microangiopathic hemolytic anemia in patients with systemic lupus erythematosus exacerbation: distinction from thrombotic thrombocytopenic purpura, prognosis, and outcome. *Arthrit. Rheumat.* 2005; 53 (6): 982-985.

[64] George JN, Vesely SK, James JA. Overlapping features of thrombotic thrombocytopenic purpura and systemic lupus erythematosus. *South Med. J.* 2007; 100 (5): 512-514.

[65] Shah AA, Higgins JP, Chakravarty EF. Thrombotic microangiopathic hemolytic anemia in a patient with SLE: diagnostic difficulties. *Nat. Clin. Pract. Rheumatol.* 2007; 3 (6): 357-62.

[66] Cheung WY. Thrombotic thrombocytopenic purpura and systemic lupus erythematosus – distinct entities or overlapping syndromes? *Transfus. Apher. Sci.* 2006; 34 (3): 263-266.

[67] Hunt BJ, Tueger S, Pattison J, Cavenagh J, D'Cruz DP. Microangiopathic haemolytic anaemia secondary to lupus nephritis: an important differential diagnosis of thrombotic thrombocytopenic purpura. *Lupus.* 2007; 16: 358-362.

[68] Chen J, Fu X, Wang Y, Ling M, McMullen B, Kulman J, Chung DW, Lopez JA. Oxidative modification of von Willebrand factor by neutrophile oxidants inhibits its cleavage by ADAMS 13. *Blood.* 2010; 115: 706-712.

[69] Lansigan F, Isufi I, Tagoe CE. Microangiopathic haemolytic anaemia resembling thrombotic thrombocytopenic purpura in systemic lupus erythematosus: the role of ADAMTS13. *Rheumatology* (Oxford). 2011; 50: 824-829.

[70] Matsuyama T, Kuwana M, Matsumoto M, Isonishi A, Inokuma S. Heterogeneous pathogenic processes of thrombotic microangiopathies in patients with connective tissue diseases. *Thromb. Haemost.* 2009; 102: 371-378.

[71] Maruoka H, Koga T, Inoue Y, Honda S, Takeo M, Fukuda T, Aizawa H. Recurrent thrombotic thrombocytopenic purpura in a patient with systemic lupus erythematosus. *Mod. Rheumatol.* 2007; 17: 426-428.

[72] Austin SK, Starke RD, Lawrie AS, Cohen H, Machin SJ, Mackie IJ. The VWF/ADAMTS13 axis in the antiphospholipid syndrome: ADAMTS13 antibodies and ADAMTS13 dysfunction. *B. J. Haematology*. 2008; 141: 536-544.

[73] Comellas-Kirkerup L, Hernandez-Molina G, Cabral AR. Antiphospholipid-associated thrombocytopenia or autoimmune hemolytic anemia in patients with or without definite primary antiphospholipid syndrome according to the Sapporo revised classification criteria: a 6-year follow-up study. *Blood.* 2010; 116 (16): 3058-3063.

[74] Pereira RMR, Velloso ERP, Menezes Y, Gualandro S, Vassalo J, Yoshinari NH. Bone marrow findings in systemic lupus erythematosus patients with peripheral cytopenias. *Clin. Rheumatol.* 1998; 17: 219-222.

[75] Voulgarelis M, Giannouli S, Tasidou A, Anagnostou D, Ziakas PD, Tziofas AG. Bone marrow histological findings in systemic lupus erythematosus with hematologic abnormalities: a clinicopathological study. *Am. J. Hematol.* 2006; 81: 590-597.

[76] Taylor KE, Chung SA, Graham RR, Ortmann WA, Lee AT, Langefeld CD, Jacob CO, Kamboh MI, Alarcon-Riquelme ME, Tsao BP, Moser KL, Gaffney PM, Harley JB, Petri M, Manzi S, Gregersen PK, Behrens TW, Criswell LA. Risk alleles for systemic lupus erythematosus in a large case-control collection and associations with clinical subphenotypes. *PLoS Genet.* 2011; 7 (2): e1001311.

[77] Strand V. Lessons learned from clinical trials in SLE. *Autoimmun Rev.* 2007; 6 (4): 209-214.

[78] Font J, Cervera R, Ramos-Casals M, Garcia-Carrasco M, Sentis J, Herrero C, Del Olmo JA, Darnell A, Ingelmo M. Clusters of clinical and immunologic features in systemic lupus erythematosus: analysis of 600 patients from a single center. *Sem. Arthrit. Rheumat.* 2004; 23 (4): 217-230.

[79] Tokano Y, Morimoto S, Amano H, Kawanishi T, Yano T, Tomyo M, Sugawara M, Kobayashi S, Tsuda H, Takasaki Y, Hashimoto H. The relationship between initial clinical manifestation and long-term prognosis of patients with systemic lupus erythematosus. *Mod. Rheumatol.* 2005; 15: 275-282.

In: Lupus: Symptoms, Treatment and Potential Complications ISBN: 978-1-62081-078-1
Editors: T. D. Marquez and D. U. Neto

Chapter VI

Interleukin-21 in Systemic Lupus Erythematosus: Pathogenic Relevance and Therapeutic Applications

Hélène Dumortier and Fanny Monneaux*
Centre National de la Recherche Scientifique,
Institut de Biologie Moléculaire et Cellulaire, Strasbourg, France

Abstract

Interleukin-21 (IL-21) is a member of the γchain-dependent cytokine family and as such, its receptor (R) is made of the common γ chain associated to the IL-21R-specific α chain. This four α-helical bundle type I cytokine was first discovered in 2000 and since then, a large number of studies have evidenced its pleiotropic functions on the immune system. IL-21 seems to be a critical regulator of T cells since it induces the development of inflammatory Th17 cells while blocking the differentiation and counteracting the activity of regulatory T cells. It also modulates CD8+ T cell, natural killer cells, as well as dendritic cell functions. Moreover, IL-21 is involved in shaping the effector function and the fate of B cells and especially their final differentiation step in plasma cells, which implies that it may be central in immune diseases that have a major B cell component. Systemic lupus erythematosus (SLE) is one of these "B-cell mediated" disease, and numerous B cell abnormalities have been described, although T cells and many other immune mediators are also known to be altered. Lupus disease is indeed characterized by the production of autoantibodies (a lot of them being specific for nuclear components) and by the subsequent formation of inflammatory immune complexes. Some of them play a crucial role in associated cutaneous lesions and in glomerulonephritis, which can in turn be fatal. Therefore, B lymphocytes are undoubtedly key players in lupus disease. As such, they constitute a privileged objective for the development of new specific biologics and every molecule that affects their function, such as IL-21, may be a valuable

* Corresponding author : UPR9021 CNRS, Institut de Biologie Moléculaire et Cellulaire, 15 rue René Descartes, 67 Strasbourg, France. Tel : +33 388417027, Fax : +33 388610680, E-mail : f.monneaux@ibmc-cnrs.unistra.fr

therapeutic target in SLE. In this review, we will provide an overview of the role of IL-21 in B cell physiology and lupus pathology, and we will discuss the possible targeting of this cytokine to treat SLE.

Introduction: Overview on Systemic Lupus Erythematosus

Systemic lupus erythematosus (SLE) is an autoimmune disease characterized by acute and chronic inflammation of various tissues of the body including joints, skin, kidneys, heart, lungs, blood vessels, and brain. Although lupus patients may have many different symptoms, some of the most common ones include extreme fatigue, painful or swollen joints (arthritis), unexplained fever, skin rashes, and kidney troubles. The course of the disease is unpredictable, with periods of illness (called *flares*) alternating with remissions. Although it is difficult to estimate how many people have lupus because symptoms of the disease vary widely and its onset is often hard to pinpoint, SLE is considered as a rare disease and the prevalence in the general population varies from 12 to 50.8 cases per 100,000 persons. The disease occurs nine times more often in women than in men, especially in women in child-bearing years ages (15 to 35), and is also more common in those of non-European descent. At the immunological and biological levels, SLE is characterized by complement deficiencies, modification of cytokine secretion, hyperglobulinemia, production of autoantibodies (autoAb) (Ab to native DNA constitute a marker of the disease) and formation of immune complexes, which play a crucial role in associated glomerulonephritis. Most patients with SLE produce Ab to components of the nucleus and these Ab often target macromolecular complexes such as the nucleosome, spliceosome, Ro/La particle and ribosome [1,2]. The precise reasons leading to autoreactivity in lupus patients are still not known, but the development of the disease is considered to be of multifactorial etiology, involving genetic susceptibility, hormonal and environmental factors.

In its worst form, lupus can be fatal: 10% of patients die from kidney disease, cardiovascular disease or infections.However, compared with previous decades, when the 4-year survival was estimated to be just 50% in the 1950s, patients with SLE today are less likely to die from the disease itself (the 15-year survival rate is now estimated to be around 80-85%). Even if at present, there is no specific cure for lupus, this notable improvement comes from the use as medication of immunosuppressive drugs such as azathioprine, methotrexate, cyclophosphamide, mycophenolate mofetil (CellCept) and methotrexate, antimalarial drugs (hydroxychloroquine) as well as steroidal and non-steroidal anti-inflammatory agents.

Multiple Roles for B Cells in SLE

Autoimmune diseases such as SLE are characterized by an impaired immune tolerance [3], B cell hyperactivity and the production of high-affinity autoAb directed against self-structures. Some of these autoAb have substantial diagnosis importance, such as anti-Sm or anti-dsDNA, which are highly specific for SLE. They can also centrally contribute to disease pathology by causing inflammatory damages upon immune complex formation and deposition in tissues such as the skin or kidneys leading to complement activation [4-6]. As the producers of autoAb, B cells have therefore long been considered as major contributors to SLE pathogenesis. In that context, we have recently shown that pathogenic autoAb specific for histone H2B can even be locally produced by plasma cells, which have homed to inflamed kidneys of lupus NZB/W mice [7]. It has also been suggested that B cell activation, somatic hypermutation and autoab production may not only occur in secondary lymphoid organs but also *in situ* in ectopic lymphoid tissues, both in tubulo-interstitial inflammation in human lupus nephritis [8] and in a mouse model of chemically-induced lupus [9]. Moreover, there is a reduction in the number of naïve B cells but a marked increase of plasma cells in the periphery of active SLE patients [10], and the expanded circulating CD27^{high} plasma cell population correlates with disease activity [11]. Overall, it is clear that autoAb and plasma cells are absolutely central to SLE pathogenesis. However, one should not forget that B cells are much more than the precursors of antibody-secreting cells and harbor other essential roles both in physiology and SLE pathology. This is supported by many evidences among which the observation of clinical discordance between serological and disease activity in some SLE patients [12], and the rather striking following one: MRL/lpr lupus mice made deficient for circulating autoAb but harboring functionally normal B cells, still develop an SLE-like disease (although milder).

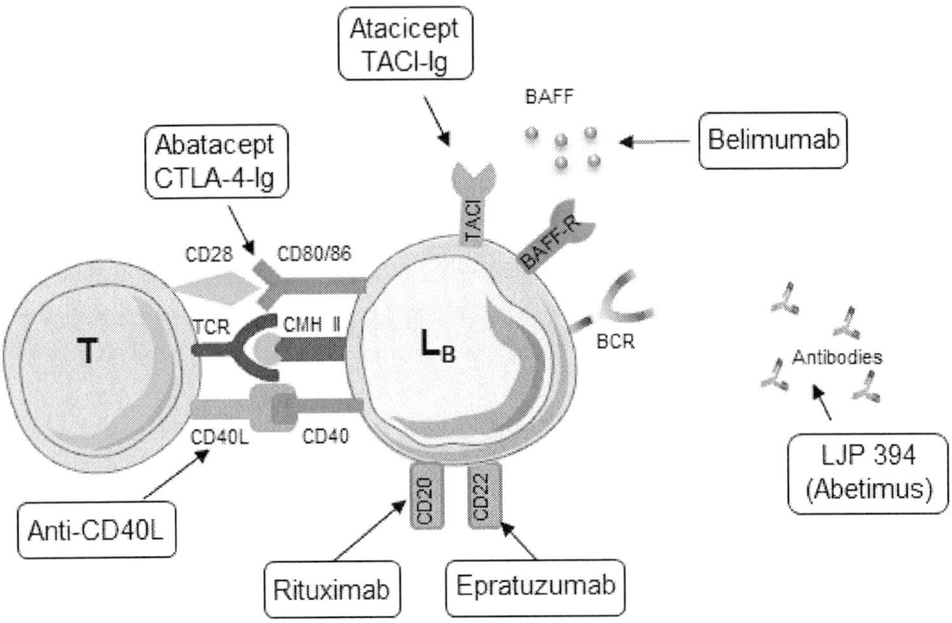

Figure 1. B-cell targeted therapies in SLE. Current therapeutic approaches targeting B cell costimulatory molecules (Rituximab, a humanized anti-CD20 Ab, and Epratuzumab, a humanized anti-CD22 Ab), co-stimulatory interaction between T and B cells (anti-CD40L Ab or Abatacept, that is a CTLA-4Ig fusion protein inhibiting the B7 pathway), autoAb production (Abetimus/LJP 394, an immunomodulating agent that aims at inducing tolerance in dsDNA-specific B cells), or molecules involved in B cell survival such as BAFF (Atacicept, a TACI-Ig fusion protein or Belimumab, a humanized anti-BLyS Ab) are represented.

Indeed, B cells can greatly participate to T cell activation through presentation of autoantigens [13] and costimulation (e.g. CD40/CD154; [14]), and contribute to (auto)immune responses through proinflammatory (e.g. IL-6, IFN-α), T cell polarizing (e.g. IFN-γ/IL-4), lymphogenic (e.g. lymphotoxin) and regulatory (e.g. IL-10) cytokines.

In conclusion, B lymphocytes are undoubtedly key players in lupus disease. As such, they constitute a privileged objective for the development of new specific biologics (reviewed in [15] and in Figure 1) and every molecule that affects their function (such as IL-21) may be a valuable therapeutic target in SLE.

IL-21 Is aCritical Regulator of B Cell Responses

IL-21: Ligand and Receptor

IL-21 is a member of the γchain(γc)-dependent cytokine family together with IL-2, IL-4, IL-7, IL-9 and IL-15. As such, its receptor (R) is made of the common γc associated to the specific IL-21R-specific α chain. This four α-helical bundle type I cytokine was first discovered in 2000 [16] and since then, a large number of studies have evidenced its pleiotropic functions on the immune system ([17]; Figure 2).

Indeed, IL-21R is expressed on a wide range of lymphohematopoietic cells, among which B lymphocytes, which all express variable levels of IL-21R during their differentiation process from progenitors to mature B cells [18-21]. Like other γc-dependent cytokines, IL-21 signals through the Janus kinase (JAK)/ signal transducers and activators of transcripts (STAT) pathway and preferentially activates STAT1 and STAT3 (and STAT5 to a lesser extent).

Involvement of the mitogen-activated protein kinases (MAPK) and phosphoinositide 3-kinases (PI3K) pathways in IL-21-induced proliferation has also been described, suggesting a cooperative effect of those 3 pathways [22-25]. Interestingly, B cells from patients harboring inactivating mutations in STAT3 fail to differentiate in immunoglobulin (Ig)-secreting cells in response to IL-21 [26].

IL-21 Controls Proliferation and Survival of Mature B Cells

The first evidence of the implication of IL-21 in B cell responses was brought when this cytokine was identified [16]. Next to its role in natural killer (NK) cell expansion and T cell stimulation, IL-21 was shown to participate to the activation and proliferation of human mature B cells costimulated through CD40.

Its function as a growth factor for naïve human B cells in combination with CD40 signaling was later confirmed by Good et al. [27] who further showed that IL-21 has greater effects than any other cytokines such as IL-4, IL-10 or IL-13. The same observation was made for murine B cells stimulated via the B cell receptor (BCR) and CD40 ([28]; Figure 2).

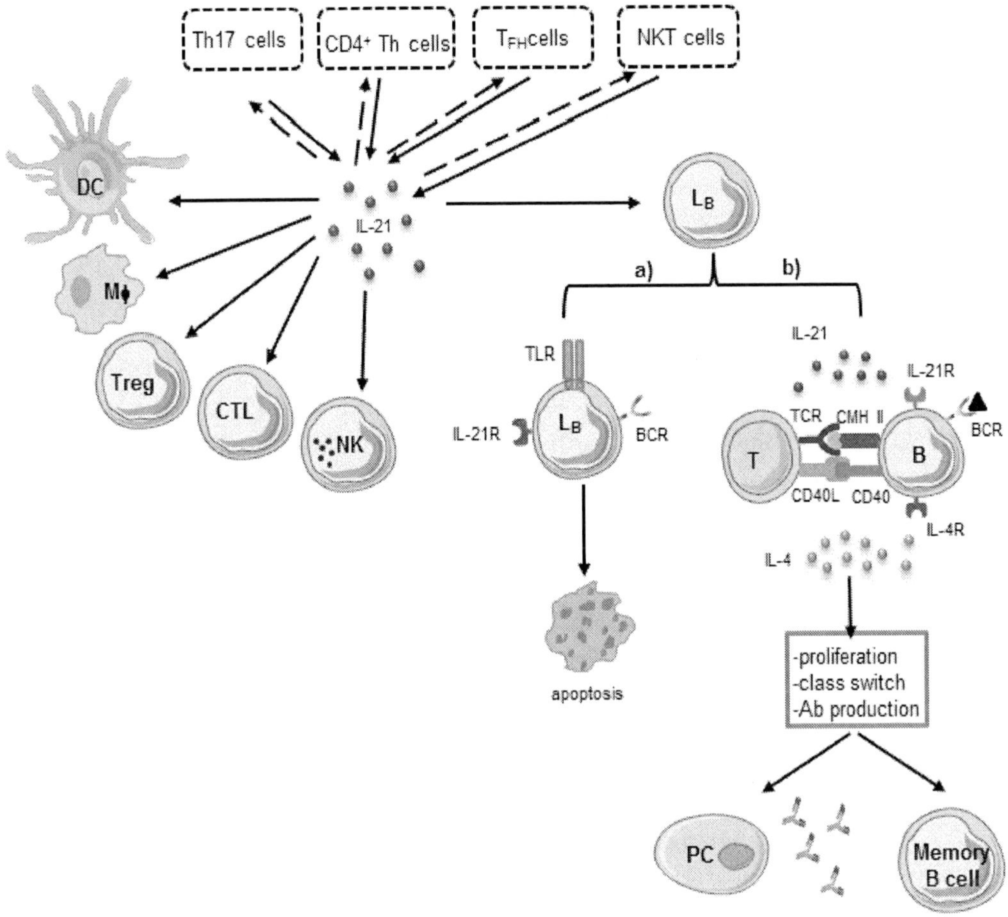

Figure 2. Main functions of IL-21. IL-21 is produced by a wide range of T cells including activated $CD4^+$ T cells, Th17 cells, T_{FH} cells and NKT cells. Once produced, IL-21 exerts pleiotropic autocrine and paracrine effects on IL-21 producers and dendritic cells, macrophages, $CD4^+CD25^+$ regulatory T cells, $CD8^+$ T cells and NK cells, respectively. Its effects on B cell function depends on the nature of the co-stimulatory signals they received. In the presence of TLR stimulation but in absence of BCR signaling, IL-21 induces B cell apoptosis (a), whereas in the presence of BCR signaling and/or T cell co-stimulation, IL-21 can induce B cell differentiation into memory B cells or plasma cells (b).DC; dendritic cells, MΦ; macrophages, NK; natural killer; PC; plasma cells, TLR; toll like receptor.

However, paradoxically, IL-21 can also induce growth arrest and exert pro-apoptotic effects, and this is a very specific characteristic of this γc-dependent cytokine.

Indeed, when combined to strong innate signals such as the toll like receptor (TLR)4 ligand lipopolysaccharide (LPS) or the TLR9 ligand CpG DNA, IL-21 does not only inhibit cell proliferation but also induces B cell death through a Bim-dependent mitochondrial pathway, as identified in murine B cells by Jin et al. ([18]; Figure 2).

Interestingly, follicular and marginal zone B cell subsets harbor similar susceptibility to IL-21-induced apoptosis [19] and CD40 signal can rescue primary B cells from TLR-induced cell death through induction of the pro-survival factor Bcl-x_L[29]. Therefore, it is clear that the outcome of B cell activation by IL-21 strongly depends on the associated costimulatory signal and that IL-21 is a key regulator of B cell fate.

IL-21 Is Central to Antibody Production and Plasma Cell Differentiation

As a major B cell regulator, IL-21 is also essential to the plasma cell differentiation and Ig secretion processes. Critical insights into those aspects came from the study of IL-21R-deficient as well as IL-21-overexpressing mice. IL-21R-deficient mice were found to harbor a higher production of IgE but lower IgG levels than wild-type animals, both in naïve mice and upon immunization (variations in IgG subclasses were observed depending on the antigen used). When combined to IL-4 deficiency, the absence of IL-21R leads to an even more strikingly impaired Ig response together with disorganized germinal centers [30]. IgE synthesis regulation by IL-21 was shown to be related to the inhibition of germline Cε transcripts in IL-4-activated mouse B cells [31]. However, Kobayashi et al. observed that IL-21 stimulates IgE synthesis by IL-4/CD40-activated human B cells [32]. Recently, the IL-21 pathway has also been identified as a critical component of the memory B cell response as secondary antigen-specific IgG responses are impaired in IL-21R-knockout mice [33]. IL-21-overexpressing animals have also been generated [28]. Both chronically (transgenic) and acutely (*in vivo* hydrodynamic-based transfection) IL-21-expressing mice show increased Ig levels (mainly IgM and IgG1) as compared to wild-type mice, and it was even demonstrated that some of these IL-21 transgenic mice spontaneously produce DNA-specific autoAb as lupus mice do [34]. Consistently with this observation regarding Ig production, IL-21 overexpression leads to increased numbers of post-switch B cells and plasma cells *in vivo*[28]. The direct impact of IL-21 on the differentiation of Ig-secreting cells was further demonstrated by *in vitro* experiments using purified B lymphocytes. In the same work, Osaki et al [28] highlighted for the first time the capacity of IL-21 to induce Blimp-1 (B lymphocyte-induced maturation protein-1) and Bcl-6 (B cell lymphoma-6), which are transcription factors intimately involved in plasma cell and germinal center cell differentiation respectively. Blimp-1 was also strongly induced when IL-21 was added to CD40/IgM-activated human peripheral blood B cells. Similar results were obtained when using poorly responsive naïve cord blood B cells [35]. Of note, Ettinger et al. [36] have described a population of IgG^+ marginal zone analogous human B cells, which are uniquely receptive to the IL-21/BAFF (B cell activating factor) combination and differentiate in $Blimp\text{-}1^+$ plasma cells in the absence of any other activation signal (antigen/costimulation), suggesting they contribute to bystander replenishment of serological memory. Indeed, fully correlating with its potent induction of Blimp-1, IL-21 was also shown to induce not only the differentiation of high numbers of plasma cells but also the production of large amounts of IgG. IL-21 has the capacity to induce up-regulation of AID (activation-induced cytidine deaminase) and class switch recombination (CSR) but not somatic hypermutation, which are two mechanisms respectively governed by the C-terminal and N-terminal part of AID [37]. Several other works have described the CSR property of IL-21, which seems to lead to different outcomes regarding isotypes and IgG subclasses, depending on the nature and original location of the studied B lymphocytes [35,38,39]. The physiologically relevant and predominant role of IL-21 in plasma cell differentiation was further evidenced in experimental settings based on T cell-B cell collaboration. Indeed, neutralization of IL-21 significantly inhibits T cell-induced naïve and memory human B cell differentiation into Ig-secreting cells [40]. Moreover, Bryant et al. [41] showed that the ability of human tonsillar follicular helper T cells to induce plasma cell differentiation is mediated by IL-21, knowing that they are a major source of this cytokine (see below).

Production of IL-21

IL-21 is not detected in normal tissues but is most notably expressed by $CD4^+$ T cells following activation with phorbol myristate acetate (PMA) and ionomycin or CD3 and CD28 ligation [16]. Among $CD4^+$ T cells, various functional subsets were shown to be capable of producing IL-21, i.e, Th1 cells, which are involved in the control of viruses and intracellular pathogens, Th2 cells, which mediate Ab responses to extracellular pathogens and Th17 cells, which mediate inflammatory processes [42]. Although IL-21 has no role in Th1 and Th2 differentiation, it is required for the generation of Th17 cells in mice and humans [43,44]. In mice, IL-21 was also shown to be secreted by *ex vivo* activated NKT cells [45]. Moreover, α-galactosylceramide (a ligand known to activate NKT cells) administration into C57BL/6 mice leads to IL-21 mRNA expression by NKT cells purified from liver and spleen. To date, no data are available regarding the IL-21 production by human NKT cells. Recently, it was shown that T follicular helper cells (T_{FH}), which localize into germinal centers (GC), produce vast amounts of IL-21 mRNA and protein both in mice [46,47] and humans [48]. T_{FH}, identified by their expression of the CXC chemokine receptor 5 (CXCR5), PD-1 (Programmed Death-1), and ICOS (Inducible T cell CO-Stimulator, especially in humans) are involved in the GC formation and function and therefore in the B cell response. To date, the production of IL-21 by $CD4^+CD25^+$ regulatory T cells has not been evidenced. Finally, $CD4^+$ T cells expressing high levels of ICOS but not CXCR5, suggesting an extrafollicular localization, was described as the major source of IL-21 in BXSB-Y*aa* and MRL-Fas^{lpr} lupus mice [49,50].

IL-21 and SLE

IL-21 Expression in Murine Models of Lupus

One of the first observations of IL-21 involved in SLE was made by Ozakietal. In 2004, whodescribedelevatedIL-21 at the transcriptional and serum protein levels, in BXSB. Y*aa*mice,which develop an SLE-like disease [28]. The elevation of IL-21 transcripts was observed in 16-week-old but not in 8-week-old BXSB. Y*aa* mice [50], indicating that the IL-21 elevation correlates with the development of the disease.

Interestingly, in IL-21 receptor (IL-21R) deficient BXSB-Y*aa* mice, levels of antinuclear Ab were significantly decreased and no splenomegaly, lymphadenopathy nor spontaneous atypical GC formation were observed. More importantly, kidneys of BXSB-Y*aa*/IL-21R-/- mice did not exhibit any pathological features, resulting in an extended lifespan [50].

Taken together, these data support a key role of IL-21 in the production of auto Ab and tissue injury. Studiesin MRL-Fas^{lpr} mouse, another model of SLE, showed a10-fold increase of IL-21 secretion by activated $CD4^+$ T cells compared to cells from controlmice [51]. Moreover,even if the addition of IL-21 enhanced *in vitro* proliferation and IgG secretion of all CD40/IgM-activated B cells, Blymphocytes from MRL-Fas^{lpr} mice were the most responsive as compared to healthy or Fas-intact MRL mice. Finally, arandommutagenesis-generated mouse, called "sanroque", unexpectedly brought some evidence of a role for IL-21 in SLE. This mouse has a mutation in anenzyme (the ubiquitinligaseroquin) that disrupts are pressor of ICOS, an essential costimulator of T_{FH}cells. Consequences are an excessive number of T_{FH} and GC reactions, high levels of IL-21 and the development to fasevere SLE-like autoimmune syndrome [52,53].

Expression of IL-21 and IL-21R in Lupus Patients

Two independent studies reported that T cells of SLE patients exhibit similar levels of IL-21R than T cells from healthy individuals [54,55]. Concerning B cells, cell surface expression of IL-21R was shown to be lower in lupus patients than controls [54,56], and this decreased expression was associated with nephritis and high titers of anti-DNA Ab [56]. However, the lowered expression level of IL-21R on B cells was not confirmed in a recent study [55]. These discrepancies may be explained by differences between B cell populations that were analyzed and between patient characteristics (disease activity, treatment), and further studies are needed to clarify this point.

Serum levels of IL-21 were found to be elevated in patients with SLE [34,54,57]. The high level of IL-21 does not seem to be associated with disease activity as defined by the SLEDAI, however the IL-21 level increased in patients with lupus nephritis and correlated with disease severity [57]. Analysis by real-time-PCR of skin biopsies taken from 3 patients with lupus revealed that IL-21 transcripts were significantly increased compared to control individuals [58].

As described above, IL-21 is mainly produced by a range of differentiated $CD4^+$Th cells, such as Th17 and T_{FH}cells. Interestingly, there is an increased proportion of IL-21-secreting T cells in lupus patients as compared to healthy individuals ($10.2 \pm 5.4\%$ *vs* $6.5 \pm 3.5\%$, $p=0.007$), which correlates with the proportion of IL-17-secreting cells ($r=0.55$, $p=0.0006$) [55]. Moreover, itwasrecentlydescribed that the frequency of circulating T_{FH} cells defined as $CD4^+CXCR5^+PD\text{-}1^{high}$T lymphocytes was significantly increased in lupus patients ($n=17$, median 1.16% among $CD4^+$Tcells) compared to healthy controls ($n=6$, median 0.33% among $CD4^+$ T cells, $p=0.0046$) [59].

PolymorphismWithinIL-21AndIL-21RGenes

The human IL-21 genemaps to 4q26-q27 chromosome, and interestingly, genome-wide association (GWA) studies have provided evidence that this chromosom alregion containing the IL-2 and IL-21 genesis associated with chronic inflammatory disorders, including celiac disease, psoriasis, diabetes, rheumatoid arthritis and SLE [60]. Several respective predisposing single-nucleotidepoly morphisms (SNPs) have been described and among these, rs6822844, in the intergenicregion between IL-21 and IL-2, has been shown to be the most significantly associated with multiple autoimmune diseases [61, 62]. However, regarding lupus patients, are cent work demonstrated that rs6822844 is only modestly associated with lupus in European ancestry (a total of 4248 lupus patients *vs* 3818 controls; Oddsratio (OR): 1.12, p=0.014) and not with African American population (1569 lupus patients *vs* 1893 controls, odds ratio: 1.13, p=0.41) ([63]; Table 1).

Using a population-basedcase-control approach (a total of 1318 independent lupuspatients and 1318 healthy controls matched forsex, ageand race), Sawalhaetal. Genotyped three SNPs in the IL-21 gene [64]. By performing association analyses, they found agenetic association with lupus and 2 of these SNPs, namely rs2221903 located within these condintron and rs907715 located with in the third in tron (Table 1).

Stratification by racerevealed that rs2221903 is associated with lupus in both European-American and African-American lupus patients (OR=1.19, p=0.044 and OR=1.63, p=0.014, respectively), while rs907715 is only associated with European-American lupus patients (OR:1.29, p=0.002). The analys is of the association between 16 confirmed susceptibility loci with lupus manifestations, revealed that the SNP rs907715 associated with haematological disorders (OR:1.13, p=0.0027; false discovery rate (FDR) <0.05)[65].

By examining gene-gene interactions in some of the previously established and confirmed susceptibility loci for lupus, and using a large set of lupus patients and controls (4248 lupus patients and 3818 healthy controls), Hughes et al. recently described a suggestive gene-gene interaction (FDR>0.05 and ≤0.25) between rs907715 in IL-21 and rs11568821 in PD-1 (interaction OR:1.16, P=0.0084) [66].

This result is particularly interesting in the lupus context, as PD-1 is expressed at high levels on mouse and human T_{FH} cells [67], and as these T_{FH}cells are clearly defined by their ability to provide help to B cells for antibody production at least partly through IL-21 secretion. Of note, in a subset of lupus patients, the levels of circulating T_{FH}cells was increased [59].

A genetic polymorphis min IL-21R was also evaluated in 2 in dependent cohorts, one composed of European individuals (2573 lupus patients and 3075 healthy controls) and the other one of Hispanic ancestry (657 lupus patients and 265 healthy controls).

Table 1. Genetic association between SNPs within IL-21 and IL-21R

SNP	Associated allele	cohort n	origin	OR (95% CI)	p	ref
IL-21						
Rs6822844	C	4248	European	1.12 (1.02-1.23)	0.014	[63]
Rs6822844	C	1569	African	1.13 (0.85-1.51)	0.41	[63]
Rs907715	G	644	European	1.29 (1.10-1.52)	0.002	[64]
Rs907715	G	366	African	1.16 (0.94-1.43)	0.18	[64]
Rs2221903	G	644	European	1.19 (1.01-1.41)	0.044	[64]
Rs2221903	G	366	African	1.63 (1.10-2.41)	0.014	[64]
IL-21R						
Rs3093301	A	2573	European	1.13 -1.05-1.23)	0.0022	[68]
Rs3093301	A	657	Hispanic	1.43 (1.13-1.80)	0.025	[68]
Rs3093301	A	3230*	European+hispanic	1.16 (1.08-1.25)	10^{-4}	[68]

*Meta-analysis; 95% CI: 95% confidence interval.

Among 17SNPs genotyped in this study, one was found to associate with lupus, namely rs3093301 in both the European-derived and Hispanic cohorts (OR:1.13, p=0.002 and OR: 1.43, p=0.0025 respectively) ([68]; Table 1).

Recently, by examining the copy number variations of Th17-related genes and possible association with SLE, Yu et al. found that genotype and allele frequencies for copy number amplification of IL-21 were significantly higher in SLE patients than in healthy individuals (938 lupus Chinese patients *vs* 1017 controls, p values for genotype and allele frequencies of 5.26×10^{-31} and 6.12×10^{-33} respectively, OR=12.24; [69]). Moreover, increased copy numbers of IL-21 correlated with elevated mRNA levels [69].

Treatment of Spontaneous Lupus Mice Using Agents Able to Block IL-21/IL-21R Signaling

Regarding the role of IL-21 on B cell differentiation and the description of elevated levels of IL-21 in lupus mice, it appeared reasonable to envisage that blocking the IL-21 signaling could influence the disease development. Neutralization of IL-21 was evaluated in lupus mice using a fusion protein consisting in the IL-21R linked to the Fc domain of a mouse IgG2a (IL-21R.Fc), which binds to IL-21 and prevents activation of its receptor.

The administration of IL-21R.Fc into 8-week-old BXSB-Y*aa* mice (400µg intraperitoneally) every 2 days during 24 weeks, led to a decline in IL-21 and in circulating IgG1 levels (but not IgG2a, IgG2b, IgG3) as measured in sera from BXSB-Y*aa* treated mice [50]. However, the levels of anti-dsDNA Ab and of antinuclear Ab were not statistically different between groups that were treated or not with the IL-21R.Fc. The protein levels tend to be lower in treated mice compared to control mice, but IL-21R.Fc administration did not statistically ameliorate life span of the animals. Overall, these data suggest that IL-21R.Fc therapy only displays a slight benefit in the BXSB-Y*aa* lupus model.

Results obtained in the MRL-Fas^{lpr}are much more promising. Indeed, 8-week-old MRL-Fas^{lpr} treated for 10 weeks with IL-21R.Fc (400µg, 3 times a week, intraperitoneally) have reduced circulating levels of anti-ds-DNA auto Ab and Ig (IgG1 and IgG2a), reduced skin lesions, proteinuria and lymphadenopathy and reduced glomerular IgG deposits [51]. Moreover, B lymphocytes from MRL-Fas^{lpr} mice that received IL-21R.Fc secrete less IgG *ex vivo* after IL-21 stimulation than B lymphocytes from control mice.

Another approach to block the IL-21/IL-21R pathway is to target the IL-21R. Recently, neutralizing Ab against the human and mouse IL-21R have been generated using phage display and analyzed for their pharmacological activity [70]. Two Ab showed potent inhibition of human and mouse IL-21R in cell-based assays, and were thus evaluated *invivo*. These Ab were administered 3 times a week for 10 weeks intraperitoneally into 12-week-old MRL-Fas^{lpr} mice.

Administration of one of these 2 neutralizing Ab significantly reduced anti-ds-DNA Ab titers and reduced IgG deposits in the kidneys when compared to control mice. These data indicate that anti-IL-21R Ab may represent another useful alternative to block the IL-21 signaling pathway in lupus.

Conclusion

Data that have been gathered to date underscore the potential involvement of IL-21 in pathogenic processes in SLE (Figure 3), both in murine models and in patients, and indicate that interfering with the action of IL-21might have a promising the rapeutic potential for SLE. However, one should be cautious with global blockade of such a pleiotropic cytokine as it may also lead to failure in mounting regular anti-pathogen/anti-cancer immune responses.

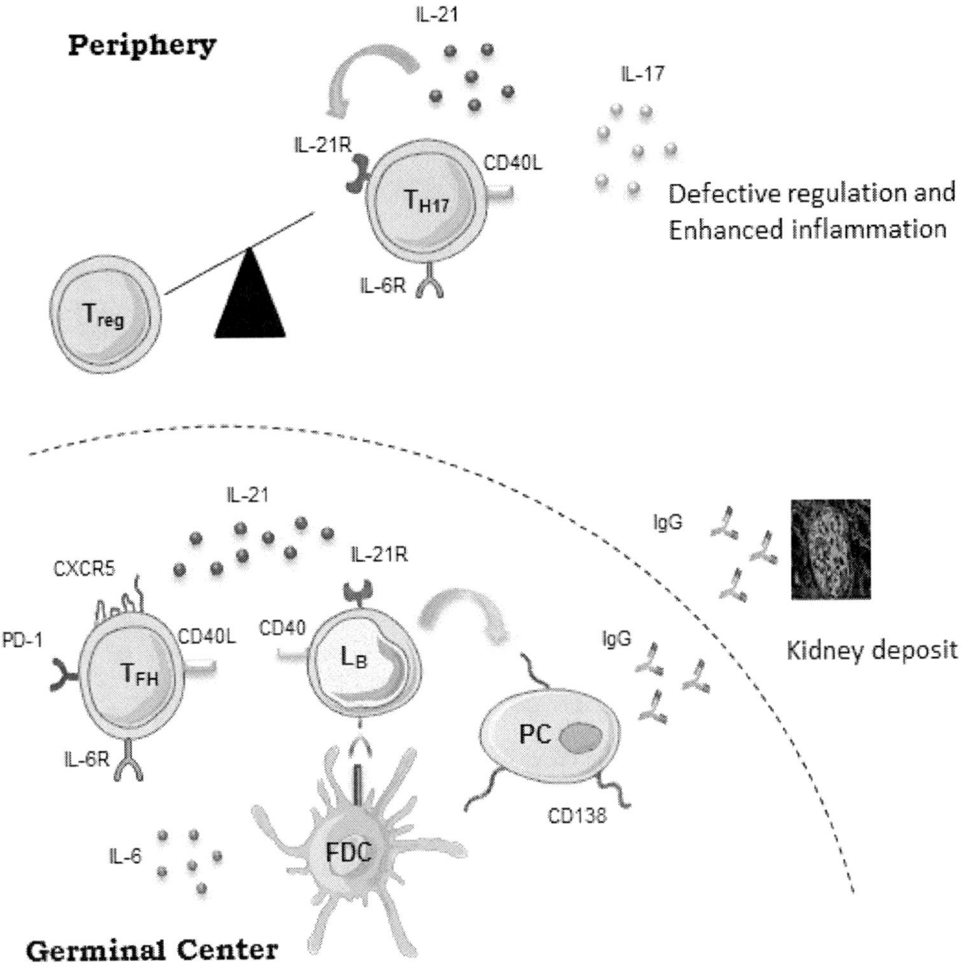

Figure 3. Schematic overview of the hypothetic role of IL-21 in SLE pathogenesis. Within germinal centers, activated T_{FH} produce high levels of IL-21 (due to an increased number of T_{FH} and/or to intrinsic defects), which in turn, drive B cells that have taken up Ag held on follicular dendritic cells (FDC) to differentiate into plasma cells. Secreted auto Abs can then get back to the circulation and reach target organs such as kidneys. In the periphery, excessive Il-21 production promotes the differentiation of Th17 cells, but inhibits the development of regulatory T cells (Tregs), resulting in enhanced secretion of proinflammatory cytokines such as IL-17 and a reduced capacity of immune cell regulation.

References

[1] Northway, J. D. and Tan, E. M. (1972) Differentiation of antinuclear anti bodies giving speckled staining patterns in immunofluorescence.*Clin. Immunol. Immunopathol.* 1, 140-154.

[2] Mattioli, M. and Reichlin, M. (1973) Physical association of two nuclear antigens and mutual occurrence of their antibodies: there lationship of the Sm and RNA protein (Mo) systems in SLEsera. *J. Immunol.* 110, 1318-1324.

[3] Yurasov, S., Wadermann, H., Hammersen, J., Tsuiji, M., Meffre, E., Pascual, V., et al. (2005) Defective B cell tolerance checkpoints in systemic lupusery the matosus. *J. Exp. Med.*201,703-711.

[4] Davidson, A. and Aranow, C.(2010) Lupus nephritis: lessons from murine models. *Nat. Rev. Rheumatol.*6,13-20.

[5] Muller, S.,Dieker,J.,Tincani,A. and Meroni,P.L.(2008) Pathogenicanti-nucleosome antibodies. *Lupus*17,431-436.

[6] Kalaaji,M., Fenton, K.A., Mortensen,E.S., Olsen,R., Sturfelt,G., Alm,P., et al.(2007) Glomerularapoptoticnucleo some sarecentraltargetstructuresfornephritogenic antibodies in human SLE nephritis. *Kidney Intern.*71, 664-672.

[7] Lacotte, S., Dumortier,H.,Décossas,M., Briand,J.-P. and Muller, S.(2010) Identification of new pathogenic players in lupus: autoantibody-secreting cells are present in nephritic kidneys of (NZBxNZW) F1mice. *J. Immunol.* 184,3937-3945.

[8] Chang,A.,Henderson,S.G.,Brandt,D.,Liu,N.,Guttikonda,R.,Hsieh,C.,etal.(2011) In situ B cell-Mediated immune responses and tubulointerstitial inflammation in human lupus nephritis.*J.Immunol.*186,1849-1860.

[9] Nacionales,D.C.,Weinstein,J.S.,Yan,X.-J.,Albesiano,E.,Lee,P.Y.,Kelly-Scumpia, K.M.,et al. (2009) B cell proliferation, somatic hypermutation, class switch recombination, and auto antibody production in ectopic lymphoid tissue in murine lupus. *J. Immunol.* 182,4226-4236.

[10] Odendahl, M.,Jacobi, A.,Hansen,A.,Feist,E., Hiepe,F.,Burmester,G.R.,et al. (2000) Disturbed peripheral B lymphocyte homeostasis in systemic lupus erythematosus. *J. Immunol.*165,5970-5979.

[11] Jacobi,A.M., Odendahl, M., Reiter,K., Bruns,A., Burmenster,G.R., Radbruch, A.,et al. (2003) Correlation between circulating CD27^{high}plasma cells and diseaseactivity in patients with systemic lupusery the matosus. *Arthritis Rheum.*48,1332-1342.

[12] Gladman, D.D., Hirani,N.,Ibanez,D. and Urowitz, M.B.(2003) Clinically active serologicallyquiescent systemic lupusery the matosus. *J. Rheumatol.*30, 1960-1962.

[13] Mamula, M.J., Fatenejad, S. and Craft,J.(1994) B cells process and present lupus auto antigens that initiate auto immune T cell responses.*J .Immunol.*152,1453-1461.

[14] Ma, J., Xu, J., Madaio, M. P., Peng, Q., Zhang, J., Grewal, I. S., et al. (1996) Auto immunelpr/lprmice deficient in CD40 ligand: spontaneousIgclassswitching with dichotomy of auto antibody responses.*J. Immunol.*157,417-426.

[15] LaCava, A. (2010)Targeting B cells with biologics in SLE. *Expert Opin. Biol. Ther.* 10,1555-1561.

[16] Parris-Novak, J., Dillon, S. R., Nelson, A., Hammond, A., Sprecher, C., Groos, J. A., et al. (2000) Inter leukin 21 and its receptor are involved in NK cell expansion and regulation of lymphocyte function. *Nature* 408,57-63.

[17] Leonard, W. J., Zeng, R. and Spolski, R. (2008) Interleukin 21: a cytokine/cytokine receptor system that has come of age. *J. Leukoc. Biol.* 84, 348-356.

[18] Jin, H., Carrio, R.,Yu, A. and Malek, T. R. (2004) Distinct activation signals determine whether IL-21 induces B cell costimulation, growth arrest, or Bim-dependent apoptosis. *J. Immunol.*173,657-665.

[19] Jin, H. and Malek,T.(2006) Redundant and unique regulation of activated mouse Blymphocytes by IL-4 and IL-21. *J. Leukoc. Biol.* 80, 1416-1423.

[20] Ozaki, K., Hishiya, A., Hatanaka, K., Nakajima, H., Wang, G., Hwu, P., et al. (2006) Over expression of interleukin 21 induces expansion of hematopoietic progenitor cells. *Int. J. Hematol.* 84, 224-230.

[21] Simard, N.,Konforte, D.,Tran, A. H.,Esufali, J., Leonard, W. J. and Paige, C. J. (2011) Analysis of the role of IL-21 in development of murine B cell progenitors in the bone marrow.*J.Immunol.* 186, 5244-5253.

[22] Habib, T., Senadheera, S., Weinberg, K. and Kaushansky, K. (2002) The common gamma chain(gammac) is are quired signaling componentt of the IL-21 receptor and supports IL-21-induced cell proliferation via JAK3. *Biochemistry* 41, 8725-8731.

[23] Konforte, D. and Paige,C.J.(2006) Identification of cellular intermediates and molecular pathways induced by IL-21 in human B cells. *J .Immunol.*177,8381-8392.

[24] Zeng, R., Spolski, R.,Casas, E.,Zhu, W.,Levy, D. E. and Leonard, W. J. (2007) The molecular basis of IL-21-mediated proliferation. *Blood* 109, 4135-4142.

[25] de Totero, D., Meazza, R., Zupo, S., Cutrona, G., Matis, S., Colombo, M., et al. (2006) Interleukin-21 receptor (IL-21R) is up-regulated by CD40 triggering and mediat es proapoptotic signals in chronicly mphocytic leukemia B cells. *Blood* 107, 3708-3715.

[26] Avery,D.T., Deenick,E.K.,Ma,C.S.,Suryani,S.,Simpson,N.,Chew,G.Y.,etal.(2010)Bcell-in trinsic signaling through IL-21 receptor and STAT3 is required for establishing long-lived antibody responses in humans. *J. Exp. Med.* 207,155-171.

[27] Good, K. L., Bryant, V. L. and Tangye, S. G. (2006) Kinetics ofhumanB cell behavior and amplific ation of proliferative responses following stimulation with IL-21. *J. Immunol.* 177, 5236-5247.

[28] Ozaki, K.,Spolski, R.,Ettinger, R.,Kim,H. P.,Wang, G.,Qi, C. F., et al. (2004) Regulation of B cell differentiation and plasma cell generation by IL-21, a novel inducer of B limp-1 and Bcl-6. *J. Immunol.* 173,5361-5371.

[29] Mehta, D. S., Wurster, A. L., Whitters, M. J., Young, D. A., Collins, M. and Grusby, M. J. (2003) IL-21 induces the apoptosis of resting and activated primary B cells. *J. Immunol.* 170, 4111-4118.

[30] Ozaki, K., Spolski, R.,Feng, C. G.,Qi, C. F.,Cheng, J.,Sher, A., et al. (2002) Acritical rolc for IL-21 in rcgulating immunoglobulin production. *Science* 298,1630-1634.

[31] Suto, A., Nakajima, H., Hirose, K., Suzuki, K.,Kagami, S., Seto, Y., et al. (2002) Interleukin 21 prevents antigen-induced IgE production by inhibiting germline C(epsilon) transcription of IL-4-stimulated B cells. *Blood* 100, 4565-4573.

[32] Kobayashi, S., Haruo, N., Sugane, K.,Ochs, H. D. and Agematsu, K. (2009) Inter leukin-21 stimulates B-cell immunoglobulin Esynthesis in human beings concomitantly

with activation-induced cytidinedeaminase expression and differentiation into plasma cells. *Hum. Immunol.* 70, 35-40.

[33] Rankin, A. L., MacLeod, H., Keegan, S., Andreyeva, T.,Lowe, L.,Bloom, L., et al. (2011) IL-21 receptor is critical for the development of memory B cell responses. *J. Immunol.* 186, 667-674.

[34] Ettinger, R., Kuchen, S. and Lipsky, P. E. (2008). The role of IL-21in regulating B-cell function in health and disease. *Immunol. Rev.* 223,60-86.

[35] Ettinger, R.,Sims, G. P.,Fairhurst, A. M.,Robbins, R.,daSilva, Y. S.,Spolski, R. et al. (2005) IL-21 induces differentiation of human naïve and memory B cells in to antibody-secreting plasma cells. *J. Immunol.* 175,7867-7879.

[36] Ettinger, R., Sims, G. P.,Robbins, R.,Withers, D.,Fischer, R. T.,Grammer, A. C., et al.(2007)IL-21 and BAFF/BLyS synergize in stimulating plasma cell differentiation from a unique population of humans plenic memory B cells. *J. Immunol.*178, 2872-2882.

[37] Shinkura, R., Ito, S.,Begum, N. A.,Nagaoka, H.,Muramatsu, M.,Kinoshita, K., et al. (2004) Separate domains of AID are required for somatic hypermutation and class-switch recombination. *Nat. Immunol.* 5, 707-712.

[38] Pène, J., Gauchat, J. F., Lécart, S., Drouet, E., Guglielmi, P., Boulay, V., et al. (2004) Cuttingedge: IL-21 is as witch factor for the production of IgG1 and IgG3 by human B cells. *J. Immunol.* 172, 5154-5157.

[39] Avery, D.T., Bryant, V.L.,Ma,C.S.,de Waal Malefyt, R. and Tangye, S.G.(2008) IL-21-induced isotypes witching to IgG and IgA by humannaive B cells is differentially regulated by IL-4. *J. Immunol.* 181, 1767-177 9.

[40] Kuchen, S.,Robbins, R.,Sims, G. P.,Sheng, C., Phillips, T. M.,Lipsky, P. E., et al.(2007) Essential role of IL-21 in B cell activation, expansion, and plasma cell generation during CD4+Tcell-B cell collaboration. *J. Immunol.*179,5886-5896.

[41] Bryant, V. L.,Ma, C. S., Avery, D. T.,Li, Y.,Good, K. L.,Corcoran, L. M. et al.,(2007) Cytokine-mediated regulation of human B cell differentiation into Ig-secreting cells:predominant role of IL-21 produced by CXCR5+T follicular helper cells. *J. Immunol.*179,8180-8190.

[42] Spolski, R. and Leonard, W. J. (2008) Interleukin-21: basic biology and implications for cancer and auto immunity. *Ann.Rev. Immunol.* 26, 57-79.

[43] Korn,T.,Bettelli,E.,Gao,W., Awasthi, A., Jager, A., Strom, T. B., et al. (2007) IL-21 initiates an alternative pathway to induce proinflammatory T(H)17 cells. *Nature* 448, 484-487.

[44] Yang,L.,Anderson,D.E.,Baecher-Allan,C.,Hastings,W.D., Bettelli, E., Oukka, M., et al. (2008) IL-21 and TGF-beta are required for differentiation of human T(H)17 cells. *Nature*454, 350-352

[45] Coquet,J.,Kyparissoudis,K.,Pellicci,D.G.,Besra,G.,Berzins,S.P.,Smyth,M.J.,Godfrey,D. I.(2007) IL-21 is produced by NKT cells and modulates NKT cell activation and cytokine production. *J. Immunol.*178,2827-2834.

[46] Nurieva, R. I., Chung, Y., Hwang, D., Yang, X. O., Kang, H. S., Ma, L., et al. (2008) Generation of T follicular helper cells is mediated by interleukin-21 but independent of T helper 1, 2 or 17 lineages. *Immunity* 29, 138-149.

[47] Vozelgang, A., McGuire, H. M., Yu, D., Sprent, J., Mackay, C. R. and King, C. (2008) A fundamental role for interleukin-21 in the generation of T follicular helper cells. *Immunity*29, 127-137.

[48] Chtanova, T., Tangye, S. G., Newton, R., Franck, N., Hodges, M. R., Rolph, M. S. and Mackay, C. R. (2004) T follicular helper cells express a distinctive transcriptional profile, reflecting their role as non-Th1/Th2 effector cells that provide help for B cells. *J.Immunol.* 173, 68-78.

[49] Odegard, J. M., Marks, B. R., DiPlacido, L. D., Poholek, A. C., Kono, D. H., Dong, C., et al. (2008) ICOS-dependent extra follicular helper T cells elicit IgG production via IL-21 in systemic autoimmunity. *J. Exp.Med.* 205, 2873-2886.

[50] Bubier, J. A., Sproule, T. J., Foreman, O., Spolski, R., Shaffer, D. J., Morse III, H. C., et al. (2009) A critical role for IL-21 receptor signalling in the pathogenesis of systemic lupus erythematosus in BXSB-Yaa mice. *Proc. Natl. Acad. Sci. US.* 106, 1518-1523.

[51] Herber, D., Brown, T. P., Liang, S., Young, D. A., Collins, M. and Dunussi-Joannopoulos, K. (2007)IL-21 has a pathogenic role in a lupus-pronemouse model and its blockade with IL-21R.Fc reduces disease progression. *J. Immunol.*178,3822-3830.

[52] Vinuesa, C. G., Cook, M. C., Angelucci, C., Athanasopoulos, V.,Rui, L.,Hill, K. M., et al. (2005) ARING-type ubiquity in ligase family member required to repress follicular helper Tcells and auto immunity. *Nature*435,452-458.

[53] Linterman, M. A.,Rigby, R. J.,Wong, R. K.,Yu, D.,Brink, R.,Cannons, J. L.,Schwartzberg, P. L., et al. (2009). Follicular helper T cells are required for systemic auto immunity. *J. Exp. Med.*206,561-576.

[54] Wong, C. K., Wong, P. T. Y., Tam, L. S., Li, E. K., Chen, D. P. and Lam, C. W. K. (2010) Elevated production of B cell chemokine CXCL13 is correlated with systemic lupus erythematosus disease activity. *J.Clin.Immunol.* 30, 45-52.

[55] Dolff, S., Abdulahad, W. H., Westra, J., Doornbos-van der Meer, B., Limburg, P. C., Kallenberg, C. G. M. and Bijl, M. (2011) Increase in IL-21 producing T-cells in patients with systemic lupus erythematosus. *Arthr.Res.Ther.* 13, R157.

[56] Mitoma, H., Horiuchi, T., Kimoto, Y., Tsukamoto, H., Uchino, A., Tamimoto, Y., et al. (2005) Decreased expression of interleukin-21 receptor on peripheral B lymphocytes in systemic lupus erythematosus. *Int.J.Mol.Med.* 16, 609-615.

[57] Wang, X. F., Yuan, S. L., Jiang, L., Zhang, X. L., Li, S. F., Guo, Y., et al. (2007) Changes of serum BAFF and IL-21 levels in patients with systemic lupus erythematosus and their clinical significance. *Xi Bao Yu Fen Mian Yi XueZaZhi* 23, 1041-1042.

[58] Caruso, R., Booti, E., Sarra, M., Esposito, M., Stolfi, C., Diluvio, L., et al. (2009) Involvement of inter leukin-21 in the epidermal hyperplasia of psoriasis. *Nat.Med.* 15, 113-1015.

[59] Simpson,N.,Gatenby,P. A.,Wilson,A.,Malik,S.,Fulcher,D. A.,Stuart,G.,etal. (2010) Expansion of circulating T cells resembling follicular helper T cells is a fixed phenotype that identifies as ubset of severe systemic lupusery the matosus. *Arthritis Rheum.* 62, 234-244.

[60] Monteleone, G., Pallone, F. and Macdonald, T. T. (2009) Interleukin-21 as a new therapeutic target for immune-mediated diseases. *Trends Pharmacol. Sci.*30, 441-447.

[61] VanHeel, D. A., Franke, L., Hunt,K. A., Gwilliam, R., Zhernakova, A., Inouye, M.,et al. (2007) Agenome-wideassociation study for celiac diseases identifies risk variants in the region harbouring IL2 a nd IL21. *Nat. Genet.*39, 827-829.
[62] Festen,E. A.,Goyette,P.,Scott,R.,Annese,V.,Zhernakova,A.,Lian,J.,etal. (2009) Genectic variants in the region harbouring IL2/IL21 associated with ulcer at ivecolitis.*Gu t*58, 799-804.
[63] Hughes, T., Kim-Howard, X., Kelly, J. A., Kaufman, K. M., Langefeld, CD., Ziegler, J., et al. (2011) Fine-mapping and trans ethnic genotyping establish IL2/IL21 genetic association with lupus and localize this genetic effect to IL21. *Arthritis Rheum.* 63,1689-1697.
[64] Sawalha, A. H., Kaufman, K. M., Kelly, J. A., Adler, A.J., Aberle, T., Kilpatrick,J.,et al.(2008) Genetic association of interleukin-21 polymorphisms with systemic lupusery the matosus. *Ann. Rheum. Dis.*67, 458-461.
[65] Sanchez ,E., Nadig,A., Richardson,B. C., Freedman,B. I., Kaufman,K. M., Kelly,J. A. , et al. (2001) Phenotypic associations of genetic susceptibility lociin systemic lupusery the matosus. *Ann. Rheum. Dis.*70,1752-1757.
[66] Hughes, T., Adler, A., Kelly, J.A., Kaufman, K.M., Williams, A., Langefeld, C.D.,et al.(2011) Evidence for gene-gene epistatic interactions among susceptibility loci for systemic lupusery the matosus. *Arthritis Rheum.*doi:10.1002/art.33354.
[67] Crotty, S. (2010) Follicular helper CD4 T cells (TFH). *Ann. Rev. Immunol.* 29,621-623.
[68] Webb, R., Merrill, J. T., Kelly, J. A., Sestak, A., Kaufman, K. M., Langefeld, C. D.,etal. (2009) Apolymorphism within IL 21R confers risk for systemic lupusery the matosus. *Arthritis Rheum.*60, 2402-2407.
[69] Yu, A., Guan, M., Peng, Y., Shao, Y., Zhang, C., Yue, X., et al. (2011) Copy number variations of interleukin-17F, inter leukin-21, and inter leukin-22 are associated with systemic lupusery the matosus. *Arthritis Rheum.* 63, 3487-3492.
[70] Vugmenyster, Y., Guay, H., Szkklut, P., Qian, M. D., Jin, M., Widom, A., et al. (2010) In vitro potency, pharmacokinetic profiles and pharmacological activity of optimized anti-IL-21R antibodies in a mouse model of lupus. *mAbs* 2, 335-346.

In: Lupus: Symptoms, Treatment and Potential Complications ISBN: 978-1-62081-078-1
Editors: T. D. Marquez and D. U. Neto

Chapter VII

Metabolic Syndrome and Inflammatory Cytokines in Systemic Lupus Erythematosus

Nailú Angélica Sinicato, Jozélio Freire de Carvalho and Simone Appenzeller*
Department of Medicine, Rheumatology Unit,
Faculty of Medical Science, State University of Campinas,
Cidade Universitária, Campinas SP, Brazil

Abstract

Systemic lupus erythematosus (SLE) is a chronic, multisystemic autoimmune disease predominantly affecting women of childbearing age. The impact of coronary heart disease (CHD) on morbidity and mortality in patients with established SLE has assumed increasing importance in their long-term management. Classic CHD risk factors and lupus-specific factors, such as antiphospholipid antibodies and nephrotic proteinuria, seem to be important in determining long-term cardiovascular risk, but the role of metabolic derangement, specifically the metabolic syndrome (MetS), is gaining increasing prominence in the literature.

One very important aspects of classical cytokines derived from inflammatory cells is their importance in the pathogenesis of the metabolic syndrome. A generally enhanced adipose tissue-derived cytokine expression may be one plausible mechanism for the inflammation–MetS relationship. MetS can be associated with increased risk of develop autoimmune inflammatory diseases like SLE.

The best treatment to MetS in SLE patients is maximizing lifestyle therapies. Statins treatment are used to reduction levels of low-density lipoprotein cholesterol (LDL-c) and one of the various immunomodulatory functions realized by statins, is to be able to

* Correspondence to: Simone Appenzeller-Department of Medicine, Faculty of Medical Science, State University of Campinas, Cidade Universitária, Campinas SP, Brazil, CEP 13083-970; FAX: +55 19 3289-1818, Email: appenzellersimone@yahoo.com

reduce atherosclerotic vascular disease in SLE by lowering immune activation in the arterial wall and by attenuating SLE activity, but this result is not unanimous.

In this chapter we will review the prevalence and importance of Mets in SLE and its implication in mortality in SLE.

Keywords: Metabolic Syndrome, Tumor necrosis factor alpha (TNF-α), systemic lupus erythematosus

Introduction

Systemic lupus erythematosus (SLE) is a chronic, multisystemic autoimmune disease predominantly affecting women of childbearing age [1]. However, 10–20% of all SLE cases occur approximately in the first two decades of life [2]. This disease is characterized by periods of remission and exacerbation [3].

The bimodal pattern of mortality, observed for over 30 years is characterized by early death due to predominantly active disease and infection, and a predominance of cardiovascular disease (CVD) in patients with more than 10 years of disease [6-8]. With improvement of life expectancy in the past decades, reaching an survival rate of over 80% in 10 years, evidence points to an increased morbidity and mortality from CVD in SLE patients [4,5]. Patients with SLE have a 5- to 6-fold increased risk for CVD, and this excess risk is especially pronounced in younger women [6].

The impact of coronary heart disease (CHD) on morbidity and mortality in patients with established SLE has assumed increasing importance in their long-term management. Classic CHD risk factors and lupus-specific factors, such as antiphospholipid antibodies and nephrotic proteinuria, seem to be important in determining long-term cardiovascular risk, but the role of metabolic derangement, specifically the metabolic syndrome (MetS), is gaining increasing prominence in the literature [7].

CVD in SLE

The reason why SLE patients are affected by CVD so frequently has been studied by many authors [8-15]. SLE is characterized by chronic inflammation and inflammation is a prominent feature of atherosclerotic lesions [5]. Although clinically manifestation of ischemic heart disease have been observed between 8% and 16% in various studies of SLE patients [15-18], the frequency of subclinical coronary artery disease (CAD) is likely to be considerably higher. Perfusion abnormalities have been reported in up to 38% of adult SLE patients [19-21] and even in 16% of children with SLE [22]. Through the use of various noninvasive methods, atherosclerosis was detected in 28-40% of SLE patients [5,23-26], and was associated with increasing age and longer disease duration [27-31].

Epidemiological observations have linked inflammation to CVD in general population [32, 33]. Clinical epidemiological observations strongly suggest that, together with classical conventional risk factors, other mechanisms (non-conventional/disease-specific factors) promote accelerated atherosclerosis in inflammatory diseases like SLE [10-14]. The excess risk observed in autoimmune disease appears to be driven by systemic inflammation that directly or indirectly damages the vasculature and promotes atherosclerosis.

Traditional Risk Factors

Traditional risk factors are factors commonly associated with predisposition to CVD in general population. Epidemiologic studies have identified several risk factors, such as smoking, diabetes mellitus, hypertension and dyslipidemia, involved in the pathogenesis of atherosclerosis in general population [34]. New risk factors, such as homocysteinemia, elevated plasma levels of lipoprotein(a) [Lp(a)], excessive iron load in the body, an imbalance between oxidant and antioxidant species and hypercoagulability have also been linked to the atherosclerosis process [34 –39]. In addition, several genetic markers of atherosclerosis and CAD, were identified, such as angiotensin-converting enzyme polymorphism and human leukocyte antigen (HLA)-DR class II genotypes [40-44].

Several studies have addressed the question of whether the frequency and level of traditional risk factors in SLE patients differ from those observed in age and sex-matched healthy controls [5, 16, 23, 45-47]. These studies have shown that traditional risk factors do not entirely count for the increase risk of CVD in SLE and only a few significant differences have been observed such as adverse lipid profile in SLE, including increased serum levels of total cholesterol, triglycerides and LDL cholesterol [33,48] (Figure 1).

MetS is considered an independent predictor of cardiovascular morbidity and mortality that identifies substantial additional cardiovascular risk beyond the sum of the individual risk factors.

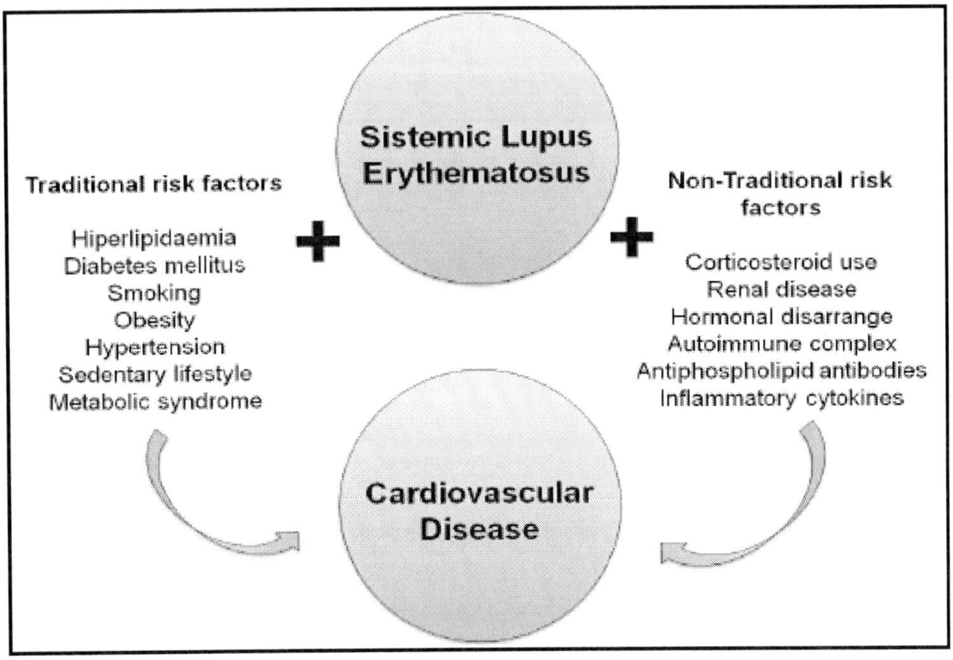

Figure 1. A diagram illustrating traditional and non-traditional risk factors for CVD.

MetS is actually defined by a cluster of different metabolic risk factors that includes atherogenic dyslipidemia, abdominal obesity, elevated blood pressure and elevated plasma glucose associated with insulin resistance and a pro-inflammatory state [3,49]. Recently, representatives from International Diabetes Federation (IDF) decided to uniform the criteria for MetS. MetS was therefore defined as the presence of 3 of 5 features: elevated waist circumference (based on population- and country-specific definitions), elevated triglycerides, reduced HDL-C, elevated blood pressure, and elevated fasting glucose levels [50] (Table 1).

The prevalence of MetS in the National Health and Nutrition Examination Survey (1999–2002) ranged from 20% to almost 40% in general population, depending on which MetS definition was used [51]. In addition to the cardiovascular risk factors that comprise the metabolic syndrome, there is a strong relationship with inflammation. Several studies have shown an increase in MetS in SLE, with prevalence ranging from 16.3% – 38.2% [3,52-56]. On important finding is that SLE patients have an increased risk for cardiovascular events even after adjustment for Framingham risk factors (hypertension, hypercholesterolemia, diabetes mellitus, older age, and postmenopausal status) [32], so it is necessary to develop other methods to determine the subgroup of SLE patients that are at highest risk for CVD disease. Although traditional risk factors as defined by the Framingham studies are important in increasing risk for atherosclerosis in SLE, they do not adequately explain the increase in cardiovascular disease [32] and this suggests that disease-related factors constitute an equal or even greater risk.

Table 1. IDF definition for Mets and references values

Indice / Definition	IDF 10-16	IDF >16
Elevated fasting glucose (mg/dL)	>100	>110
Elevated blood pressure (mmHg) or antihypertensive drug treatment	>130/ >85	>130/ >85
Triglycerides (mg/dL)	>150	>150
Reduced HDL-C (mg/dL)	< 40 male < 50 female	< 40 male < 50 female
Central Obesity: waist to hip ratio (cm)	> 90 male > 80 female	> 102 male > 88 female
Albumin excretion	not included	not included
BMI	not included	not included

Non-Traditional Risk Factors

The non-traditional factors present in SLE are Lupus-specific including renal disease [45, 57-59] and corticosteroid use (duration or the cumulative dose of prednisone) [5,17,23,26,60] (Figure 1). It is known that nephritis and corticosteroid therapy are able to aggravate hyperlipidemia, hypertension and obesity [16].

The presence of antiphospholipid antibodies [45,61-64], as well as anti - oxLDL antibodies have been associated with angina and myocardial infarction [5,45,65-67]. Other disease-related factors are the formation of autoimmune complex, pro-inflammatory cytokines and hormonal disarrange [45, 68, 69].

SLE can be considered an independent risk factor for CHD and disease-specific factors but the results available to date are too inconsistent to allow any definite conclusions as to the role of inflammatory mediators in premature atherosclerosis [70].

The data available to date are conflicting does not allow any conclusions about the pathophysiology of accelerated atherosclerosis in SLE patients or about possible preventive measures beyond the treatment of traditional risk factors. Prospective studies are necessary in order to address both of these issues [16].

CVD Features and Cytokines Involved on SLE

Inflammation

The mechanism of inflammation occurs in a response for stimuli of infection, tissue injury and tissue malfunction or homeostatic imbalance. Not much is known about mechanisms of systemic chronic inflammation, particularly in chronic infections and autoimmune diseases [71].

Inflammation can be caused by exogenous (microbial) or endogenous (cell, tissue and plasma derived components), but the physiological mechanisms involved in inflammatory conditions are not clearly understood [71]. It is known that inflammatory cytokines can stimulate the hypothalamic-pituitary-adrenal (HPA), resulting in an increase in glucocorticoid levels that will affect some immune and inflammatory processes [72,73]. We can say that inflammation is able to induce obesity and insulin resistance on the other hand there seems to be a positive feedback because researchers believe that obesity may promote low-grade inflammation [72, 74].

Chronic subclinical inflammation may be an intrinsic part of the MetS, and several studies have shown that a proinflammatory state is an important component to this disease [75]. In SLE patients, the metabolic syndrome was associated with higher levels of inflammation (CRP) and can provide a link between inflammation and increased cardiovascular risk [48].

Obesity

Obesity represents an expansion of adipose tissue mass [76], with an increasing prevalence, has become the most common metabolic disorder in the developed world [77]. The adipose tissue can be considered pathogenic when in excess and numerous adipocytes secrete products which have recently been described that play a role in carbohydrate and lipid metabolism [76]. Obesity also can be considered a low intensity chronic inflammation state [78]. The large number of adipocytes present in obesity attracts increased number of monocytes to infiltrate the tissue; such bond may be the cause of the release of inflammatory cytokines on this process. The accumulation of fat and the systemic inflammation are associated with hypertension, dyslipidemia and atherosclerosis, all compounds of MetS [79,80]. In this way obesity is accompanied by generalized inflammation, characterized by increased plasma c-reative protein (CRP) levels as well as by dys-regulated cytokine production by monocytes, lymphocytes and other immune cells [81]. A group [82] demonstrated that obesity, LDL-c>100mg/dL, older age at lupus diagnostic, higher damage index and nephrotic proteinuria were independently associated with MetS and concluded that some of those factors, especially LDL-c >100mg/dl and age at lupus diagnosis, have been associated with atherosclerosis in lupus patients.

In addition to that, the adipose tissue secrete a variety of cytokines (leptin, adiponectin, resistin, visfatin, IL-6, IL10, TNF-α and resistin) with autocrine/paracrine and endocrine functions that influence body weight and glucose/lipid metabolism [83].

A generally enhanced adipose tissue-derived cytokine expression may be another plausible mechanism for the inflammation–MetS relationship [84] and so MetS can be associated with increased risk of develop autoimmune inflammatory diseases like SLE [84].

Cytokines

Cytokines are definite by regulatory proteins secreted by white blood cells and a variety of other cells on the body [85]. One of the very important aspects of classical cytokines derived from inflammatory cells is their importance in the pathogenesis of the MetS [86].

Among the cytokines released by monocytes on adipose tissue were the ILs´s; IL-10 which has an atheroprotective function, IL-6 which stimulate the release of fatty acids and overproduction of C-reactive protein (CRP), a protein that appears in systemic inflammation and can be a strong predictor for CVD [68]. And inflammatory cytokines like TNF-α which is produced in a large scale by adipose tissue [87] and skeletal muscle [88] and may act in an autocrine manner to modification insulin transduction inhibiting glucose transport, causing in elevated levels, insulin resistance [87]. Studies about TNF-α administration showed that this treatment can causes an increase serum level of triglycerides and very low density lipoproteins in rats and humans [89-91]. Studies with TNF- α blockers in rheumatoid arthritis showed that they can interfere positively on mechanisms on development of atherosclerosis process as well as reduce the cardiovascular risk in this disease [92].

SLE patients presents high TNF-α levels, one of the main inhibitors of adipocytokines production; however it was noted that there is an increase in adipocytokine mainly in SLE patients with renal involvement regardless of the TNF- α of the patient [71].

Others proinflammatory cytokines that are also involved in the development of atherosclerosis are increased in SLE such asinterferon-γ (IFN- γ) [93], IL-12 [94] and IL-18 [95]. There is strong evidence that this cytokines may play a role in the pathogenesis of SLE, independently of the age of onset [96, 97].

Adiponectin is an adipocytokine that acts mainly on skeletal muscle and liver, and increases insulin sensitization. In animals models with induced SLE this adipocytokines can enhance insulin sensibility and could protect against CVD [98]. So it has been suggested that levels of adiponectin may have a protective role in the development of atherosclerosis because adiponectin inhibits proinflammatory cytokines production [99-104].

The release of adipocytokines has the ability to influence and change and vascular endothelial function, favoring hypertension and atherosclerosis. This mechanism could be an explanation for the relationship between obesity and cardiovascular phenotypes [86]. The high level of inflammatory cytokines existing on chronic inflammation may inhibit the production of adipocytokines. Decreased concentration of adipocytokines can be observed along the presence of metabolic syndrome, CVD, and with increasing obesity [98].

Relationship between SLE Treatment in Patients with MetS

Traditional treatment of SLE was established in use of corticosteroids (prednisone, methylpredinisolone, hydrocortisone and dexamethasone), nonsteroidal antiinflammatory drugs, antimalarials (chloroquine and hydroxychloroquine (HCQ)), and immunosuppressive drugs (cyclophosphamide, mycophenolate mofetil, azathioprine and cyclosporine). Studies suggest that steroid treatment using at leats one year can prevent atherosclerosis by decreasing the risk of a CVD [105]. Immunossupressive drugs like cyclosporine can inhibit vascular smooth muscle proliferation [106], and antimalarial had a supposed antilipemic effect [107].

It is well known that glucocorticoids have deleterious side effects with regards to cardiovascular risk and MetS components. Glucocorticoids promote hypertriglyceridemia and insulin resistance and are associated with a higher cholesterol plasma level, higher blood pressure and weight change in lupus patients [106,108]. Researchers [82] found no association of prednisone use and MetS, in accordance with other authors [109,110]. However, another study [52] observed that prednisone use >10 mg/d presented risk factor to MetS (OR:3.7; 95%IC:0.14-0.92). Intravenous methylprednisolone has been previously associated to MetS diagnosis and components in lupus patients [52,111]. So, higher doses of prednisone and intravenous methylprednisolone could be reflective of disease activity and lupus severity [108].

On the other hand, studies proved that HCQ therapy, an immunomodulator, are able to reduce serum cholesterol, triglycerides and fibrinogen and to increase HDL. In addition, hydroxychoroquine therapy reduces the insulin resistance in SLE. The current use of HCQ seemed to be protective against MetS, which remained significant in a multivariate analysis (OR:0.192; 95% CI, 0.061–0.605) [56]. Another study showed that HCQ use was also protective against MetS (OR:0.13; P=0.015) [53].

What Is the Best Treatment to MetS in SLE Patients?

The best treatment to MetS in SLE patients is maximizing lifestyle therapies. It is well established that weight loss is beneficial for treating all of the components of the MetS, including excessive adiposity, dyslipidemia, hypertension, insulin resistance, and hyperglycemia [112].

Statins treatment is the most effective strategies used to reduce CVD and reduce levels of serum lipids and low-density lipoprotein cholesterol (LDL-c). New data identified that statins can have an anti-inflammatory and immune modulator function associated with improvement of endothelial function [113,114]. It has already been showen that SLE patients are most frequently stricken by precocious and aggressive atherosclerotic disease and one of the various immunomodulatory functions realized by statins, is to be able to reduce atherosclerotic vascular disease in SLE by lowering immune activation in the arterial wall and by attenuating SLE activity, but this result is not unanimous and no solid confirmation of this hypothesis is available [115]. Studies demonstrade that activity measured by SLEDAI were lower after a therapy with statins [116,117]. And also a prominent suppression of TNFα in patients treated supposing that statin therapy might be one mechanism to led an improvement of endothelial function [117].

It´s not clear how statins can reduce inflammatory but are suggested that the mechanism may involve inhibition of adhesion molecules and the recruitment of inflammatory cells [118]. Statins reduce expression of adhesion molecules and thereby attenuate adhesion and extravasation. Furthermore, they inhibit expression of major histocompatibility complex class II and costimulatory molecules by antigen-presenting cells and prevent antigen presentation to CD4 T cells [119]. By virtue of the various immunomodulatory functions exerted by statins, they may be able to reduce atherosclerotic vascular disease in SLE by reducing immune activation within the arterial wall and also by attenuating lupus activity [115]. Making the decision whether or not to initiate statin therapy in SLE dependent on the 10-year cardiovascular risk estimate exceeding 10–20%, does not take lupus into account as a risk factor and will result in under treatment [115]. Thus, Statin treatment should be considered more often in patients with SLE, even more so in the presence of concomitant risk factors for CVD.

No evidence was found that atorvastatin reduces subclinical measures of atherosclerosis or disease activity over 2 years in patients with SLE in a double-blind study with 200 SLE patients. This study also does not observe any reduce on biochemical measures of inflammation on this SLE population as observed on general population trials [120].

Although low-dose aspirin is frequently recommended to patients with MetS [121,122], there are no specific studies of the use of aspirin or other antiplatelet agents for the primary prevention of CVD in individuals with the MetS specifically. Long-term use of aspirin therapy has been advocated in the secondary prevention of CVD [123], and some have recommended aspirin in high-risk patients with the MetS, especially those with CVD [122]. Until there are more data, however, the use of aspirin in the primary prevention of CVD should remain as an "individual clinical judgment" [123,124].

Conclusion and Perspective Future

The MetS is characterized by an increase in circulating factors that shift the homeostatic balance from an antithrombotic to a prothrombotic state associated to inflammatory state [125]. Coagulation changes that have been reported to be associated with the metabolic syndrome include increases in circulating fibrinogen, Factor VII, PAI-1 and platelet defects. These factors have been implicated both in atherogenesis itself and in the thrombosis that can complicate atherosclerotic lesions. Both undoubtedly predispose to major cardiovascular events. In addition, 30 a 50% of the SLE patients present antiphospholipid antibodies that increase the thrombotic risk. So, treatment with statins, aspirin or clopidogrel should be considered more often in patients with SLE. Another interesting point is the better understanding about inflammatory citokines and the real function of the adipocytokines in SLE and its relationship with insulin resistance, inflammation and MetS. So, adipocytokines may provide a mechanistic link among impaired insulin sensitivity, obesity, chronic inflammation, and atherosclerosis. Future studies are necessary to evaluate individualized therapeutic regimes that take into account cardiovascular risk.

Acknowledgments

Grants: Fundação de Amparo à Pesquisa do Estado de São Paulo (FAPESP 08/020917-0 and 2009/06049-6 and 2009/15286-1), Conselho Nacional Pesquisa Desenvolvimento-Brasil CNPq (300447/2009-4)

References

[1] Danchenko N, Satia JA, Anthony MS. Epidemiology of systemic lupus erythematosus: a comparison of worldwide disease burden. *Lupus* 2006;15:308–18.

[2] Lee PP, Lee TL, Ho MH, Wong WH, Lau YL. Recurrent major infections in juvenile-onset systemic lupus erythematosus--a close link with long-term disease damage. *Rheumatology* (Oxford). 2007;46:1290-6.

[3] Chung, C. P., Avalos I., Oeser, A., et al. High prevalence of the metabolic syndrome in patients with systemic lupus erythematosus: association with disease characteristics and cardiovascular risk factors. *Ann. Rheum. Dis.* 2007;66:208-214.

[4] Merrell M, Shulman LE. Determination of prognosis in chronic disease, illustrated by systemic lupus erythematosus. *J. Chronic. Dis.* 1955;1:12-32.

[5] Svenungsson E, Jensen-Urstad K, Heimburger M, Silveira A, Hamsten A, HamstenU, et al. Risk factors for cardiovascular disease in systemic lupus erythematosus. *Circulation* 2001;104:1887–93.

[6] Gladman DD, Urowitz MB. Prognosis, mortality and morbidity in systemic lupus erythematosus. In: Wallace DJ, Hahn BH, eds. Dubois' lupus erythematosus. 7th ed. Philadelphia: Lippincott Williams and Wilkins, 2007:1333-53.

[7] Parker B, Bruce IN.The Metabolic Syndrome in Systemic Lupus Erythematosus· *Rheum. Dis. Clin. N. Am.* 2010;36:81–97.

[8] Esdaile JM, Abrahamowicz M, Grodzicky T, et al. Traditional Framingham risk factors fail to fully account for accelerated atherosclerosis in systemic lupus erythematosus. *Arthritis. Rheum.* 2001;44:23331–7.

[9] Haque S, Bruce IN. Therapy insight: systemic lupus erythematosus as a risk factor for cardiovascular disease. *Nat. Clin. Pract. Cardiovasc. Med.* 2005;2:423–30.

[10] Ross R. Atherosclerosis-an inflammatory disease. *N. Engl. J. Med.* 1999;340:115–26.

[11] Willerson JT, Ridker PM. Inflammation as a cardiovascular risk factor. *Circulation.* 2004;109:2–10.

[12] Sattar N, McCarey DW, Capell H, McInnes IB. Explaining how "high-grade" systemic inflammation accelerates vascular risk in rheumatoid arthritis. *Circulation.* 2003;108:2957–63.

[13] Ridker PM, Cushman M, Stampfer MJ, Tracy RP, Hennekens CH. Inflammation, aspirin, and the risk of cardiovascular disease in apparently healthy men. *N. Engl. J. Med.* 1997;336:973–9.

[14] Abou-Raya A, Abou-Raya S. Inflammation: a pivotal link between autoimmune diseases and atherosclerosis. *Autoimmun. Rev.* 2006;5:331–7.

[15] Badui E, Garcia-Rubi D, Robles E, et al. Cardiovascular manifestations in systemic lupus erythematosus. Prospective study of 100 patients. *Angiology.* 1985;36:431–41.

[16] Borchers AT, Keen CL, Shoenfeld Y, Gershwin ME. Surviving the butterfly and the wolf: mortality trends in systemic lupus erythematosus. *Autoimmun. Rev.* 2004;3: 423–53.

[17] Petri M, Perez-Gutthann S, Spence D, Hochberg MC. Risk factors for coronary artery disease in patients with systemic lupus erythematosus. *Am. J. Med.* 1992;93:513–9.

[18] Gladman DD, Urowitz MB. Morbidity in systemic lupus erythematosus. *J. Rheumatol.* 1987;14:223–6.

[19] Bruce IN, Gladman DD, Ibanez D, Urowitz MB. Single photon emission computed tomography dual isotope myocardial perfusion imaging in women with systemic lupus erythematosus: II. Predictive factors for perfusion abnormalities. *J. Rheumatol.* 2003;30:288–91.

[20] Sella EM, Sato EI, Leite WA, Oliveira Filho JA, Barbieri A. Myocardial perfusion cintigraphy and coronary disease risk factors in systemic lupus erythematosus. *Ann. Rheum. Dis.*. 2003;62:1066–70.

[21] Hosenpud JD, Montanaro A, Hart MV, et al. Myocardial perfusion abnormalities in asymptomatic patients with systemic lupus erythematosus. *Am. J. Med.* 1984;77: 286–92.

[22] Gazarian M, Feldman BM, Benson LN, Gilday DL, Laxer RM, Silverman ED. Assessment of myocardial perfusion and function in childhood systemic lupus erythematosus. *J. Pediatr.*. 1998;132:109–16.

[23] Manzi S, Selzer F, Sutton-Tyrrell K, et al. Prevalence and risk factors of carotid plaque in women with systemic lupus erythematosus. *Arthritis. Rheum.* 1999;42:51–60.

[24] Roman MJ, Shanker BA, Davis A, et al. Prevalence and correlates of accelerated atherosclerosis in systemic lupus erythematosus. *N. Engl. J. Med.* 2003;349:2399–406.

[25] Asanuma Y, Oeser A, Shintani AK, et al. Premature coronary-artery atherosclerosis in systemic lupus erythematosus. *N. Engl. J. Med.* 2003;349:2407–15.

[26] Manger K, Kusus M, Forster C, et al. Factors associated with coronary artery calcification in young female patients with SLE. *Ann. Rheum. Dis.*. 2003;62:846–50.

[27] Font J, Ramos-Casals M, Cervera R, et al. Cardiovascular risk factors and the long-term outcome of lupus nephritis. *QJM.* 2001;94:19–26.

[28] Bono L, Cameron JS, Hicks JA. The very long-term prognosis and complications of lupus nephritis and its treatment. *QJM.* 1999;92:211–8.

[29] Reveille JD, Bartolucci A, Alarcon GS. Prognosis in systemic lupus erythematosus. Negative impact of increasing age at onset, black race, and thrombocytopenia, as well as causes of death. *Arthritis. Rheum.* 1990;33:37–48.

[30] Nossent JC. Course and prognostic value of systemic lupus erythematosus disease activity index in black Caribbean patients. *Semin. Arthritis. Rheum.* 1993;23:16–21.

[31] Jacobsen S, Petersen J, Ullman S, et al. Mortality and causes of death of 513 Danish patients with systemic lupus erythematosus. *Scand. J. Rheumatol.* 1999;28:75–80.

[32] Esdaile JM, Abrahamowicz M, Grodzicky T, et al. Traditional Framingham risk factors fail to fully account for accelerated atherosclerosis in systemic lupus erythematosus. *Arthritis. Rheum.* 2001;44:23331–7.

[33] Haque S, Bruce IN. Therapy insight: systemic lupus erythematosus as a risk factor for cardiovascular disease. *Nat. Clin. Pract. Cardiovasc. Med.* 2005;2:423–30.

[34] Mehta JL, Saldeen TGP , Rand K. Interactive Role of Infection, Inflammation and Traditional Risk Factors in Atherosclerosis and Coronary Artery Disease. *JACC.* 1998;31:1217-1225.

[35] D'Angelo A, Selhub J. Homocysteine and thrombotic disease. *Blood* 1997;90:1–11.

[36] Rhoads GG, Dahlen GH, Berg K, Morton NE, Dannenberg AL. Lp(a) lipoprotein as a risk factor for myocardial infarction. *JAMA* 1986;74:758.

[37] Dahlen GH. Lipoprotein (a) atherosclerosis and thrombosis. *Prog. Lipid. Res.* 1991;30:189.

[38] Steinberg D, Parthasarthy S, Carew TE, Khoo JC, Witztum JL. Beyond cholesterol: modification of low-density lipoprotein that increase its atherogenicity. *N. Engl. J. Med.* 1989;320:915–24.

[39] Hamsten A, de-Faire U, Walldius G, et al. Plasminogen activator inhibitor in plasma: risk factor for recurrent myocardial infarction. *Lancet* 1987;2:3–9.

[40] Meyers DG. The iron hypothesis—does iron cause atherosclerosis? *Clin. Cardiol.* 1996;19:925–9.

[41] Cambien F, Polrier O, Lecerf L, et al. Deletion polymorphism in the gene for angiotensin-converting enzyme is a potent risk factor for myocardial infarction. *Nature* 1992;359:641– 4.

[42] Ohlishi M, Fuji K, Minamino T, et al. A potent genetic risk factor for restenosis. *Nature Genet.* 1993;5:324 –5.

[43] Dahlen GH, Slunga L, Lindblom B. Importance of Lp(a) lipoprotein and HLA genotypes in atherosclerosis and diabetes. *Clin. Genet.* 1994;46:46 –56.

[44] Dahlen GH, Boman J, Birgander LS, Lindblom B. Lp(a) lipoprotein, IgG, IgA and IgM antibodies to Chlamydia pneumoniae and HLA class II genotype in early coronary artery disease. *Atherosclerosis* 1995;114:165–74.

[45] Zeller CB, Appenzeller S. Cardiovascular Disease in Systemic Lupus Erythematosus: The Role of Traditional and Lupus Related Risk Factors, *Current Cardiology Reviews*, 2008, 4, 116-122.

[46] Roman MJ, Shanker BA, Davis A, et al. Prevalence and correlates of accelerated atherosclerosis in systemic lupus erythematosus. *N. Engl. J. Med* 2003; 349: 2399-406.

[47] Asanuma Y, Oeser A, Shintani AK, et al. Premature coronaryartery atherosclerosis in systemic lupus erythematosus. *N. Engl. J. Med.* 2003; 349: 2407-15.

[48] Leong KH et al. Lipid profiles in patients with Systemic lupus erythematosus. *J. Rheumatol.* 1994;21: 1264–1267.

[49] Chakraborty S, Zawieja S, Wang W, Zawieja DC., Muthuchamy M.Lymphatic system: a vital link between metabolic syndrome and inflammation. *Ann. N.Y. Acad. Sci.* 2010;1207:94–102.

[50] Alberti KGMM., Eckel RH., Grundy SM., Zimmet P Z., Cleeman JI, Donato KA., Fruchart JC, James WPT., Loria CM. Smith SC Jr. Harmonizing the Metabolic Syndrome: A Joint Interim Statement of the International Diabetes Federation Task Force on Epidemiology and Prevention; National Heart, Lung, and Blood Institute; American Heart Association; World Heart Federation; International Atherosclerosis Society; and International Association for the Study of Obesity. *Circulation* 2009;120;1640-45.

[51] Cheung BM, Ong KL, Man YB, Wong LY, Lau CP, et al. Prevalence of the metabolic syndrome in the United States national health and nutrition examination survey 1999–2002 according to different defining criteria. *J. Clin. Hypertens* 2006;8:562–70.

[52] Negrón AM, Molina MJ, Mayor AM, Rodríguez VE, Vilá LM. Factors associated with metabolic syndrome in patients with systemic lupus erythematosus from Puerto Rico. *Lupus* 2008;17: 348–54.

[53] Bellomio V, Spindler A, Lucero E, et al. Metabolic syndrome in Argentinean patients with systemic lupus erythematosus. *Lupus* 2009; 18: 1019–25.

[54] Mok CC, Poon WL, Lai JPS, Wong CK, Chiu SM, Wong CK, Lun SWM, Ko GTC, Lam CWK, Lam CS. Metabolic syndrome, endothelial injury, and subclinical atherosclerosis in patients with systemic lupus erythematosus. *Scand. J. Rheumatol.* 2010;39:42-49.

[55] Sabio JM, Zamora-Pasadas M, Jiménez-Jáimez J, Albadalejo F, Vargas-Hitos J, Rodríguez del Águila MDM, Hidalgo-Tenorio C, Gonzalez-Gay MA, Alonso JJ. Metabolic syndrome in patients with systemic lupus erythematosus from Southern Spain. *Lupus* 2008;17:849–59.

[56] Vilar MJ, Azevedo GD, Gadelha RG, et al. Prevalence of metabolic syndrome and its components in Brazilian women with systemic lupus erythematosus: implications for cardiovascular risk. *Ann. Rheum. Dis.* 2006;65:362.

[57] Kitagawa Y, Gotoh F, Koto A, Okayasu H. Stroke in systemic lupus erythematosus. *Stroke* 1990; 21:1533-9.

[58] Manger K, Kusus M, Forster C, et al. Factors associated with coronary artery calcification in young female patients with SLE. *Ann. Rheum. Dis.* 2003; 62: 846-50.

[59] Font J, Ramos-Casals M, Cervera R, et al. Cardiovascular risk factors and the long-term outcome of lupus nephritis. *QJM* 2001;94: 19-26.

[60] Rahman P, Gladman DD, Urowitz MB. Premature coronary artery disease in systemic lupus erythematosus in the absence of corticosteroid use. *J. Rheumatol.* 2000; 27: 1323- 5.

[61] Emeson EE, Shen ML, Bell CG, et al. Inhibition of atherosclerosis in CD4 T-cell-depleted and nude (nu/nu) C57BL/6 hyperlipidemic mice. *Am. J. Pathol.* 1996; 149: 675-685.

[62] Vaarala O, Manttari V, Mannienen, et al. Anti-cardiolipin antibodies and risk of myocardial infarction in a prospective cohort of middle-aged men. *Circulation* 1995; 91: 23-27.

[63] Sherer Y, Shemesh J, Tenenbaum A, et al. Coronary calcium and anti-cardiolipin antibody are elevated in patients with typical chest pain. *Am. J. Cardiol.* 2000; 86:1306-1311.

[64] Sherer Y, Tenebaum A, Blank M, et al. Coronary artery disease but not coronary calcification is associated with elevated levels of cardiolipin, 2-glycoprotein-I, and oxidized-LDL antibodies. *Cardiology* 2001; 95: 20-24.

[65] George J, Harats D, Gilburd B, et al. Atherosclerosis-related markers n systemic lupus erythematosus patients: the role of humoral immunity in enhanced atherogenesis. *Lupus* 1999; 8: 220-226.

[66] Doria A, Shoenfeld Y, Wu R. Risk factors for subclinical atherosclerosis in a prospective cohort of patients with systemic lupus erythematosus. *Ann. Rheum. Dis.* 2003; 62: 1071-1077.

[67] Hayem G, Nicaise-Roland P, Palazzo E, et al. Anti-oxidized lowdensitylipoprotein (OxLDL) antibodies in systemic lupus erythematosus with and without antiphospholipid syndrome. *Lupus* 2001; 6-351.

[68] Skamra C, Ramsey-Goldman R. Management of cardiovascular complications in systemic lupus erythematosus. *Int. J. Clin. Rheumtol.* 2010; 5: 75–100.

[69] Frostegard J. SLE, atherosclerosis and cardiovascular disease. *J. Intern. Med.* 2005; 257: 485-95.

[70] Bruce IN. Not only but also: factors that contribute to accelerated atherosclerosis and premature coronary heart disease in systemic lupus erythematosus. *Rheumatology* 2005;44:1492–502.

[71] Ruslan Medzhitov Origin and physiological roles of inflammation. *Nature* 2008;454:428-435.

[72] Leticia Martín-Cordero, Juan J García, Maria D Hinchado and Eduardo Ortega The interleukin-6 and noradrenaline mediated inflammation-stress feedback mechanism is dysregulated in metabolic syndrome: Effect of exercise. *Cardiovascular Diabetology* 2011;10:42.

[73] Besedovsky HO, Del Rey A: Physiology of psychoneuroimmunology: A personal view. *Brain Behav. Immun.* 2007, 21:34-44.

[74] Wellen KE, Hotamisligil GS: Inflammation, stress, and diabetes. *J. Clin. Invest.* 2005, 115:1111-1119.

[75] Festa A, D'Agostino R Jr, Howard G, Mykkänen L, Tracy RP, Haffner SM. Chronic subclinical inflammation as part of the insulin resistance syndrome: the Insulin Resistance Atherosclerosis Study (IRAS). *Circulation.* 2000;102:42-7.

[76] Kern PA, Ranganathan S, Li C, Wood L, Ranganathan G. Adipose tissue tumor necrosis factor and interleukin-6 expression in human obesity and insulin resistance . *Am. J. Physiol. Endocrinol. Metab.*2001;280: 745–751.

[77] Uysal KT, Wiesbrock SM, Hotamisligil GS. Functional Analysis of Tumor Necrosis Factor (TNF) Receptors in TNF-a-Mediated Insulin Resistance in Genetic Obesity. *Endocrinology* 1998 139: 4832-4838.

[78] Bays HE, González-Campoy JM, Bray GA, Kitabchi AE, Bergman DA, Schorr AB, Rodbard HW, Henry RR. Pathogenic potential of adipose tissue and metabolic consequences of adipocyte visceral adiposity. *Expert Rev. Cardiovas. Ther.* 2008; 6: 343-368.

[79] Hermsdorff HHM, Monteiro JBR. Gordura Visceral, Subcutânea ou Intramuscular: Onde Está o Problema? *Arq. Bras. Endocrinol. Metab.* 2004; 48:803-811.

[80] Fantuzzi G, Mazzone T. Adipose Tissue and Atherosclerosis: Exploring the Connection. *Arterioscler. Thromb. Vasc. Biol.* 2007; 27;996-1003.

[81] Ouchi N, Kihara S, Funahashi T, Matsuzawa Y, Walsh K. Obesity, adiponectin and vascular inflammatory disease. *Curr. Opin. Lipidol.* 2003; 14:561-566.

[82] Telles RW, Lanna CCD, Ferreira GA, Ribeiro AL. Metabolic syndrome in patients with systemic lupus erythematosus:association with traditional risk factors for coronary heart diseaseand lupus characteristics. *Lupus* 2010;19:803-809.

[83] Zhou X, Stemme S, Hansson GK. Evidence for a local immune response in atherosclerosis. CD4+ T cells infiltrate lesions of apolipoprotein-E-deficient mice. *Am. J. Pathol.* 1996;149:359-66.

[84] Stemme S, Faber B, Holm J, Wiklund O, Witztum JL, Hansson GK. T lymphocytes from human atherosclerotic plaques recognize oxidized low density lipoprotein. *Proc. Natl. Acad. Sci.* 1995;92:3893-7.

[85] Turnbull AV, Rivier CL. Regulation of the hypotalamic-pituitary-adrenal axis by cytokines: actions and mechanisms of action. *Physiological reviews.* 1999;79:1-72.

[86] Guzik TJ, Mangalat D, Korbut R. Adipocytokines - novel link between inflammation and vascular function? *J. Physiol. Pharmacol.* 2006;57:505-28.

[87] Saghizadeh M, Ong JM, Garvey WT, Henry RR, Kern PA: The expression of TNF alpha by human muscle: relationship to insulin resistance. *J. Clin. Invest.* 1996;97:1111–16.

[88] Hotamisligil GS, Arner P, Caro JF, Atkinson RL, Spiegelman BM: Increased adipose tissue expression of tumor necrosis factor-alpha in human obesity and insulin resistance. *J. Clin. Invest.* 1995;95:2409 –15.

[89] Semb H., Peterson J., Tavernier J., Olivecrona T., Multiple effects of tumor necrosis factor on lipoprotein lipase in vivo *J. Biol. Chem.* 1987 15;262:8390-4.

[90] Grunfeld C., Gulli R., Moser A. H., Gavin L. A., Feingold K. R. Effect of tumor necrosis factor administration in vivo on lipoprotein lipase activity in various tissues of the rat. *J. Lipid. Res.* 1989;30:579-85.

[91] Feingold KR, Soued M, Staprans I, Gavin LA, Donahue ME, Huang BJ, Moser AH, Gulli R, Grunfeld C.Effect of tumor necrosis factor (TNF) on lipid metabolism in the diabetic rat. Evidence that inhibition of adipose tissue lipoprotein lipase activity is not required for TNF-induced hyperlipidemia. *J. Clin. Invest.* 1989 83:1116-21.

[92] Seriolo B, Ferrone C, Cutolo M. Longterm anti-tumor necrosis factor-alpha treatment in patients with refractory rheumatoid arthritis: relationship between insulin resistance and disease activity. *J. Rheumatol.* 2008;35:355-7.

[93] Whitman SC, Ravisankar P, Elam H, Daugherty A. Exogenous interferon-_ enhances atherosclerosis in apolipoprotein E_/_ mice. *Am. J. Pathol.* 2000;157:1819 –1824.

[94] Davenport P, Tipping PG. The role of interleukin-4 and interleukin-12 in the progression of atherosclerosis in apolipoprotein E deficient mice. *Am. J. Pathol.* 2003;163:1117–1125.

[95] Whitman SC, Ravisankar P, Daugherty A. Interleukin-18 enhances atherosclerosis in apolipoprotein E (_/_) mice through release of interferon-_. *Circ. Res.* 2002;90:34–38.

[96] Jiménez-Morales S, Velázquez-Cruz R, Ramírez-Bello J, Bonilla-González E, Romero-Hidalgo S, Escamilla-Guerrero G, et al. Tumor necrosis factor-alpha is a common

genetic risk factor for asthma, juvenile rheumatoid arthritis, and systemic lupus erythematosus in a Mexican pediatric population. *Hum. Immunol.* 2009;70:251-6.

[97] Tayal V. and Kalra BS. Cytokines and anti-cytokines as therapeutics—an update. *Eur. J. Pharmacol.* 2008;579:1–12.

[98] Giamila Fantuzzi. Adiponectin and inflammation: Consensus and controversy. *J. Allergy Clin. Immunol.* 2008;121:2.

[99] Marjon Al, Lawrence Ng, Tyrrell P, Bargman J, Bradley T, Silverman E. Adipokines as novel biomarkers in paediatric systemic lupus erythematosus. *Rheumatology* 2009;48:497–501.

[100] Rothenbacher D, Brenner H, Marz W, Koenig W. Adiponectin, risk of coronary heart disease and correlations with cardiovascular risk markers. *Eur. Heart J.* 2005;26: 1640–6.

[101] Hashimoto N, Kanda J, Nakamura T et al. Association of hypoadiponectinemia in men with early onset of coronary heart disease and multiple coronary artery stenoses. *Metabolism* 2006;55:1653–7.

[102] Kobashi C, Urakaze M, Kishida M et al. Adiponectin inhibits endothelial synthesis of interleukin-8. *Circ. Res* 2005;97:1245–52.

[103] Tsatsanis C, Zacharioudaki V, Androulidaki A et al. Adiponectin induces TNF-alpha and IL-6 in macrophages and promotes tolerance to itself and other pro-inflammatory stimuli. *Biochem. Biophys. Res. Commun.* 2005;335:1254–63.

[104] Kim KY, Kim JK, Han SH et al. Adiponectin is a negative regulator of NK cell cytotoxicity. *J. Immunol.* 2006;176:5958–64.

[105] Wållberg-Jonsson S, Johansson H, Ohman ML, Rantapää-Dahlqvist S. Extent of inflammation predicts cardiovascular disease and overall mortality in seropositive rheumatoid arthritis. A retrospective cohort study from disease onset. *J. Rheumatol.* 1999;26(12):2562-71.

[106] Bruce IN, Urowitz MB, Gladman DD, Hallett DC. Natural history of hypercholesterolemia in systemic lupus erythematosus. *J. Rheumatol.* 1999;26(10):2137-43.

[107] Ardoin SP, Sandborg C, Schanberg LE. Management of dyslipidemia in children and adolescents with systemic lupus erythematosus. *Lupus* 2007;16:618-26.

[108] Petri M. Detection of coronary artery disease and the role of traditional risk factors in the Hopkins Lupus Cohort. *Lupus* 2000; 9: 170–75.

[109] Davis SE, Burns PB, Chung KC. The outcomes of outcome studies in plastic surgery: a systematic review of 17 years of plastic surgery research. *Plast Reconstr. Surg.* 2007;120:2059-65.

[110] Zonana-Nacach A, Santana-Sahagu´n E, Jime´nez-Balderas FJ, Camargo-Coronel A. Prevalence and factors associated with metabolic syndrome in patients with rheumatoid arthritis and systemic lupus erythematosus. *J. Clin. Rheumatol.* 2008; 14: 74–77.

[111] Bultink IEM, Turkstra F, Diamant M, Dijmans BAC, Voskuyl E. Prevalence of and risk factors for the metabolic syndrome in women with systemic lupus erythematosus. *Clin. Exp. Rheumatol.* 2008; 26: 32–38.

[112] Pasanisi F, Contaldo F, de Simone G, Mancini M. Benefits of sustained moderate weight loss in obesity. *Nutr. Metab. Cardiovasc. Dis.* 200111:401–406.

[113] Kwak B, Mulhaupt F, Myit S, Mach F. Statins as a newly recognized type of immunomodulator. *Nat. Med.* 2000;6:1399–402.

[114] Shovman O, Levy Y, Gilburd B, Shoenfeld Y. Antiinflammatory and immunomodulatory properties of statins. *Immunol. Res.* 2002;25:271–8.
[115] van Leuven SI, Mendez-Fernandez YV, Stroes ES, Tak PP, Major AS. Statin therapy in lupus-mediated atherogenesis: two birds with one stone? *Ann. Rheum. Dis.*. 2011;70:245-8.
[116] Ferreira GA, Navarro TP, Telles RW, Andrade LEC, Sato,E. I. "Atorvastatin therapy improves endothelialdependent vasodilation in patients with systemic lupus erythematosus: an 8 weeks controlled trial," *Rheumatology* 2007; 46:1560–65.
[117] Kotyla P. J., Sliwinska-Kotyla B., Kucharz E. J., et al. "TNF- α as a potential target in the treatment of systemic lúpus erythematosus: a role for the HMG-CoA reductase inhibitor simvastatin," *Journal of Rheumatology* 2006; 33:2361–63.
[118] Takemoto M, Liao JK. Pleiotropic effects of 3-hydroxy-3-methylglutaryl coenzyme A reductase inhibitors. *Arterioscler. Thromb. Vasc. Biol.* 2001;21:1712-19.
[119] Greenwood J, Steinman L, Zamvil SS. Statin therapy and autoimmune disease: from protein prenylation to immunomodulation. *Nat. Rev. Immunol.* 2006;6:358 – 70.
[120] Petri, MA; Kiani, AN; Post, W; Christopher-Stine, L; Magder, LS. Lupus Atherosclerosis Prevention Study (LAPS) *Ann. Rheum. Dis.* 2011;70:760–765.
[121] Sowers JR. Recommendations for special populations: diabetes mellitus and the metabolic syndrome. *Am. J. Hypertens* 2003;16:41–45.
[122] Shields TM, Hennekens CH. Management of metabolic syndrome: aspirin. *Endocrinol. Metab. Clin. North Am* 2004;33:577–93.
[123] Hennekens CH, Dyken ML, Fuster V. Aspirin as a therapeutic agent in cardiovascular disease: a statement for healthcare professionals from the American Heart Association. *Circulation* 1997,96:2751–53.
[124] Grundy SM, Cleeman JI, Daniels SR, et al. Diagnosis and management of the metabolic syndrome: an American Heart Association/National Heart, Lung, and Blood Institute Scientific Statement. *Circulation* 2005;112:2735–52.
[125] De Pergola, G. Pannacciulli, N. Coagulation and fibrinolysis abnormalities in obesity. *J. Endocrinol. Invest.* 2002;25:899–904.

In: Lupus: Symptoms, Treatment and Potential Complications ISBN: 978-1-62081-078-1
Editors: T. D. Marquez and D. U. Neto

Chapter VIII

Pulmonary Hypertension in Systemic Lupus Erythematosus

Javier A. Cavallasca[1], Cecilia A. Costa[1], Maria del Rosario Maliandi[2] and Jorge L. Musuruana[1]
[1]Section of Rheumatology and Autoimmune Diseases. Hospital J. B. Iturraspe
[2]Section of Rheumatology, Sanatorio Garay, Santa Fe, Argentina

Definition

Pulmonary arterial hypertension (PAH) is defined as a sustained elevation of pulmonary arterial pressure to more than 25 mm Hg at rest or to more than 30 mm Hg with exercise, with a mean pulmonary-capillary wedge pressure and left ventricular end-diastolic pressure of less than 15 mm Hg.

Classification

The World Health Organization (WHO) classified pulmonary hypertension (PH) into five groups on the basis of mechanisms, rather than associated conditions (Table 1). However, the pathogenesis of most forms of PAH is unknown. All five WHO categories of PH can be found in patients with Systemic Lupus Erythematosus (SLE).

Pulmonary Manifestations in SLE

The most common pulmonary manifestation attributable to SLE is pleural disease (pleural effusion and pleurisy), but other pulmonary involvement can be seen, as well as parenchymal diseases (acute lupus pneumonitis, acute respiratory distress syndrome, diffuse alveolar hemorrhage, chronic interstitial pneumonitis, shrinking lung syndrome), pulmonary vascular disease (acute reversible hypoxemia, pulmonary embolism, pulmonary arterial hypertension), diaphragmatic dysfunction, and upper airway dysfunction.

Epidemiology

Pulmonary hypertension in patients with SLE has been described since 1973. Estimates of the prevalence of PAH in SLE vary from 0.5 to 43%, depending on the cohort studied and the method of diagnosis used.

Patients are predominantly women of child-bearing potential: aged from 18 to 40 years with a 10 to 1 ratio of female over male.

Table 1.

Group I: Pulmonary arterial hypertension
• Idiopathic (primary)
• Familial
Related conditions: collagen vascular disease, congenital systemic-to-pulmonary shunts, portal hypertension, HIV infection, drugs and toxins, thyroid disorders, glycogen storage disease, Gaucher's disease, hereditary hemorrhagic telangiectasia, hemoglobinopathies, myeloproliferative disorders, splenectomy.
• Associated with significant venous or capillary involvement
Pulmonary veno-occlusive disease
Pulmonary-capillary hemangiomatosis
• Persistent pulmonary hypertension of the newborn.
Group II: Pulmonary venous hypertension
• Left sided atrial or ventricular heart disease
• Left sided valvular heart disease
Group III: Pulmonary hypertension associated with hypoxemia
• Cronic obstructive pulmonary disease
• Intersticial lung disease
• Sleep-disordered breathing
• Alveolar hypoventilation disorders
• Chronic exposure to high altitude
• Developmental abnormalities
Group IV: pulmonary hypertension due to chronic thrombotic disease, embolic disease, or both
• Thromboembolic obstruction of proximal pulmonary arteries
• Thromboembolic obstruction of distal pulmonary arteries
• Pulmonary embolism (tumor, parasites, foreing material)
Group V: Miscellaneous
Sarcoidosis, pulmonary Langerhan's cell histiocytosis, lymphangiomatosis, compression of pulmonary vessels (adenopathy, tumor, fibrosing mediastinitis)

Pathogenesis

The causal relationship between SLE and PAH is still unknown. However, small vessel inflammation and/or vasculitis, sustained vasoconstriction, in situ thrombosis, and/or thromboembolism, all features of SLE, may damage and reduce the pulmonary vascular bed and lead to PAH.

There is an imbalance between vasoconstrictors and vasodilators in SLE-PAH. Increased concentrations of endothelin-1, a potent vasoconstrictor, cause hypoxia, which may originate structural changes in the vessels increasing pressures that progress to PAH. There is also an imbalance between prostacyclin (vasodilator) and thromboxane A2 (vasoconstrictor) shifted towards the last one, that results in endothelial dysfunction, vascular damage, and remodeling. Antiphospolipid antibodies and antiendothelial cell antibodies; important source of IL-6; have also been associated with vascular injury, ensuing intimal and medial proliferation and in situ thrombosis. The striking correlation between the presence of Raynaud´s phenomenon and SLE-PAH suggests that pulmonary arterial vasospasm may also be involved in the pathogenesis. On the other hand, hypoxia and fibrosis caused by interstitial lung disease originate higher pressures in pulmonary arteries leading to PAH.

Histological examination revealed in small pulmonary arteries and arterioles the presence of acute fibrinoid necrosis, thrombotic lesions, vasculitis, chronic intimal fibrosis, medial hypertrophy, alteration of elastic laminae, periadventitial fibrosis, aneurysmal dilation, and plexiform lesions, which are virtually identical to the alterations seen in patients with idiophatic PAH (iPAH).

Clinical Manifestations

Symptoms are similar to iPAH and include shortness of breath, fatigue, diminished exercise tolerance and in advanced states they progress to symptoms of cardiac failure; distended jugular veins, peripheral oedema, a loud pulmonary second heart sound, hepatomegaly and ascites. Unfortunately, the disease process is usually far advanced with irreversible changes of the pulmonary vasculature by the time symptoms or signs develop.

Raynaud´s phenomenon is a frequent manifestation in this patients group, some authors have reported that this clinical manifestation correlates with pulmonary artery systolic pressure (PASP). The duration of SLE and the extrapulmonary activity of SLE do not correlate with the development of PAH, and PAH can be a presenting manifestation of SLE.

Early diagnosis, therefore, depends on additional methods of screening.

Diagnostic Methods

Doppler echocardiography is the preferred screening detection method, pulmonary embolism should be excluded with a ventilation/perfusion (VQ) scan or pulmonary angiography. Right heart catheterization is necessary to confirm pulmonary arterial hypertension especially in those patients with a Doppler echocardiography that showed moderate- severe PAH.

Autoantibodies

All the patients with SLE- PAH are positive for antinuclear antibodies (ANA). Some other autoantibodies have been associated with PAH in SLE, frequently present are the antiphospholipid antibodies (Anticardiolipin Antibodies and Lupus anticoagulant), with a high relation SLE-PAH patients 83% (positive) versus 25% (negative).

Antiendothelial antibodies, anti SM antibodies, antibodies to ribonuclear protein (RNP) and rheumatoid factor (RF); are also linked to SLE –PAH patients, although is unknown if they are an epiphenomenon or have a pathogenic role.

Pregnancy

The majority of SLE patients are in childbearing age. Pregnancy is contraindicated in SLE patients with active disease. PAH is an absolute contraindication for pregnancy, as the physiological, cardiovascular, and pulmonary changes that occur during pregnancy can exacerbate the condition. However, several viable treatment options are available to improve the outcomes for both the mother and infant. Targeted pulmonary vasodilators demonstrated benefits in these group of patients.

Treatment

At the moment there are no consensus guidelines for the treatment of SLE-PAH; instead, standard treatment of iPAH would benefit SLE-PAH patients. General measures may be used including anticoagulation (although there is no evidence in SLE-PAH, there is a survival benefit in iPAH). Supplemental oxygen and diuretics may be prescribed when hypoxia and right heart failure are present. Calcium channel blockers use is controversial.

Immunosuppressive Therapy

Although direct injury mediated by immunologic factors has not yet been clearly reported, the presence of deposits of antinuclear antibodies, anti DNA, rheumatoid factor, immunoglobulins and complement fractions on the pulmonary vessels in PAH suggests an immune basis. Cyclophosphamide decrese the synthesis of immunoglobulins and immunocomplexes.

Based on studies of cyclophosphamide plus prednisolone therapy in patients with SLE-PAH, it would seem that mild SLE (DELETE SLE) PAH can benefit from immunosuppresion alone, whereas more severe SLE (DELETE SLE) PAH requires vasodilators in combination with immunosuppression. As relapses are no rare, the need of an immunosuppressive maintenance regimen similar that recommended for other serious involvement could be considered. Anti CD20 therapy reduces circulating levels of SLE autoantibodies, which presumably reduces formation of immune complexes and complement activation that may be directly cytotoxic. There is little evidence to use Rituximab in patients with severe or refractory disease. The experience suggests that Rituximab is a safe and efficacious option, which improves clinical and hemodynamic indices for more than a year.

Sildenafil

Sildenafil inhibits phosphodiesterase type 5, an enzyme that metabolizes cyclic guanosine monophosphate (cGMP) thereby enhancing the cGMP mediated relaxation and growth inhibition of smooth muscle in the lung vasculature. Multiple case reports show the benefits in these patients. In a randomized trial of PAH asociated with connective tissue diseases, where 23% of patients had SLE, the use of Sildenafil 20 mg TID improves exercise capacity, hemodynamic measures, and functional class with an acceptable tolerability profile.

Prostanoids

Prostacyclin stimulates the production of cyclic adenosine monophosphate, which leads to smooth muscle relaxation, inhibition of smooth muscle cell growth, and inhibition of platelet aggregation, producing vasodilatation. Several prostanoid formulations are available for treatment of PAH. Intravenous Epoprostenol has been shown to be effective in a randomized trial of patients suffering from Scleroderma spectrum. It has been shown that Epoprostenol treatment can improve exercise capacity, symptoms and haemodynamics. However, no improvement in survival was observed. There are reports describing a benefit from Epoprostenol in patients with SLE-PAH. In a small group of 6 SLE –PAH patients, Epoprostenol use was associated with mean pulmonary artery pressure decreased pulmonary vascular resistance and a improve of New York Heart Association (NYHA) functional class.

Endothelin Receptor Antagonists

Endothelin is a potent vasoconstrictor and smooth muscle mitogen, secreted by the pulmonary endothelium. It produces PAH by binding to two receptors, endothelin A (ETA) and endothelin B (ETB). It is also considered as a key pathogenic mediator of PAH secondary to connective tissue disease (CTD). Circulating levels of endothelin correlate with disease severity. Bosentan is an oral, dual endothelin A/B receptor antagonists and in several studies have showed clinical efficacy in patient with primary or associated PAH and CTD . In post-hoc analysis of the CTD subgroup from studies of Bosentan efficacy, eight patients with SLE were included. Patients who were treated with Bosentan were stable during the 6-minute walking distance test in contrast with the placebo group. In an uncontrolled study of patient with scleroderma and SLE with PAH, long-term treatment with Bosentan improved exercise capacity and pulmonary hemodynamics. Ambrisentan is a selective endothelin A receptor antagonist, that has been evaluated in randomized placebo controlled, double-blind, trials (ARIES-1 and ARIES-2). In both studies, patients had idiopathic PAH or PAH associated with CTD, HIV infection, or anorexigen use and the primary endpoint was the change in 6-minute walk distance from baseline to week 12. At 12 weeks, the six-minute walk distance increased in all ambrisentan groups. Improvements in secondary end points such as time to clinical worsening, functional class, and symptom assessments, and B-type natriuretic peptide measurements were also seen. Bosentan and Ambrisentan could cause transient elevation of liver transaminases, so these laboratory tests should be monitored at least monthly for as long as the patient is taking them. They have been associated with small decreases in hemoglobin and are highly teratogenic.

Transplantation

Althoug there are considerable experience about renal transplant in SLE patients, heart-lung transplantation in PAH-SLE patients is not frequent.

However there are reports of lung or heart-lung transplant in SLE patients with severe PAH that has resulted in long term survival.

Prognosis

The natural course of PAH is gradually progressive over time and has a profound influence on the prognosis of patients with SLE. Preliminary data suggest that SLE patients have a significantly better prognosis than Scleroderma patients (3-year survival rate of 74 vs 47%). However, some authors reported that PAH is actually the third most common cause of death in SLE following infection and organ failure.

This can be explained by the improvement in treatment of severe complications (kidney, brain, heart) in SLE over the years, while SLE-PAH is still a challenge and often is not possible to get good outcomes, producing high morbidity and mortality.

Conclusion

The association between PAH and SLE is not rare and is a devastating complication. More studies are needed in order to improve treatments and get better outcomes.

References

[1] Gaine SP, Rubin LJ. Primary pulmonary hypertension. *Lancet* 1998; 352:719-25.

[2] Harrison W, Loscalzo J. Pulmonary Arterial Hypertension. *N Engl J Med* 2004; 351:1655-65.

[3] Kamen DL, Strange C. Pulmonary Manifestations of Systemic Lupus Erythematosus. *Clin Chest Med* 2010; 31: 479-488.

[4] Fahey PJ, Utell MJ, Condemi JJ, et al. Raynaud's phenomenon of the lung. *Am J Med* 1984; 76:263-269.

[5] Yokoi T, Tomita Y, Fukaya M, et al. Pulmonary hypertension associated with systemic lupus erythematosus: predominantly thrombotic arteriopathy accompanied by plexiform lesions. *Arch Pathol Lab Med.* 1998 ;122:467-70.

[6] Quadrelli SA, Alvarez C, Arce SC, et al. Pulmonary involvement of systemic lupus erythematosus: analysis of 90 necropsies. *Lupus* 2009; 18: 1053-1060.

[7] Asherson RA. Pulmonary hypertension in systemic lupus erythematosus. *J Rheumatol.* 1990; 17: 414-415.

[8] Asherson RA, Higenbottam TW, Dinh Xuan AT, et al. Pulmonary hypertension in a lupus clinic: experience with twenty-four patients. *J Rheumatol.* 1990; 10:1292-8.

[9] Distler O, Pignone A. Pulmonary arterial hypertension and rheumatic diseases – from diagnosis to treatment. *Rheumatology.* 2006; 45:22-25.

[10] 10.Huang S, DeSantis ER. Treatment of pulmonary arterial hypertension in pregnancy. *Am J Health Syst Pharm.* 2007;64:1922-6.

[11] Jais X, Launay D, Yaici A et al. Immunosuppressive Therapy in Lupus – and Mixed Connective Tissue Disease – Associated Pulmonary Arterial Hypertension. A retrospective analysis of twenty-three cases. *Arthritis Rheum* 2008; 58:521-531.

[12] Gonzalez-Lopez L, Cardona Muñoz EG, Celis A, et al. Therapy with intermittent pulse cyclophosphamide for pulmonary hypertension associated with systemic lupus erythematosus. *Lupus* 2004; 13: 105-112.

[13] Hennigan S, Channick RN, Silverman GJ. Rituximab treatment of pulmonary arterial hypertension associated with systemic lupus erythematosus: a case report. *Lupus.* 2008; 17: 754-756.

[14] Cea-Calvo L, Escribano Subías P, Tello de Menesses R, et al. Sildenafil as a substitute for subcutaneous prostacyclin in pulmonary hypertension. *Arch. Bronconeumol.* 2003;39:476-7.

[15] Badesch DB, Hill NS, Burgess G, et al. Sildenafil for pulmonary arterial hypertension associated with connective tissue disease. *J Rheumatol.* 2007;34:2417-22.

[16] Molina J, Lucero E, Luluaga S, et al Systemic lupus erythematosus-associated pulmonary hypertension: good outcome following sildenafil therapy. *Lupus.* 2003;12:321-3.

[17] Robbins IM, Gaine SP, Schilz R, et al. Epoprostenol for treatment of pulmonary hypertension in patients with systemic lupus erythematosus. *Chest.* 2000;117:14-8.

[18] Channick RN, Simonneau G, Sitbon O, et al. Effects of the dual endothelin-receptor antagonist bosentan in patients with pulmonary hypertension: a randomised placebo-controlled study. *Lancet.* 2001;358:1119-23.

[19] Rubin LJ, Badesch DB, Barst RJ,et al. Bosentan therapy for pulmonary arterial hypertension. *N Engl J Med.* 2002;346:896-903.

[20] Cozzi F, Montisci R, Marotta H, et al. Bosentan Therapy of pulmonary arterial hypertension in connective tissue diseases: *Eur J Clin Invest.* 2006; 36(Suppl 3):49-53.

[21] Denton CP, Humbert M, Rubin L et al. Bosentan treatment for pulmonary arterial hypertension related to connective tissue disease: a subgroup analysis of the pivotal clinical trials and their open-label extensions. *Ann Rheum Dis*. 2006; 65:1336-1340.

[22] Galiè N, Olschewski H, Oudiz RJ,et al Ambrisentan in Pulmonary Arterial Hypertension, Randomized, Double-Blind, Placebo-Controlled, Multicenter, Efficacy Studies (ARIES) Group. Ambrisentan for the treatment of pulmonary arterial hypertension: results of the ambrisentan in pulmonary arterial hypertension, randomized, double-blind, placebo-controlled, multicenter, efficacy (ARIES) study 1 and 2. *Circulation*. 2008;117:3010-9.

[23] Chen LJ, Chang HC, Lu LY, et al. Prolonged survival after single lung transplantation for pulmonary hypertension secondary to systemic lupus erythematosus. *J Chin Med Assoc*. 2004;67:248-51.

[24] Levy RD, Guerraty AJ, Yacoub MH, et al. Prolonged survival after heart-lung transplantation in systemic lupus erythematosus. *Chest*. 1993;104:1903-5.

[25] Condliffe R, Kiely DG, Peacock AJ, et al. Connective tissue disease-associated pulmonary arterial hypertension in the modern treatment era. *Am J Respir Crit Care Med*. 2009 ;179:151-7.

[26] Kim WU, Min JK, Lee SH, et al. Causes of death in Korean patients with systemic lupus erythematosus: a single centre retrospective study. *Clin Exp Rheumatol* 1999; 17:539–545.

In: Lupus: Symptoms, Treatment and Potential Complications ISBN: 978-1-62081-078-1
Editors: T. D. Marquez and D. U. Neto

Chapter IX

Dual Roles for Antibodies in Lupus Nephritis

*Marilyn Diaz**
Somatic Hypermutation Group,
Laboratory of Molecular Genetics,
National Institute of Environmental Health Sciences,
National Institutes of Health, Research Triangle Park,
North Carolina, US

Abstract

Pathogenic antibodies in Systemic Lupus Erythematosus (SLE) are known to play a major role in initiating and exacerbating the disease through the formation of immune complexes that are deposited in kidney glomeruli. It is apparent that the IgG isotype and an antibody specificity to nuclear components, particularly double-stranded DNA, is associated with increased pathogenesis of autoantibodies.

The role of autoreactive IgM is less clear. Through a series of experiments, we have demonstrated that IgM is not only not pathogenic in mice with a lupus-like syndrome (MRL/lpr) but that it is actually protective.

Passive transfer experiments using anti-dsDNA IgM antibodies prevented development of lupus nephritis in these mice. The cells secreting protective antibodies displayed a different repertoire of immunoglobulin heavy chain variable region usage, suggesting the possibility of a distinct population of B cells that secrete these antibodies. The possibility of IgM therapy or differential activation of a putative B cell population secreting protective antibodies is discussed.

* Somatic Hypermutation Group, Laboratory of Molecular Genetics, National Institute of Environmental Health Sciences, National Institutes of Health, Research Triangle Park, North Carolina 27709, USA. Tel: 919-541-4740; Fax: 919-541-7593; Email: diaz@niehs.nih.gov.

The Origins of Pathogenic Antibodies in Autoimmunity

B lymphocytes of the immune system contribute to primary and secondary immune responses by producing antibodies that mark pathogens for destruction by other components of the immune system. The key to B cell responses is the recognition of foreign antigens. To this end, the B cell repertoire and immune response is orchestrated via three mechanisms of somatic genetic alteration that enhance diversity as well as specificity of the immunoglobulin (Ig) receptor: 1) V(D)J recombination 2) Ig somatic hypermutation (SHM), and 3) class switch recombination (CSR). V(D)J recombination generates the pre-immune highly diverse B cell repertoire and is independent of antigen (pre-immune repertoire. SHM and CSR are the key contributors to B cell specificity and antibody effector function during immune responses and play a major role in the generation of pathogenic antibodies in autoimmunity.

SHM and CSR are activated following exposure to a particular pathogen and occur in germinal center B cells, a transient lymphoid structure formed in secondary lymphoid tissues [1-4]. CSR is the mechanism responsible for the generation of downstream isotypes from IgM such as IgG, IgA and IgE [5]. SHM introduces mutations into the DNA encoding the variable (V) regions of Ig receptors [1]. These mutations in combination with selection for high affinity variants lead to the formation of B cells that secrete high affinity antibodies to a specific antigen [6-7]. Those B cells constitute the memory B cell compartment that contributes to a swift, high affinity recall response upon re-exposure to a particular pathogen.

When not regulated properly, the germinal center reaction and its components can lead to the production of autoreactive B cells that contribute to autoimmune disorders. This happens when mutations that enhance autoreactivity are incidentally introduced by the SHM mechanism leading to the formation of autoreactive memory B cells [8-10]. It is presumed that these cells are normally eliminated from the germinal center through apoptosis but that this process may be defective in autoimmune patients. Activated autoreactive B cells secrete high affinity pathogenic IgG antibodies that can cause tissue damage in autoimmunity [9]. Indeed, systemic autoimmune disorders such as lupus are characterized by hypermutated, class-switched autoantibodies [11-12]. Understanding the relative contribution of the germinal center reaction to autoimmune disease is pivotal to the development of novel therapies to this disease.

Pathogenic Antibodies in Lupus

Systemic Lupus Erythematosus (SLE), is a systemic autoimmune disease characterized by the production of autoantibodies and immune complex deposition in various tissues, particularly the kidney glomeruli [13]. Hallmark autoantibodies of SLE recognize nuclear cellular components, in particular double-stranded DNA (dsDNA) are mostly of the IgG isotype and highly are mutated, suggesting that they originate from memory B cells. MRL-Faslpr/lpr (MRL/lpr) mice develop a systemic autoimmune syndrome that shares many characteristics of SLE and is an accepted experimental model of the disease [14-15]. Like the human disease, the MRL/lpr syndrome is characterized by polygenic inheritance, the presence of circulating autoantibodies, particularly to nuclear components, and lupus nephritis development through glomerular disease, mononuclear cell infiltration, and immune complex deposition. MRL/lpr mice also develop splenomegaly and lymphadenopathy, with mononuclear cell infiltration in lungs, liver, and other tissues. Multiple factors have been implicated in the development of this disease such as cytokine regulation, complement defects, defective apoptosis, and particularly, a breakdown in lymphocyte tolerance (for review see 16).

Several pieces of evidence conclusively demonstrated an active role for autoantibodies and B cells in the lupus-like syndrome. These included the development of transgenic mice rendered autoimmune by the generation of B-cells with autoreactive specificities, the identification of defects associated specifically with B-cell tolerance, and studies demonstrating that B cells play multiple (key) roles in the development of the lupus syndrome associated with MRL/lpr mice, both as secretors of autoantibodies and as cells that can stimulate autoreactive T lymphocytes [16-18]. That immunoglobulin G (IgG) autoantibodies are required for kidney damage is suggested by the reduction in glomerular injury in mice that are deficient in FcRc and FccRIII [19]. Furthermore, we demonstrated that the kidney pathology associated with MRL/lpr mice is critically dependent on the presence of the activation-induced deaminase (AID) protein that triggers the generation of somatically mutated, high-affinity, isotype switched autoantibodies [20]. IgG antibodies, particularly those that recognize nuclear components such as dsDNA, are critical to the development of lupus nephritis and other aspects of the syndrome.

We examined AID deficiency in MRL/lpr mice. We found that AID-deficient MRL/lpr mice had dramatically decreased nephritis and experienced a dramatic increase in survival suggesting an important role for affinity maturation in the syndrome [20]. That the survival levels exceeded those of mice lacking secreted antibodies, also suggested an additional factor besides loss of IgG contributed to survival.

Anti-DsDNA IgM Protects against Lupus Nephritis

Paradoxically, we identified this factor to be also antibodies that recognize dsDNA , but that were of the IgM isotype [21]. Indeed, passive transfer experiments using anti-dsDNA IgM antibodies prevented development of lupus nephritis in these mice [21]. These surprising results suggest that autoreactive IgM is protective, rather than pathogenic in lupus nephritis. We also found evidence that anti-dsDNA IgM protects through an IgG mediated process, likely by preventing the formation of pathogenic IgG-bearing immune complexes, their deposition in kidney glomeruli, and/or the inflammatory cascade that ensues. MRL/lpr mice that received the protective antibodies had minimal or no evidence of glomerulonephritis that correlated with decreased apoptotic material in the kidneys and reduced kidney infiltration by inflammatory cells, such as macrophages [21]. Interestingly, the cells secreting protective antibodies displayed a different repertoire of immunoglobulin heavy chain variable region usage, suggesting the possibility that a distinct population of B cells secretes protective antibodies.

If so, differentially activating these cells to secrete protective IgM may be of therapeutic benefit in SLE. We are currently identifying the mechanism of IgM protection in lupus nephritis and in other aspects of the autoimmune syndrome in MRL/lpr mice with two long term goals in mind: to define the B cell population secreting protective IgM antibodies and to identify equivalent protective IgM autoantibodies in humans that may lead to novel therapies for SLE.

Conclusion

Antibodies play a pivotal role in the development of lupus nephritis. As pathogenic agents, high affinity autoreactive IgG antibodies significantly contribute to the glomerulonephritis associated with the lupus syndrome of MRL/lpr mice through the formation of immune complexes and their deposition in kidney glomeruli. Therefore, a therapeutic goal may be to lower the levels of these antibodies in SLE patients. One such approach could target AID levels or activity, as this molecule is required for both isotype switching to IgG and the generation of high affinity antibodies [22]. Indeed, there is evidence that too much AID activity may contribute to autoimmunity in several mouse models of lupus [23-24].

In contrast to pathogenic IgG, anti-dsDNA IgM is protective against lupus nephritis. This discovery may provide the basis for a novel therapy that is based in autoreactive IgM. However, in addition to antibody-based therapy, the possibility that a dedicated B cell population that secretes protective antibodies exists and could be differentially activated in SLE patients to prevent lupus nephritis is an exciting prospect for therapy. However, the existence of this population has not been proven, and our laboratory is aggressively pursuing this possibility. Finally, previous studies have found a correlation between high circulating levels of IgG to IgM ratio and an increased probability of lupus nephritis development in SLE patients [25]. This finding fits well with the notion that IgM and IgG autoantibody play opposite roles in lupus nephritis and If true, determining this ratio may help patients and their care providers better determine the probability for future kidney involvement, a serious complication of SLE.

References

[1] Weigert MG, Cesari IM, Yonkovich SJ, Cohn M. Variability in the lambda light chain sequences of mouse antibody. *Nature,* 1970;228:1045-7.

[2] Berek C, Berger A, Apel M. Maturation of the immune response in germinal centers. *Cell*, 1991;67:1121-9.

[3] Eisen HN, Siskind GW. Variations in affinities of antibodies during the immune response. *Biochemistry*, 1964;3:996-1008.

[4] Klinman NR. The mechanism of antigenic stimulation of primary and secondary clonal precursor cells. *J. Exp. Med.*, 1972;136:241-60.

[5] Muramatsu M, Kinoshita K, Fagarasan S, Yamada S, Shinkai Y, Honjo T. Class switch recombination and hypermutation require activation-induced cytidine deaminase (AID), a potential RNA editing enzyme. *Cell*, 2000;102:553-63.

[6] Clarke SH, Huppi K, Ruezinsky D, Staudt L, Gerhard W, Weigert M. Inter- and intraclonal diversity in the antibody response to influenza hemagglutinin. *J. Exp. Med.*, 1985;161:687-704.

[7] Shlomchik MJ, Marshak-Rothstein A, Wolfowicz CB, Rothstein TL, Weigert MG. The role of clonal selection and somatic mutation in autoimmunity. *Nature*, 1987; 328:805-11.

[8] Radic MZ, Mascelli MA, Erikson J, Shan H, Shlomchik M, Weigert M. Structural patterns in anti-DNA antibodies from MRL/lpr mice. *Cold Spring Harb. Symp. Quant. Biol.*, 1989;54 Pt 2:933-46.

[9] Shlomchik M, Mascelli M, Shan H, Radic MZ, Pisetsky D, Marshak-Rothstein A *et al.* Anti-DNA antibodies from autoimmune mice arise by clonal expansion and somatic mutation. *J. Exp. Med.*, 1990;171:265-92.

[10] van Es JH, Gmelig Meyling FH, van de Akker WR, Aanstoot H, Derksen RH, Logtenberg T. Somatic mutations in the variable regions of a human IgG anti-double-stranded DNA autoantibody suggest a role for antigen in the induction of systemic lupus erythematosus. *J. Exp. Med.,* 1991;173:461-70.

[11] Winkler TH, Fehr H, Kalden JR. Analysis of immunoglobulin variable region genes from human IgG anti-DNA hybridomas. *Eur. J. Immunol.,* 1992;22:1719-28.

[12] Wellmann U, Letz M, Herrmann M, Angermuller S, Kalden JR, Winkler TH. The evolution of human anti-double-stranded DNA autoantibodies. *Proc. Natl. Acad. Sci. U S A*, 2005;102:9258-63.

[13] Eisenberg R. Why can't we find a new treatment for SLE? *J. Autoimmun,* 2009; 32:223-30.

[14] Theofilopoulos AN, Dixon FJ. Murine models of systemic lupus erythematosus. *Adv. Immunol.*, 1985; 37:269-390.

[15] Andrews BS, Eisenberg R A, Theofilopoulos AN, Izui S., Wilson CB, McConahey PJ, Murphy, ED, Roths JB, Dixon FJ. Spontaneous murine lupus-like syndromes: clinical and immunopathological manifestations in several strains. *J. Exp. Med.* 1978; 148: 1198-1215.

[16] von Boehmer H, Melchers F. Checkpoints in lymphocyte development and autoimmune disease. *Nat. Immunol.* 2010; 11:14-20.

[17] Chan O, Shlomchik MJ. A new role for B cells in systemic autoimmunity: B cells promote spontaneous T cell activation in MRL-lpr/lpr mice. *J. Immunol.*, 1998; 160:51-9.

[18] Chan OT, Hannum LG, Haberman AM, Madaio MP, Shlomchik MJ. A novel mouse with B cells but lacking serum antibody reveals an antibody-independent role for B cells in murine lupus. *J. Exp. Med.*, 1999;189:1639.

[19] Ravetch JV, Bolland S. IgG Fc receptors. *Annu. Rev. Immunol.,* 2001;19:275-90.

[20] Jiang C, Foley J, Clayton N, Kissling G, Jokinen M, Herbert R *et al.* Abrogation of lupus nephritis in activation-induced deaminase-deficient MRL/lpr mice. *J. Immunol.,* 2007;178:7422-31.

[21] Jiang C, Zhao ML, Scearce RM, Diaz M. Activation-induced deaminase-deficient MRL/lpr mice secrete high levels of protective antibodies against lupus nephritis. *Arthritis Rheum.*, 2011;63:1086-1096.

[22] Hsu HC, Yang P, Wu Q, Wang JH, Job G, Guentert T, Li J, Stockard CR, Le TV, Chaplin DD, Grizzle WE, Mountz JD. Inhibition of the catalytic function of activation-

induced cytidine deaminase promotes apoptosis of germinal center B cells in BXD2 mice. *Arthritis Rheum.* 2011; 63:2038-2048.

[23] Zan H, Zhang J, Ardeshna S, Xu Z, Park SR, Casali P. Lupus-prone MRL/faslpr/lpr mice display increased AID expression and extensive DNA lesions, comprising deletions and insertions, in the immunoglobulin locus: concurrent upregulation of somatic hypermutation and class switch DNA recombination. *Autoimmunity.* 2009; 42:89-103.

[24] Hsu HC, Wu Y, Yang P, Wu Q, Job G, Chen J, Wang J, Accavitti-Loper MA, Grizzle WE, Carter RH, Mountz JD. Overexpression of activation-induced cytidine deaminase in B cells is associated with production of highly pathogenic autoantibodies. *J. Immunol.* 2007; 178:5357-5365.

[25] Forger F, Matthias T, Oppermann M, Becker H, Helmke K. Clinical significance of anti-dsDNA antibody isotypes: IgG/IgM ratio of anti-dsDNA antibodies as a prognostic marker for lupus nephritis. *Lupus* 2004;13:36–43.

In: Lupus: Symptoms, Treatment and Potential Complications ISBN: 978-1-62081-078-1
Editors: T. D. Marquez and D. U. Neto

Chapter X

Treatment of Systemic Lupus Erythematosus with Intravenous Immunoglobulins: Case Studies

J. Rovensky*[1,2]*, A. Tuchynova*[1]*, E. Strakova*[3]*,
***K. Köhler*[3] *and S. Blazickova*[4]**
[1]National Institute of Rheumatic Diseases, Piestany, Slovakia
[2]Institute of Physiotherapy, Balneology and Medical Rehabilitation in Piestany, University of St. Cyril and Methodius, Trnava, Slovakia
[3]Out-patient office for rheumatology, Presov
[4]Faculty of Health and Social Care, University of Trnava, Trnava, Slovakia

Abstract

Systemic lupus erythematosus (SLE) is an autoimmune disease with a varied clinic picture, chronic course and exacerbation tendency as well as many complications resulting from the underlying disease and the immunosuppressive therapy administered. In case of an insufficient effect of immunosuppressive treatment or its contraindication other therapeutic processes are searched that would enable mastering the disease activity. In the paper we describe two case reports of female patients with SLE with polyorgan involvement and infectious complications that were successfully treated by administering intravenous immunoglobulins.

Keywords: Systemic lupus erythematosus – intravenous immunoglobulins

Introduction

SLE is an autoimmune disorder with varied clinical symptoms, chronic course and exacerbation, as well as with complications resulting from the underlying disease and from the immunosuppressive therapy applied. Administration of intravenous immunoglobulins (IVIG) is considered to be an efficient and safe immunomodulatory therapy of SLE. Several studies confirmed the efficacy of IVIG administration in resistant form of SLE, lupus glomerulonephritis, hemolytic anemia, thrombocytopenia, neurological complications, antiphospholipid syndrome and secondary immunodefficiency [1].

Case Study 1

Thirty-six-years old female patient with history of histologically verified discoid form of SLE in 1992, developing epizodic arthritis of small joints of the hands, wrists and ankles in spring 2008. The condition was originally diagnosed as rheumatoid arthritis and therapy with prednisone and antimalarial drugs was introduced. In February 2009 skin vasculitis of hand fingers appeared, methotrexate was added to the therapy. In July 2009 the patient was admitted to the local internal clinics with septic fever, weight loss of 12 kg, hemorrhagic gastritis verified by gastrofibroscopy, progressive anemia and thrombocytopenia.

On August 5th 2009 she was transferred to the National Institute of Rheumatic Diseases with a suspicion of a systemic connective tissue disorder. In the foreground of the clinical findings on admission were manifestations of cutaneous vasculitis in fingers, suffusions in the lower extremities, leg edema, wound in the right leg and a developing decubitus in the lumbosacral area. The patient had since admission elevated body temperature (below 38.5°C). On the chest x-ray, pleural effusions were found, additional examinations identified ascites, esophageal candidosis. Polyresistant strains *Klebsiella pneumoniae* and *Pseudomonas aeruginosa* were cultivated in the throat swab. *Klebsiella pneumoniae* was found also in the urine sample and in the sample from the leg wound.

Laboratory findings revealed a high humoral activity (ESR 97/147, CRP 50.7 mg/L), pancytopenia (hemoglobin 76 g/L, leukocytes 3.2 x 10^9/L, platelets 20 x 10^9/L), hypoproteinemia (total proteins 61.3 g/L, albumine 18.3 g/L), positive D-dimer (>5000 mg/mL), antithrombin III 62.1%, high titres of autoantibodies – ANA speckled pattern, anti-DNP 113.8 U/mL, anti-ds DNA 300 U/mL, ENA SSA/Ro 300 U/mL, SSB/La 300 U/mL, CH50 43, expression of HLA-DR on monocytes 25%. The finding in urine was positive (Ery 70, Leu 45, quantitative proteinuria 1.26g/24h), with decreased glomerular filtration without nitrogen retention.

Based on the clinical picture and laboratory findings we confirmed the diagnosis of SLE with pancytopenia, polyserositis, nephritis, high activity of autoantibodies, hypercoagulable state, secondary immunodeficiency and following secondary infection. Considering the severe thrombocytopenia at the beginning of hospitalization, we administered pulses of methylprednisolone (4 x 500mg and 4 x 250 mg) together with combined antimicrobial and antimycotic therapy.

Considering the clinical manifestations of the underlying disease – nephritis, thrombocytopenia (in which a consumptive coagulopathy played a probable role) and secondary bacterial infection, we administered to the patient intravenous immunoglobulins (dose 400 mg/kg body weight/day over 5 days).

When applying the therapy during hospitalization, we noticed a decrease in humoral activity, normalization of platelet count, decrease in D-dimer and normalization of antithrombin III.

After patient's dismissal, the therapy with prednisone continued, in October 2009 azathioprine was added to the therapy. With the aforementioned treatment the inflammatory activity decreased, as well as the level of autoantibodies, proteinuria disappeared, hemoglobin and platelets normalized, the level of the total complement increased slightly. Due to leukopenia, therapy with azathioprine was terminated and cyclosporine A was added to the therapy.

Case Study 2

A 26-years old female patient, diagnosed with SLE in February 2009, in the 5th month of pregnancy. Clinical picture included butterfly erythema, Raynaud's phenomenon and edema of the legs. In laboratory findings, increase in the nitrogen catabolites (creatinine 373.4 μmol/L), anemia (hemoglobin 86 g/L), thrombocytopenia (127 x 10^9/L), positivity of ANA, anti-ds DNA, anti-nucleosome and anti-histone antibodies and features of nephritic syndrome (quantitative proteinuria 10.1 g/24h) were observed. Due to the rapid progress of renal insufficiency the pregnancy was terminated and pulse therapy with prednisolone and cyclophosphamide was started in a 4-weeks interval.

After the first cycle of the pulse therapy, hemodialysis was necessary in March 2009 due to oliguria and progressive retention of nitrogen catabolites. Because of persisting proteinuria, intravenous immunoglobulins in a dose of 50 mg/kg body weight/day were applied over 5 days in April 2009. During the therapy, the inflammatory parameters decreased (ESR from 60 to 42/h), proteinuria diminished (quantitative proteinuria 8.6 g/24h) and anti-ds DNA antibodies disappeared. In the following time, intravenous pulse therapy with methylprednisolone and cyclophosphamide, as well as the oral therapy with prednisone continued. Hemodialysis could be completed in August 2009, because of the improvement of the renal parameters.

In October 2009, a day after the 7th pulse had the patient an epileptic paroxysm. The brain MRI finding was suspect for SLE. At the same time the butterfly erythema accentuated, body temperature raised, cough appeared and the chest x-ray revealed a picture of central bronchopneumonia. The patient was treated with antiepileptics, antibiotics and at the same time with intravenous immunoglobulins in a total dose of 40 g followed by decrease in body temperature, remission of skin rash, decrease of inflammatory markers, leukocytosis, proteinuria (2.19 g/24h, creatinine 120.3 μmol/L). After the treatment of the infection, intravenous pulse therapy with prednisolone and cyclophosphamide continued. The clinical status of the patient is stabilized.

Discussion

The efficacy and safety of intravenous immunoglobulins were already described in several studies. The question about their indication as well as about their administration and dose remains still discussed. One of the indications of treatment with IVIG in SLE is the resistant form of lupus glomerulonephritis. IVIGs are usually administered for 5 days in the dose of 400 mg/kg body weight. The effect occurs within few days and lasts for several weeks after the last infusion [8]. Several authors confirmed the efficacy of IVIG in the therapy of lupus nephritis by improvement of the nephritic syndrome [4, 10], as well as by improvement of the histological findings or transition to a milder form of glomerulonephritis proven by kidney re-biopsy [5]. In the same time, decrease of autoantibodies, increase of C3, C4 and total complement, improvement of thrombocytopenia, hemoglobin concentration and decrease of serum creatinine levels could be observed in these patients [2]. The administration of low doses of IVIGs (approx. 0.5 mg/kg body weight) was efficient on several clinical features of SLE, followed by a decrease in SLEDAI score. However, these doses did not influence the thrombocytopenia, alopecia or vasculitis [9]. In our second patient, the low doses of IVIGs led to a partial improvement of the urine findings, to a decrease of inflammatory reactants and disappearance of antibodies. During reactivation of the underlying disease in the form of CNS lupus, higher doses of IVIGs were administered, which led to a more marked decrease of proteinuria. Presence of severe thrombocytopenia and leukopenia is another indication of IVIGs administration in SLE [1, 6]. Improvement of blood count could be observed in our both patients after IVIGs administration.

Problematic remains the therapy of patients with antiphospholipid syndrome and recurrent spontaneous abortion. Pericone et al. [7] describe in their study a successful high-dose therapy with IVIGs in 12 patients with recurrent spontaneous abortions. In these patients a decrease of clinical activity and levels of autoantibodies could be observed, whereby their pregnancies were terminated successfully. Zandmann et al. [12] describe a successful administration of IVIGs in various clinical features of SLE – autoimmune hemolytic anemia, pancytopenia, pneumonitis, myocarditis, CNS impairment during SLE. Combined pulse therapy with methylprednisolone, cyclophosphamide and 3 cycles of IVIGs in a patient with pericardial effusion, cardiac failure and pancytopenia led to an improvement of cardiac findings [11]. Karim [3] described the efficacy of IVIGs in patient with reactivated SLE accompanied by sepsis.

Conclusion

IVIG represent a safe and efficient therapy of several clinical symptoms of SLE as well as of SLE accompanied by secondary infection. Their administration led to improvement of several clinical and laboratory parameters in combination with immunosuppressive therapy, as well as in the period before the immunosuppressive therapy could be applied.

References

[1] Corvetta A, Della Bitta R, Gabrielli A, Spaeth PJ, Danieli G: Use of high-dose intravenous immunoglobulin in systemic lupus erythematosus: report of three cases. *Clin. Exp. Rheumatol.* 7: 295-299, 1989.

[2] Francioni C, Galeazzi M, Fioravanti A, Gelli R, Megale F, Marcolongo R: Long-term i.v. Ig treatment in systemic lupus erythematosus. *Clin. Exp. Rheumatol.* 12: 163-168, 1994.

[3] Karim MY, Pisoni CN, Khamashta MA: Update on immunotherapy for systemic lupus erythematosus--what's hot and what's not! *Rheumatology* (Oxford) 48: 332-341, 2009.

[4] Levy Y, Sherer Y, George J, Rovensky J, Lukac J, Rauova L, Poprac P, Langevitz P, Fabbrizzi F, Shoenfeld Y: Intravenous immunoglobulin treatment of lupus nephritis. *Semin. Arthritis Rheum.* 29: 321-327, 2000.

[5] Lin CY, Hsu HC, Chiang H: Improvement of histological and immunological change in steroid and immunosuppressive drug-resistant lupus nephritis by high-dose intravenous gamma globulin. *Nephron* 53: 303-310, 1989.

[6] Maier WP, Gordon DS, Howard RF, Saleh MN, Miller SB, Lieberman JD, Woodlee PM: Intravenous immunoglobulin therapy in systemic lupus erythematosus-associated thrombocytopenia. *Arthritis Rheum.* 33: 1233-1239, 1990.

[7] Perricone R, De Carolis C, Kröegler B, Greco E, Giacomelli R, Cipriani P, Fontana L, Perricone C: Intravenous immunoglobulin therapy in pregnant patients affected with systemic lupus erythematosus and recurrent spontaneous abortion. *Rheumatology* (Oxford) 47: 646-651, 2008.

[8] Rauova L, Lukac J, Levy Y, Rovensky J, Shoenfeld Y: High-dose intravenous immunoglobulins for lupus nephritis: A salvage immunomodulation. *Lupus* 10: 209-213, 2001.

[9] Sherer Y, Kuechler S, Jose Scali J, Rovensky J, Levy Y, Zandman-Goddard G, Shoenfeld Y: Low dose intravenous immunoglobulin in systemic lupus erythematosus: analysis of 62 cases. *Isr. Med. Assoc. J.* 10: 55-57, 2008.

[10] Sugisaki T, Schiwachi S, Yonekura M et al. High-dose intravenous gamma globulin for membranous nephropathy, membranoproliferative glomerulonephritis and lupus nephritis. *Fed. Proc.* 41: 692, 1982.

[11] van der Laan-Baalbergen NE, Mollema SA, Kritikos H, Schoe A, Huizinga TW, Bax JJ, Boumpas DT, van Laar JM: Heart failure as presenting manifestation of cardiac involvement in systemic lupus erythematosus. *Neth. J. Med.* 67: 295-301, 2009.

[12] Zandman-Goddard G, Levy Y, Shoenfeld Y: Intravenous immunoglobulin therapy and systemic lupus erythematosus. *Clin. Rev. Allergy. Immunol.* 29: 219-228, 2005.

In: Lupus: Symptoms, Treatment and Potential Complications ISBN: 978-1-62081-078-1
Editors: T. D. Marquez and D. U. Neto

Chapter XI

APRV (Airway Pressure-Release Ventilation) as Supportive Management for Diffuse Alveolar Hemorrhage with Systemic Lupus Erythematosus

Yoshio Ozaki and Shosaku Nomura
First Department of Internal Medicine, Kansai Medical University, Fumizono-cho, Moriguchi City, Osaka, Japan

Abstract

Diffuse alveolar hemorrhage (DAH), is a rare pulmonary complication of collagen-vascular diseases, including systemic lupus erythematosus (SLE). As the pathogenetic mechanism of DAH remains unclear, no established treatment is available. However, DAH is potentially fatal.

Similar to adult respiratory distress syndrome (ARDS), DAH patients develop severe hypoxemia caused by wide alveolar collapse. Patients may require management with mechanical ventilation in the intensive care unit.

The properties of the alveolar-capillary barrier are abnormal during acute lung injury, such as DAH. DAH patients develop severe hypoxemia. It is generally treated with immunosuppressive agents. However, the effects take several weeks. Therefore, mechanical ventilation is used to support these patients until the treatments are effective. DAH lungs include healthy tissue, recruitable tissue, and diseased tissue that are unresponsive to pressure changes. Most of the ventilation used during conventional management of these patients may be directed at recruitable and probably healthier units, resulting in their overdistention, which is thought to be one of the causes of ventilator-associated lung injury.

Airway pressure release ventilation (APRV) is one mode of ventilation that may achieve recruitment and improve oxygenation while maintaining acceptable peak airway pressures. APRV applies a continuous airway pressure (P_{high}) identical to continuous positive airway pressure (CPAP) to maintain adequate lung volume and promote alveolar recruitment. APRV adds a time-cycled release phase to a lower set pressure (P_{low}).

In addition, spontaneous breathing can be integrated and is independent of the ventilator cycle. By allowing patients to breathe spontaneously during APRV, dependent lung regions may be preferentially recruited without the need to raise the applied airway pressure. APRV has been used to treat acute lung injury, such as ARDS.

Introduction

Diffuse alveolar hemorrhage (DAH), is a rare pulmonary complication of collagen-vascular diseases, including systemic lupus erythematosus (SLE). As the pathogenetic mechanism of DAH remains unclear, no established treatment is available. However, DAH is potentially fatal. Similar to adult respiratory distress syndrome (ARDS), DAH patients develop severe hypoxemia caused by wide alveolar collapse. Patients may require management with mechanical ventilation in the intensive care unit (ICU).

The properties of the alveolar-capillary barrier are abnormal during acute lung injury, such as ARDS. ARDS patients develop severe hypoxemia.

No drugs are available to control microvascular permeability, so it is necessary to treat the cause of the disease. In addition, mechanical ventilation is used to support these patients until the treatments are effective. ARDS lungs include healthy tissue, recruitable tissue, and diseased tissue that unresponsive to pressure changes. Most of the ventilation used during conventional management of these patients may be directed at recruitable and probably more healthy units, resulting in their overdistention, which is thought to be one of the causes of ventilator-associated lung injury (VALI) [1].

Airway pressure release ventilation (APRV) is one mode of ventilation that may achieve recruitment and improve oxygenation while maintaining acceptable peak airway pressures [2]. APRV applies a continuous airway pressure (P_{high}) identical to continuous positive airway pressure (CPAP) to maintain adequate lung volume and promote alveolar recruitment. APRV adds a time-cycled release phase to a lower set pressure (P_{low}).

In addition, spontaneous breathing can be integrated and is independent of the ventilator cycle. By allowing patients to breathe spontaneously during APRV, dependent lung regions may be preferentially recruited without the need to raise the applied airway pressure [3]. APRV has been used to treat acute lung injury, such as ARDS.

APRV and DAH

APRV was originally described in 1987 by Downs and Stock [2] as animal experiment data, and then reported by Garner et al. as clinical crossover trial data [4]. APRV has been used to treat acute lung injury, such as ARDS. Conventional mechanical ventilation often causes exclusion outside the alveoli surfactant due to excessive pressure, which causes collapse of normal alveoli. Successful alveolar recruiting pressure depends on the yield or threshold opening pressure of lung units.

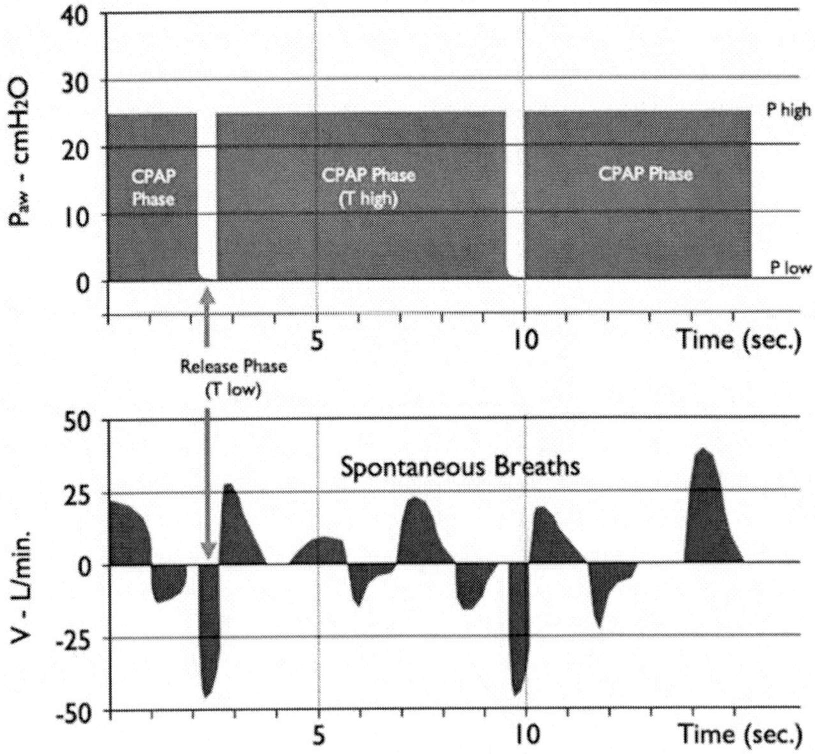

Figure 1. Airway pressure release ventilation (APRV), Paw: airway pressure, P_{high}: continuous airway pressure equivalent to CPAP level, CPAP: continuous positive airway pressure, T_{high}: duration of P_{high}, T_{low}: lower set pressure.

In addition, the time-dependent nature of recruitment should also be considered. A long P_{high} aspect (Figure 1), which is a feature of APRV, not only maintains elevated airway pressure but also supplies gas from the side sub-ventilation road such as Kohn hole and Lambert 's canal, and results in a delay to recruitment [3].

Moreover, the highest airway pressure can be kept low although P_{high} is set higher in APRV compared with conventional ventilation [3]. APRV provides a constant degree of mechanical assistance, as it combines mechanical ventilation with spontaneous breathing and therefore should decrease the workload on the respiratory muscles [5].

DAH has been reported to develop in association with collagen-vascular diseases, such as SLE and microscopic polyangiitis [6]. The main cause of DAH on collagen-vascular diseases is capillaritis, and alveolar collapse occurs because blood fills the alveolar space [7]. DAH is a frequent complication in microscopic polyangiitis with an incidence rate of 20% – 40%, and the mortality rate is about 30% [8]. Its frequency in patients with SLE is low (1% – 4%). However, mortality rates of this complication in SLE is over 30% [8]. There is still no established treatment for DAH. Intensive immunosuppressive treatment with high-dose corticosteroids, cyclophosphamide, and plasmapheresis may decrease mortality. These administering becomes treatment of the causative disorder. However, mechanical ventilation support becomes indispensable for recruitment and to stop bleeding in the pulmonary alveoli. Collapse of the pulmonary alveoli occurs in the lungs of DAH patients as well as those with ARDS. There is a risk of hyperextension of healthy pulmonary alveoli, and it may cause

VALI. Moreover, DAH may occur as a complication while treating SLE. The increased vulnerability of tissue by long-term administration of cortical steroid may increase the risk of VALI. Infection, mechanical ventilation, and creatinine levels are risk factors associated with increased mortality [9]. The period of mechanical ventilation use in DAH patients should be kept as short as possible.

Cases

Patient 1

A 36-year-old woman was referred to our hospital due to dyspnea, massive hemoptysis, and fever. She had a history of Raynaud's phenomenon and proteinuria for a few weeks. Chest radiography showed bilateral diffuse infiltrates and an increased cardiothoracic index, and computed tomography (CT) findings were consistent with DAH (Figures 2a and e).

A diagnosis of DAH due to SLE was made based on bronchoscopy with lavage revealing bloody return, hemosiderin-laden macrophages, chest X-ray, anti-nuclear antibody, anti-dsDNA antibody, hypocomplementemia, proteinuria, and facial erythema. Intravenous methylprednisolone was given at a dose of 1000 mg/day for 3 days. The patient required monitoring in the ICU and intubation due to her hypoxemia (Table 1).

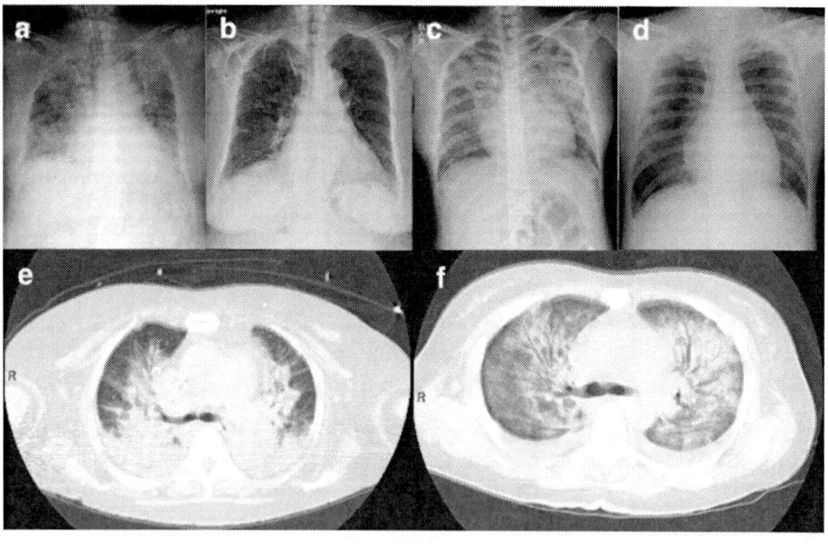

Figure 2. Chest X-ray (CXR) and computed tomography (CT), (a) CXR of patient 1 at onset of DAH. (b) CXR of patient 1 five days after onset of hemoptysis. (c) CXR of patient 2 at onset of DAH. (d) CXR of patient 2 fourteen days after onset of hemoptysis. (e) Chest CT of patient 1 at onset of DAH. (f) Chest CT of patient 2 at onset of DAH. CXR and chest CT scans of all patients demonstrated extensive infiltrative shadow with air bronchograms in the bilateral lung fields (a, c, e, f). Rapid improvements of the infiltrative shadows were observed on CXR with supportive therapy by APRV (b, 5th day; d, 14th day).

Mechanical ventilation with APRV (P_{high} was 25 cmH_2O, T_{high}; duration of P_{high} was 4.5 sec., T_{low}; duration of P_{low} was 0.6 sec., FiO_2 was 50%) was applied (Table 2), and the DAH improved with normalization of chest X-ray abnormality (Figure 2b) in only 5 days.

Table 1. Laboratory findings of patients before and after onset of DAH

		Patient 1		Patient 2	
		before	onset	before	onset
WBC	10^2/μL (35 - 100)	41	95	102	188
RBC	10^4/μL (370 - 510)	282	245	334	220
Hb	g/dL (11.3 - 15.4)	8.1	6.8	10.3	6.8
Ht	% (34.0 - 46.2)	25.2	21.4	28.0	20.1
PLT	10^4/μL (14 - 34)	20.4	19.5	18.7	16.4
BUN	mg/dL (8 - 20)	14	40	22	52
Creat	mg/dL (0.4 - 0.8)	0.95	0.97	0.90	1.09
LDH	U/L (112 - 230)	470	621	182	339
CRP	mg/dL (< 0.3)	1.063	6.220	0.800	7.261
Blood Gas Analysis			O_2 8L		O_2 10L
pH	(7.35 - 7.45)		7.473		7.391
pCO_2	mmHg (35 - 45)		28.6		28.7
pO_2	mmHg (80 - 100)		55.1		49.6
HCO_3	mEq/L (21 - 27)		20.5		17.0
BE	mM/L (-2 - 2)		-2.7		-7.1
$SatO_2$	% (94 - 100)		82.6		88.0

Patient 2

A 46-year-old woman with a 10-year history of SLE was admitted with high fever, hemoptysis, and rapid progressive dyspnea. She had been administered 7.5 mg/day of prednisolone. DAH was diagnosed based on bloody bronchoalveolar lavage fluid, chest X-ray, and CT (Figures 2c and f). The results of laboratory evaluation were: CRP 7.261 mg/dL, hemoglobin (Hb) 6.8 g/dL (Table 1).

Methylprednisolone pulse therapy was performed for her vasculitis under mechanical ventilatory support with APRV (P_{high} 30 cmH_2O, T_{high} 4.5 sec., T_{low} 0.6 sec., FiO_2 50%) because of severe hypoxemia (Table 1). Consolidation on chest X-ray and C-reactive protein levels improved rapidly (Figure 2d). DAH occurred three times with tapering of prednisolone. However in all three episodes, DAH treatment was supported with APRV (Table 2) and she was maintained without mechanical ventilatory support for 7 – 10 days after the onset of hemoptysis.

Table 2. Clinical course and APRV settings

Patient 1	Day 1	Day 2	Day 3	Day 4	
FiO_2 (%)	50	30	30		
T_{high} (sec.)	4.5	4.5	5.5	CPAP	Extubation
T_{low} (sec.)	0.6	0.6	0.6		
P_{high} (cmH_2O)	25	15	10		

Patient 2, 1st. Episode	Day 1	Day 2	Day 3	Day 4	Day 5	Day 6	Day 7	Day 10
FiO_2 (%)	50	30	30	30	30	30		
T_{high} (sec.)	4.5	6.4	6.4	6.4	6.4	7.4	CPAP	Extubation
T_{low} (sec.)	0.6	0.6	0.6	0.6	0.6	0.6		
P_{high} (cmH_2O)	30	30	28	25	24	22		

2nd. Episode	Day 1	Day 2	Day 3	Day 4	Day 7
FiO_2 (%)	50	30	30		
T_{high} (sec.)	4.5	5.5	8.5	CPAP	Extubation
T_{low} (sec.)	0.5	0.5	0.5		
P_{high} (cmH_2O)	30	25	22		

3rd. Episode	Day 1	Day 2	Day 3	Day 4	Day 5	Day 7
FiO_2 (%)	40	40	40	30		
T_{high} (sec.)	4.5	4.5	4.5	6.5	CPAP	Extubation
T_{low} (sec.)	0.5	0.5	0.5	0.5		
P_{high} (cmH_2O)	25	25	25	20		

T_{high}, duration of P_{high}; T_{low}, lower set pressure; P_{high}, continuous airway pressure equivalent to CPAP level; CPAP, continuous positive airway pressure.

Kobayashi *et al.* reported that lung opacities and hypoxemia clearly improved within 65 days and 125 days, respectively, in 13 DAH episodes of collagen-vascular disease treated with intensive immunosuppressive agents supported by conventional ventilation [7]. Of the shown cases supported with APRV, improvements were achieved in a very short time. Especially, consolidation on chest X-ray disappeared in only three days in case 2. The time to extubation of 4 episodes of these patients was 7.0 days on average. Moreover, case 1 was extubated on only the fourth day, which would have had an excellent influence on prognosis. Hemorrhage from the capillary may physically stop bleeding by APRV, which maintained a higher mean airway pressure than conventional ventilation. Patients with severe SLE have the complication of disseminated intravascular coagulation or thrombocytopenia, occasionally. APRV is advantageous for arrest of hemorrhage, and it is therefore applicable in SLE patients with DAH during mechanical ventilation.

Subcutaneous emphysema and mediastinal emphysema were frequent complications in SLE patients treated with APRV. Case 1 without emphysema had untreated SLE. She has never administrated of corticosteroid. It is presumed that emphysema complicated with APRV may have been due to increased vulnerability of tissue caused by long-term administrating of corticosteroid. However, the emphysema recovered early after weaning from ventilatory support. The recruitment of alveolar collapse and arrest of hemorrhage from the capillary can be done by APRV in a short time. It provides insight into the possible beneficial effects of APRV, which can shorten the period of ICU management for DAH with collagen-vascular diseases.

References

[1] Dreyfuss D and Saumon G, *Am J Respir Crit Care Med.* 157, 294 (1998).

[2] Downs JB and Stock MC, *Crit Care Med.* 15, 459 (1987).

[3] Habashi NM, *Crit Care Med.* 33 S228 (2005).

[4] Garner W, Downs JB, Stock MC and Räsänen J, *Chest.* 94, 779 (1988).

[5] Hering R, Zinserling J, Wrigge H, Varelmann D, Berg A, Kreyer S and Putensen C, *Chest.* 128, 2991 (2005).

[6] Green RJ, Ruoss SJ, Kraft SA, Duncan SR, Berry GJ and Raffin TA, *Chest.* 110, 1305 (1996).

[7] Kobayashi S and Inokuma S, *Intern Med.* 48, 894 (2009).

[8] Zamora MR, Warner ML, Tuder R and Schwarz MI, *Medicine (Baltimore).* 76, 192 (1997).

[9] Sengul E, Eyıleten T, Ozcan A, Yılmaz MI and Yenıcesu M, *Rheumatol Int.* 31, 1085 (2011).

Index

A

B

C

D

E

F

G

H

I

J

K

L

M

N

O

P

Q

R

S

T